Palliative Care in Respiratory Disease

Edited by
Claudia Bausewein, David C. Currow and
Miriam J. Johnson

Editor in Chief
Robert Bals

This book is one in a series of *ERS Monographs*. Each individual issue provides a comprehensive overview of one specific clinical area of respiratory health, communicating information about the most advanced techniques and systems required for its investigation. It provides factual and useful scientific detail, drawing on specific case studies and looking into the diagnosis and management of individual patients. Previously published titles in this series are listed at the back of this *Monograph*.

ERS Monographs are available online at www.erspublications.com and print copies are available from www.ersbookshop.com

Continuing medical education (CME) credits are available through many issues of the *ERS Monograph*. Following evaluation, successful *Monographs* are accredited by the European Board for Accreditation in Pneumology (EBAP) for 5 CME credits. To earn CME credits, read the book of your choice (it is clearly indicated on the online table of contents whether CME credits are available) then complete the CME question form that is available at www.ers-education.org/e-learning/cme-tests.aspx

Managing Editors: Rachel White and Catherine Pumphrey
European Respiratory Society, 442 Glossop Road, Sheffield, S10 2PX, UK
Tel: 44 114 2672860 | E-mail: Monograph@ersj.org.uk

Published by European Respiratory Society ©2016
September 2016
Print ISBN: 978-1-84984-071-2
Online ISBN: 978-1-84984-072-9
Print ISSN: 2312-508X
Online ISSN: 2312-5098
Printed by Latimer Trend and Company Limited, Plymouth, UK

C O P E
Member since 2009
JM04643

This journal is a member of and subscribes to the principles of the Committee on Publication Ethics

MIX
Paper from responsible sources
FSC® C013436
FSC www.fsc.org

THOMSON REUTERS BOOK CITATION INDEX INDEXED

ERS | monograph

Contents

Palliative Care in Respiratory Disease

Number 73
September 2016

Preface

Robert Bals

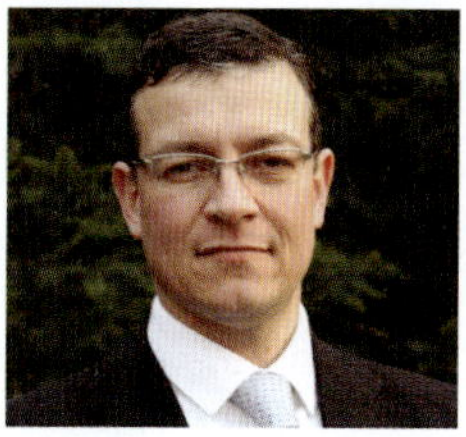

Palliative care has developed in the last decades. While many of its concepts have been part of respiratory medicine for a long time, the concept of structured palliation for patients with lung diseases is still evolving. The term "palliative care" describes a multidisciplinary approach to offer relief to patients with severe diseases for which causal therapy is limited. Historically, palliative care in its basic form has always been a part of medicine, but many of its aspects have taken a back seat due to the development of technical medicine at the beginning of the 20th century. Modern palliative care has been linked to the hospice movement, an important root of which can be seen in the St Christopher's Hospice, founded by Cicely Saunders in London in 1967. In the last decades, the field has undergone many developments in its methods and structures.

While the primary focus of palliative care has been on patients with cancer, this view has widened and palliation is seen today to be an integral part of the care of patients with many other diseases. In fact, numerous lung diseases currently cannot be cured and progress to a stage where symptom load drastically reduces the quality of life of the patient. While most respiratory physicians deal with aspects of palliation every day, palliative medicine is rarely integrated in a systematic curriculum for medical students or residents. In addition, palliative care as part of a structured programme is in many cases only available at more specialised centres.

This *ERS Monograph* focuses on palliative care for patients with lung diseases. The first section covers general items, such as definitions, epidemiology and access structures. The second section provides detailed information on individual symptoms and care in special settings, such as in low-resource settings, and the third section focuses on care of the dying.

The Guest Editors, Claudia Bausewein, David C. Currow and Miriam J. Johnson, have worked very successfully to select these

 Print ISBN: 978-1-84984-071-2. Online ISBN: 978-1-84984-072-9. Print ISSN: 2312-508X. Online ISSN: 2312-5098.

topics and to integrate these aspects into a comprehensive book on the current knowledge. I thank the Guest Editors and all authors for their work on this excellent book. I am sure that this comprehensive review will be useful for the clinical practice of a broad range of respiratory physicians and improve the care of our patients.

Disclosures: R. Bals has received grants from the German Research Ministerium and the Deutsche Forschungsgemeinschaft. He has also received personal fees from GSK, AstraZeneca, Boehringer Ingelheim and CSL Behring.

Guest Editors

Claudia Bausewein

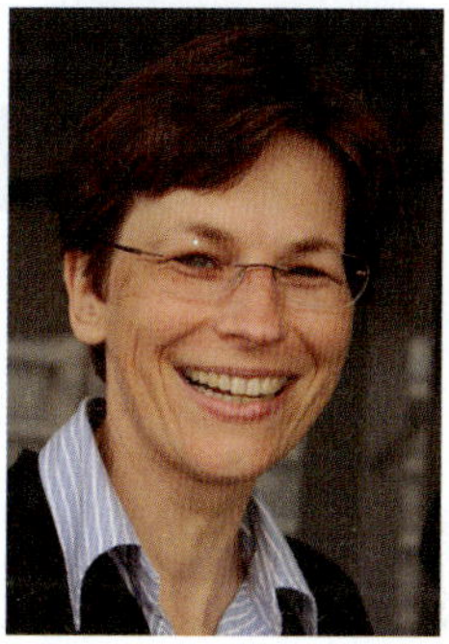

Claudia Bausewein is Professor for Palliative Medicine at Ludwig-Maximilians-University Munich (Munich, Germany) and is Director of the Dept of Palliative Medicine at Munich University Hospital. Her medical background is internal medicine and she has been involved in palliative care in Germany for more than 25 years.

She worked as Consultant in Palliative Medicine at the University of Munich and as a senior clinical research fellow in the Cicely Saunders Institute at King's College London (London, UK), where she obtained her PhD in 2009.

Claudia Bausewein is national co-lead for the German Guideline for Palliative Care and was a member of the European Association for Palliative Care Board of Directors from 2011 to 2015 and vice president of the German Association for Palliative Medicine from 2004 to 2010.

Her research interests focus on breathlessness in advanced malignant and non-malignant disease, outcome measurement in palliative care and complexity in palliative care. Her methodological expertise covers systematic reviews, cross-sectional and longitudinal studies, surveys, clinical trials and evaluation of complex interventions. She heads a multiprofessional and multidisciplinary research team, including medicine, pharmacy, psychology, sociology, health services research and statistics. Her research is funded by the German Ministry of Research, the German Cancer Aid and various charities. She has published widely and is collaborating with various national and international groups.

 Print ISBN: 978-1-84984-071-2. Online ISBN: 978-1-84984-072-9. Print ISSN: 2312-508X. Online ISSN: 2312-5098.

David C. Currow

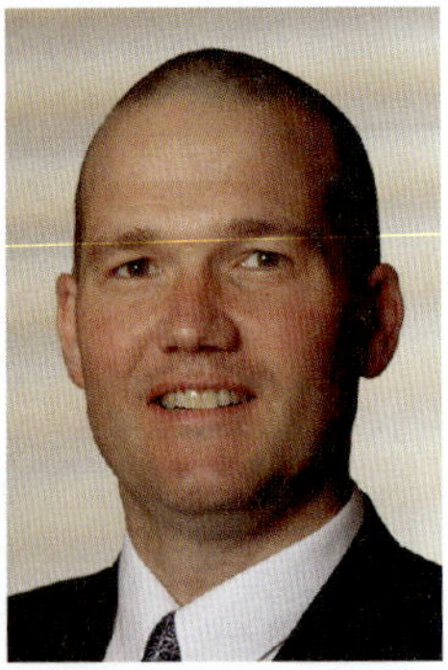

David C. Currow is an internationally recognised expert in supportive and palliative care, with a particular emphasis on chronic breathlessness and in improving health service delivery. He has a strong track record in competitive research funding (National Institutes of Health (Bethesda, MD, USA), National Health and Medical Research Council (Canberra, Australia) and Cancer Council (Sydney, Australia)) and publishing research that influences practice and policy. He leads the Palliative Care Clinical Studies Collaborative (Adelaide, Australia), the world's largest palliative care phase III clinical studies collaborative. This has generated several randomised, placebo-controlled trials of off-label use of off-patent medications frequently used in symptom control internationally. He is also a leader in the Palliative Care Outcomes Collaborative (Wollongong, Australia), a national programme for point-of-care data collection and service improvement in palliative care. He was a leader in the creation of the first patient-defined section of the Australian Pharmaceutical Benefits Scheme (the palliative care section).

He is frequently an invited plenary speaker at international conferences. He continues to supervise doctoral candidates from a variety of clinical backgrounds. He is senior associate editor of the *Journal of Palliative Medicine* and is on the editorial boards of *Journal of Oncology Practice*, *Journal of Pain and Symptom Management* and *BMJ Supportive and Palliative Care*. He was the 2015 recipient of the Tom Reeve National Award for Outstanding Contribution to Cancer Care from the Clinical Oncological Society of Australia, a team member winning the 2012 National Team Award for Postgraduate Education from the Australian Learning and Teaching Centre, the 2012 Alumni Medal from the University of Newcastle (Newcastle, Australia) for professional excellence and was a joint winner of the 2015 *Medical Journal of Australia*/Medical Defence Association National Research Award.

Miriam J. Johnson

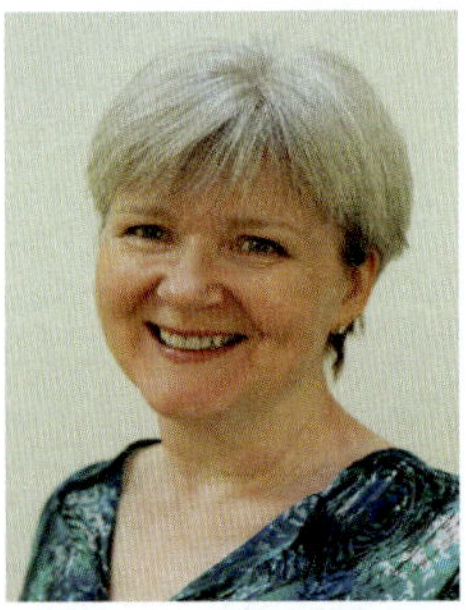

Miriam J. Johnson is Professor of Palliative Medicine at Hull York Medical School, Director of the Wolfson Palliative Care Research Centre and Co-Director of the Supportive care, Early Diagnosis and Advanced disease research group at the University of Hull (Hull, UK). Her clinical and research interests include mechanisms and management of breathlessness and inequalities in palliative care service provision, *e.g.* for people with non-malignant disease such as heart failure and respiratory disease. The projects employ a wide range of research methodologies (clinical trials of drug or complex interventions, qualitative studies, observational, secondary data analysis and data linkage studies) and collaborative partners are involved across different disciplines and countries. She has published widely and holds grants from a variety of bodies (National Institute for Health Research (London, UK), National Health and Medical Research Council (Canberra, Australia), The Dunhill Medical Trust (London, UK), Marie Curie Cancer Care/ Cancer Research UK (London, UK), Yorkshire Cancer Research (Harrogate, UK) and the British Heart Foundation (London, UK)).

She is palliative care specialty joint lead for the Yorkshire and Humber Clinical Research Network (Sheffield, UK). She has also set up one of the UK's first integrated palliative care services for people with heart failure.

Introduction

Claudia Bausewein[1], David C. Currow[2] and Miriam J. Johnson[3]

As the patterns of well-being and illness change across the community, so the way people experience impaired health continues to change. These changes lead to the need for focus on a range of issues, including symptoms that have not enjoyed sufficient attention. CRD, with its cardinal and debilitating symptom of chronic breathlessness, is one such area. Many millions of people around the world suffer from CRD. They experience a prolonged symptom burden, often for decades, which affects every area of their lives and the lives of their family and friends, and which affects their ability to contribute to their communities. This comes at a huge personal and societal cost.

As many respiratory diseases are preventable, public health measures are, quite rightly, a key priority for implementation and research. In addition, much appropriate effort and resources support the quest to find interventions that will cure, or at least ameliorate, the causative pathologies. However, the complex supportive and palliative care needs experienced by people with CRD, often from early on in their disease course, have been poorly recognised and not addressed systematically within clinical practice or research priorities. Despite the progressive and life-limiting nature of many CRDs, access to holistic assessment and management by the usual care team, access to palliative care services, advance care planning with its challenging conversations, optimisation of functional independence as the disease progresses, excellent symptom control during the course of the disease and when dying, and support for families during and after death, are areas of stark inequalities in care compared to people with cancer.

There are several reasons, although not excuses, for this discrepancy. First, palliative care services in many high-income countries have grown up in association with cancer. Thus, the original model of palliative care was one of exhaustion of disease-directed treatments followed by a handing over to palliative care for the very end-stage of life and care of the dying. This model of care is clearly not fit-for-purpose for people with respiratory diseases given the trajectory of many: disease-directed treatments do not have such a clear "use by" date. With the advent of multiple lines of cancer treatment, this traditional model has also become outmoded in oncology palliative care. A more integrated model seems to be more appropriate, with extended team working and involvement of palliative care earlier on in the disease trajectory in response to problems rather than prognosis. However, the non-cancer world has not caught up with this change (and indeed, there are many

[1]Dept of Palliative Medicine, LMU Munich, Munich University Hospital, Munich, Germany. [2]Palliative and Supportive Services, Flinders University, Adelaide, Australia. [3]Wolfson Palliative Care Research Centre, Hull York Medical School, University of Hull, Hull, UK.

Correspondence: Miriam J. Johnson, Wolfson Palliative Care Research Centre, Hull York Medical School, Hertford Building, University of Hull, Hull, HU6 7RX, UK. E-mail: Miriam.johnson@hyms.ac.uk

 Print ISBN: 978-1-84984-071-2. Online ISBN: 978-1-84984-072-9. Print ISSN: 2312-508X. Online ISSN: 2312-5098.

oncology services which have not either); thus, palliative care is thought of as something only for people who are dying very soon, and probably of cancer. Secondly, the situation is compounded by difficulties in definitions, with terms such as "terminal care", "EOL care", "palliative" and "hospice" meaning different things to different people in different healthcare settings around the world.

In this *ERS Monograph*, the World Health Organization definition of palliative care is used, with its focus on optimising quality of life for people with progressive life-limiting illness through impeccable assessment of symptoms and other concerns throughout their illness, care of the dying and family support. This approach works in response to people's needs rather than being limited either by diagnosis or prognosis, and can be initiated at the time it is recognised that the person has a life-limiting illness. In the first section, the issue of palliative care for people with respiratory diseases will be discussed in the context of the epidemiology of the diseases themselves, the palliative care needs resulting from the diseases and how palliative care services can be modelled and delivered.

The second section focuses on the key symptom of breathlessness. Most clinicians only see people who have acute breathlessness, or see chronic breathlessness as an inevitable consequence of the underlying disease process, which, itself, is not worthy of clinical attention. Most people with chronic breathlessness only seek help for the symptom when it worsens acutely. The brief encounters that clinicians have with people who experience chronic breathlessness belies the overwhelming impact that such breathlessness has on millions of people every moment of the day around the world. Although their breathlessness may improve marginally after acute exacerbations, the lived reality for these people is that of severe breathlessness at rest or on minimal exertion, often for years at life's end.

The predominant cause of such breathlessness remains respiratory disease, with the contribution of tobacco, workplace exposures and domestic smoke from fires in ill-ventilated dwellings being key contributors to this burden of suffering.

As this symptom burden continues to evolve and grow, so has the evidence base for defining and treating this pervasive and debilitating symptom. As is so often the case, the real challenge is not the development of new knowledge that can help to relieve the suffering caused by chronic breathlessness, but ensuring the widespread uptake of that new knowledge into clinical practice and policy. The pervasive nihilism that people with CRDs should silently tolerate chronic breathlessness should be defeated as a matter of urgency. People with chronic breathlessness should be demanding better symptom control and clinicians should be actively offering ways to minimise the impact of this life-changing, long-term disability.

Finally, in the third section, the issue of caring for people with advanced disease and those who are dying is tackled head on. The response to the less clear trajectory of respiratory diseases has been to avoid the issue and, especially, to avoid conversations that discuss progression of disease or plans for future care. This is often for fear of upsetting the patient, exacerbated by lack of training in advanced communication and symptom management skills, and clinical service configurations that mitigate against exploring patients' concerns, hopes or expectations. Sadly, the experience of patients and families is then one of poor knowledge and understanding of their disease, treatments and goals of care, poor involvement in their plans of care, and poor symptom control. When they come to die, they die by default in an acute care facility, still receiving invasive medical treatments, with poor access to the people they love at the time they need them most.

People with CRD deserve a better deal. This *ERS Monograph* brings together the state-of-the-art in palliative care in this field, with the aim of helping clinicians and researchers provide that better deal and redress the balance after many years of serious neglect.

Disclosures: D.C. Currow is an unpaid advisory board member for Helsinn Pharmaceuticals. He is also a paid consultant and received payment for intellectual property with Mayne Pharma, and is a consultant with Specialised Therapeutics Australia Pty Ltd. M.J. Johnson has worked as a clinical consultant to Mayne Pharma and received institutional payment.

List of abbreviations

BMI	body mass index
CHF	chronic heart failure
CNS	clinical nurse specialist
COPD	chronic obstructive pulmonary disease
CRD	chronic respiratory disease
DALYs	disability-adjusted life-years
ED	emergency department
EOL	end of life
ESRD	end-stage renal disease
FEV_1	forced expiratory volume in 1 s
FVC	forced vital capacity
GP	general practitioner
ICU	intensive care unit
ILD	interstitial lung disease
IPF	idiopathic pulmonary fibrosis
LST	life-sustaining treatment
MDP	Multidimensional Dyspnea Profile
NIV	noninvasive ventilation
NPPV	noninvasive positive pressure ventilation
NRS	numerical rating scale
NSCLC	nonsmall cell lung cancer
PEOLC	palliative and end-of-life care
RCT	randomised controlled trial
SCLC	small cell lung cancer
VAS	visual analogue scale

Chapter 1

Definitions and policy

Joshua B. Kayser[1], Kim Mooney-Doyle[2] and Paul N. Lanken[1]

Palliative care aims to provide enhanced quality of life for patients with serious and life-limiting illnesses. It thus focuses on controlling symptoms and supporting patients and family caregivers. Palliative care is a patient-/family-centred multidisciplinary process based on the ethical principles of beneficence (benefiting the patient) and respect for the patient's dignity and autonomy (self-determination). Palliative care should maximise quality of life for patients with advanced stages of respiratory diseases in the months, or even years, preceding death, and should reflect the preferences of patients and their families relating to how, where and when death will occur. Palliative care for patients with respiratory diseases can be challenging. Such patients have clinical courses that may vary from a prolonged recurrent waxing and waning course to a rapidly downhill course. Additionally, patients with advanced respiratory diseases may require repeated hospitalisations, including the need for aggressive LSTs with assisted ventilation in ICUs. This necessitates discussions and decisions related to withholding and withdrawing life support. Because differences in national and local cultures impact clinical practices in forgoing life support, the decision making process regarding the latter should take into account the relevant cultural context. This is especially important when considering the creation and adaptation of global healthcare policy in palliative care.

This chapter introduces the subject of providing PEOLC to patients with respiratory diseases. It includes descriptions of recent epidemiology related to respiratory illness and dying and death, a brief history of palliative care and hospices, definitions of commonly used terms in discussions of PEOLC (table 1), relevant bioethical context and models of decision making among healthcare providers and patients and families, and how palliative care is provided. Finally, it also characterises global variations in PEOLC with the aim of better understanding global policy efforts to improve the delivery and outcomes of palliative care.

Epidemiology of PEOLC

Few things in life are certain, but one undeniable truth is that everyone who lives ultimately dies. The National Vital Statistics Report for deaths in the USA indicates that nearly 2.6 million deaths were registered in the USA in 2013 [3]. The corresponding estimated

[1]Pulmonary, Allergy and Critical Care Division, Dept of Medicine, Dept of Medical Ethics and Health Policy, Perelman School of Medicine, University of Pennsylvania, Philadelphia, PA, USA. [2]Centers for Global Women's Health and Health Equity Research, University of Pennsylvania School of Nursing, Philadelphia, PA, USA.

Correspondence: Joshua B. Kayser, Pulmonary, Allergy and Critical Care Division, Dept of Medicine, Dept of Medical Ethics and Health Policy, Perelman School of Medicine, University of Pennsylvania, Cpl. Michael J. Crescenz Veterans Administration Medical Center, 3900 Woodland Ave, 8B115, Philadelphia, PA 19104, USA. E-mail: joshua.kayser@va.gov

 Print ISBN: 978-1-84984-071-2. Online ISBN: 978-1-84984-072-9. Print ISSN: 2312-508X. Online ISSN: 2312-5098.

Table 1. Terms and definitions related to PEOLC

Palliative care	From the 2002 WHO definition [1], palliative care is the active total care that aims to improve the quality of life of patients, and their families, with progressive, life-limiting illness through the prevention and relief of suffering by means of impeccable assessment and treatment of pain and other problems, such as physical, psychosocial and spiritual. Palliative care may be incorporated alongside disease-directed treatments from the point of diagnosis. It aims to help patients live as actively as possible until the time of their death, and helps family carers cope during the illness and after death into bereavement. Palliative care may be provided by all clinicians caring for patients with progressive disease in all health and social care settings, at least with regard to basic skills, with specialists able to provide care for those with complex and persistent problems. The provision of palliative care is in response to patient and carer concerns rather than requiring a prognostic trigger in relation to estimated time of death. Domains of palliative care include supportive care, advance care planning, EOL care (care in the last months of life), care of the dying and bereavement care.
Specialist palliative care	A multiprofessional clinical specialty in which health and social care professionals are identified as having special competence in the field of palliative care and this is their core business; palliative medicine specialists may be board certified in certain countries. Specialist palliative care may be provided in hospitals, community settings or stand-alone palliative care units (which may be called specialised palliative care units or hospices).
Hospice care	This is a term used variably in different countries. In the UK, it is generally used to describe a specialist palliative care unit that provides inpatient care beds and a variety of community and outpatient services. Patients may be referred according to need rather than prognosis, and can access inpatient spells for assessment and management of acute complex symptoms with consequent discharge home, or respite, or care of the dying. Patients continue to be able to access the full range of clinical support available on the National Health Service. In the USA, "hospice" usually refers to community-based specialist palliative care focused on relief of symptoms for patients in advanced stages of their illness and support for their family carers, *e.g.* more likely than not expected to result in death within a few months.
Supportive care	Symptomatic treatment of the different forms of suffering and pain including physical, spiritual, emotional, psychological and moral distress throughout the illness from pre-diagnosis.
EOL or terminal care	Care of patients with life-limiting diseases preceding death. Variable time periods are used to define EOL, *e.g.* in the UK it refers to the last 12 months of life and in the USA typically to the last 6 months of life.
Care of the dying	Care of actively dying patients with focus on relief of suffering and maximising dignity in the last hours or days of life.
Bereavement care	Supportive care for family and friends who are grieving the loss of their loved ones.

Definitions in this table draw on the 2002 World Health Organization (WHO) definition of palliative care [1] and a systematic review by Van Mechelen *et al.* [2].

number of deaths worldwide at that time was 55 million [4]. However, while the inevitability of death is unfailing, time has transformed the human experience of how one dies. Throughout much of recorded history, death was random and unpredictable, afflicting people of all ages. Most died at home, commonly of infectious diseases. In recent history, with the advent of public health efforts, such as sanitation, vaccination and the use of antibiotics, death has become more predictable, preferentially afflicting the very young and the elderly. In the industrialised world, infection has been supplanted by cancer and chronic illness as the primary causes of death. For example, as of 2013, infection, (specifically influenza and pneumonia) ranked as the eighth leading cause of death in the USA with its associated 57 000 deaths representing <5% of the 1.3 million deaths attributed to heart disease, cancer and chronic lower respiratory diseases, which were the top three causes of death in the USA in 2013. Sepsis was the only other infectious cause of death to rank in the top 15 [3]. According to the World Health Organization (WHO), all communicable diseases combined only account for ~25% of all deaths worldwide [5]. By comparison, the WHO fact sheet on CRD indicated there are over 65 million people worldwide living with moderate to severe COPD, corresponding to over 3 million deaths (5%) annually [6]. In their report on noncommunicable diseases in 2010, they predicted a 15% global increase in all noncommunicable disease deaths between 2010 and 2020 [7]. These statistics suggest that, in the present and future, far more patients will struggle with chronic, progressive illness for extended periods prior to ultimately succumbing to their disease than in the past.

Another notable trend over the past 50 years relates to how medical care is provided and where death occurs. Few patients receive healthcare directly in their homes, as was common in previous centuries. Additionally, life-sustaining technologies have shifted the location of death for many people to healthcare institutions. In essence, disease and death have become less communal. Sick patients often seek medical care in isolation and are far more likely to die in hospitals, with the focus on curative rather than palliative interventions. This change in location associated with nonpalliative goals of care may reflect how various societies and cultures generally regard sickness and the dying process, *i.e.* events not to be witnessed or even discussed.

However, the patient experiences of living with disease and the dying process have occurred without conversations among stakeholders about the manner in which care should be provided to support patients and families with serious and advanced diseases and how that care should be funded. Indeed, funding for PEOLC is often limited, and may be structured such that choosing a primarily palliative approach may dictate that patients forgo simultaneous curative or restorative interventions. The Worldwide Palliative Care Alliance estimated that over 20 million people (*i.e.* 37% of all deaths worldwide) could benefit from palliative care, with the vast majority (69%) being adults of 60 years of age or older. Although utilisation of palliative care is rapidly increasing, the growth is predominantly in industrialised societies, specifically in European, Western Pacific and North American regions [5]. Not only is the growth of palliative care less robust in other areas of the world, but, importantly, these increases in utilisation do not take into account the timing of palliative care. Significant variability exists in terms of providing supportive care for patients living with chronic illness as opposed to EOL care for patients dying of their disease. As such, the potential exists not only to expand palliative care efforts in less economically advanced regions of the world but also to ensure efforts to provide high-quality supportive care and symptom relief in addition to ensuring that patients receive appropriate and desired care at the EOL.

It has been over a decade since Angus *et al.* [8] first described the epidemiology of EOL care in the USA in 1999: one in five Americans died in an ICU and nearly 40% of all USA deaths occurred in a hospital. In light of the ageing US population, this portended a future shortfall in hospital and ICU capacity. In the intervening years, it is difficult to argue that much has changed. For example, according to US Medicare data from a 2013 publication by Teno *et al.* [9], although the number of deaths in hospitals decreased by 8% between 2000 and 2009, ICU utilisation by patients in their last month of life increased by 5%. Similarly, although hospice enrolment doubled over that time period, nearly two-thirds of those enrollees utilised hospice services for fewer than 4 days. Additionally, 40% of hospice referrals were preceded by ICU hospitalisation and were accompanied by numerous transitions of care in the last 3 days of life, again acknowledging the lack of early integration of palliative care prior to the EOL [9].

These statistics are not unique to the USA. A 2016 study by Bekelman *et al.* [10] retrospectively compared site of death, healthcare utilisation and hospital costs for patients of 65 years of age of older dying with cancer in 2010 in seven North American and European countries. They found that a range of 40–50% of patients in the non-US countries died in acute care hospitals (*versus* 22.2% in the USA) [10]. However, non-US patients were far less likely than US patients to utilise the ICU in the last 180 days of life (<18% *versus* 40.3%, respectively), with hospital expenditures ranging from around US $9000 to US $22 000 per capita [10].

The statistics are similarly sobering with regard to the lack of early palliative care to relieve the burdens of disease that exist prior to the EOL. For example, a 2010 study comparing COPD and cancer patients demonstrated that patients with COPD had similar disease burdens to cancer patients but survived five times longer (median survival 107 days in cancer *versus* 589 days in COPD), meaning that COPD patients suffer from symptoms of disease for years leading up to death [11]. Unfortunately, attempts to improve symptoms of respiratory illness in the years preceding death, in particular breathlessness, the defining characteristic of respiratory disease, have garnered insufficient attention when compared with efforts to improve EOL care [12]. While both are tremendously important, it will be critical for leaders of the field of respiratory medicine to ensure that any advancements in the provision of high-quality EOL care are accompanied by efforts to integrate palliative care earlier in disease in order to minimise burdens and enhance quality of life.

History and models of palliative care

The term "palliative care" was coined in 1973 by Balfour Mount, a Surgeon of the Royal Victoria Hospital in Montreal, Canada [13], and may be defined as a focus on the relief of suffering in patients with serious and advanced illness (table 1). In practice, palliative care providers seek to maximise quality of life for such patients and their families or other caregivers. A common misconception is that palliative care is synonymous with hospice or EOL care, when in fact palliative care is not limited to the terminally ill and can occur in parallel to curative and life-prolonging treatments (figure 1). The field of palliative care developed as a response to societal changes, resulting in the idea that death could be prevented, obscured or controlled, rather than being the natural order of things. Early practitioners of palliative care sought to re-emphasise and recognise death as an acceptable and natural outcome rather than a failure, and to focus primarily on relief of suffering rather than cure of disease [16].

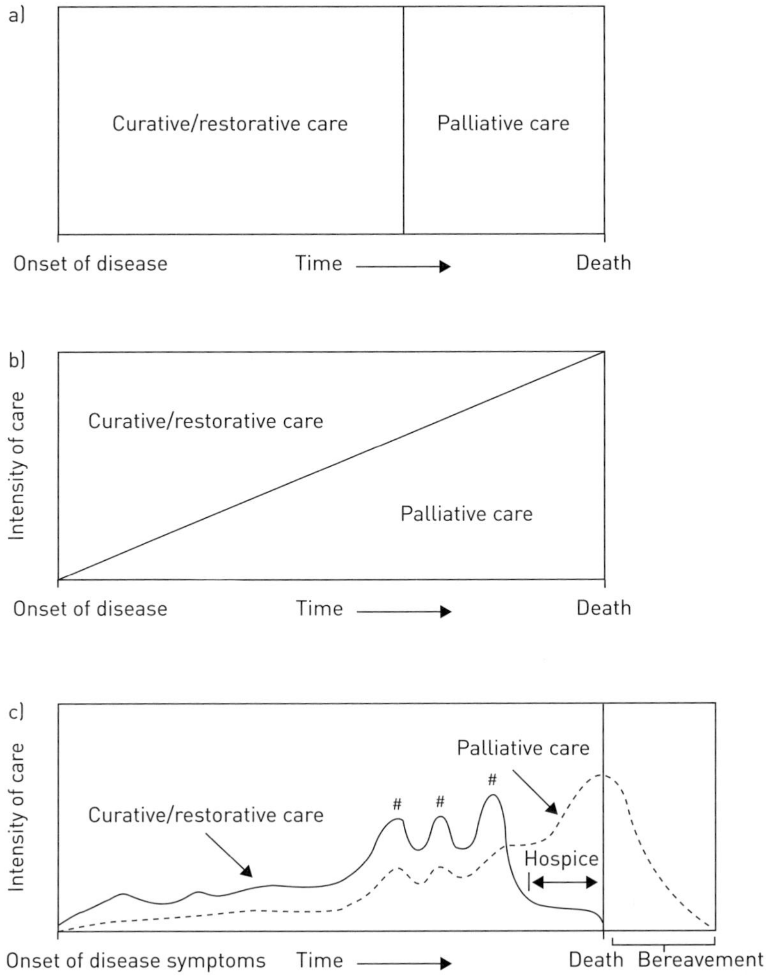

Figure 1. Schematic models of palliative care in relation to provision of curative or restorative care. a) Traditional dichotomous model, *i.e.* "all or nothing", in terms of the period of providing only curative/restorative care followed by the period of providing only palliative care. b) Overlapping model. c) Individualised model. #: periods of high intensity curative/restorative care, such as hospitalisations for lower respiratory tract infections. Reproduced and modified from [14] with permission. Originally modified from [15].

Although not synonymous with hospice care, the origins of the practice of palliative care can be traced back to the hospice movement, which began in the 1960s. The term "hospice" originates from the Latin word *hospitium*, meaning hospitality. Descriptions of the first hospices as places of care for the dying can be found in texts from medieval times. The history of modern hospice and palliative medicine is equally rich. In 1969, Elisabeth Kübler-Ross, a Swiss-American psychiatrist, published her seminal work, *On Death and Dying*, within which she first categorised five stages of grief and underscored the inadequate consideration given to suffering at the EOL [17]. Around the same time, Cicely Saunders, both a nurse and a physician, established St Christopher's Hospice in London, UK. She would later go on to write another influential book, *Living with Dying: a Guide to Palliative Care*, published in 1995 [18]. The first American hospice was established by the nurse Florence Wald in 1974 in New Haven, CT, USA. This was followed by the first palliative medicine programme introduced by Balfour Mount in Montreal in 1975. 12 years later, in 1987, hospice and palliative medicine became recognised as an official medical specialty in the UK, followed by numerous countries around the world. It took nearly 20 more years before the USA finally established hospice and palliative medicine as a medical specialty in 2006 [16].

Goals of palliative care and hospice

If the goal of a hospice is to provide relief of suffering and support to patients and their families at the EOL, then palliative care can be seen as an expansion of the early hospice movement to develop similar comprehensive support services and enhance the quality of life for those with advanced disease over the intervening months or even years preceding death (figure 2). In the last decade, numerous international societies have published guidelines and recommendations for the provision of palliative care, including the American Thoracic Society [14], the Society of Critical Care Medicine [19] and the American Academy of Hospice and Palliative Medicine [20]. Recently in the USA, the Institute of Medicine issued a report detailing the state of healthcare for patients dying in the USA, and included substantive recommendations for the approach to death and dying in the future, including early integration of palliative care into routine healthcare for patients with advanced diseases to improve quality of life and death, as illustrated in figure 1c [14, 21]. Similar statements and guidelines have been published by institutions in other countries, including the European Respiratory Society and European Society of Intensive Care Medicine [22–25]. All of these organisations have advocated for improved communication and adoption of a shared decision making model for patients with advanced illness. Shared decision making is a collective process of communication between clinicians and the patient or surrogates to determine what decisions need to be made, to engage in dialogue to clarify preferences, to ensure understanding medical interventions and to achieve consensus in those decisions [26–28].

Ethical principles of medical decision making

For physicians and other healthcare professionals, medical decision making has been closely linked to the professional obligation to adhere to the four core principles of bioethics:

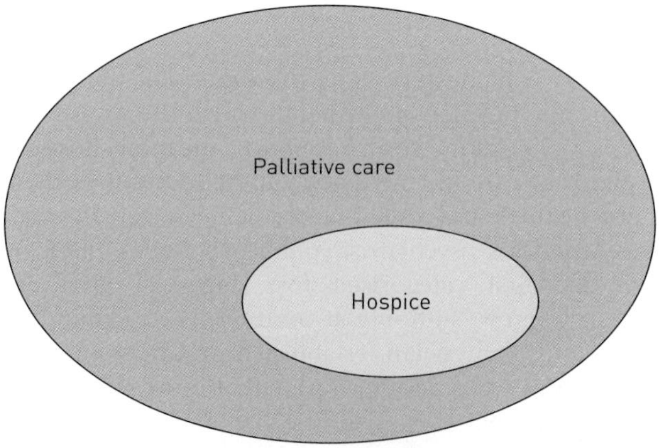

Figure 2. Hospice care is a component of a broader palliative care approach to serious respiratory illnesses.

autonomy, beneficence, non-maleficence and justice. In Western civilisation, autonomy, derived from the Greek *autos* ("self") and *nomos* ("law") [29], has traditionally been seen as the pre-eminent principle among the four. Autonomy can be defined as the right of a patient to be the primary determinant of what medical interventions and treatments he or she will receive: in essence, the right to self-determination, including the right of refusal. Beneficence refers to the ethical duty for medical professionals to promote the well-being of their patients, which dates from Hippocratic times. Non-maleficence, the corollary of beneficence, is embodied in the traditional maxim *primum non nocere* ("first do no harm"). Lastly, justice refers to the fair distribution of healthcare, and the essence of the principle of distributive justice arises from the Greek philosopher Aristotle's formal annunciation: "Equals must be treated equally, and unequals must be treated unequally" [30]. These four guiding principles provide a practical ethical framework to aid in the medical decision making process. However, in practice, these principles often come into conflict with each other (*e.g.* providing beneficent care may not respect a patient's autonomy). Furthermore, the complexities of modern medical practice, in particular when dealing with vulnerable populations, such as patients with advanced and terminal respiratory illness, have prompted some ethicists to argue for an expansion of the ethical lens through which we view decision making beyond the four basic ethical principles [31]. Additional duties include the obligations to communicate effectively, to provide culturally competent care and to understand the patient experience in sickness, including the nature of suffering. In this respect, palliative care providers may possess a unique skill set with which to explore this expanded template.

Medical decision making

The spectrum of medical decision making extends from the directed or paternalistic model of the physician as decision maker at one end to the informative, autonomy-driven model of physician as information provider with the patient or surrogate making EOL decisions at the other end (table 2). Shared decision making falls within these two bookends, with variable degrees of collaboration between provider and patient or surrogate. Experts have argued that good shared decision making necessitates that healthcare providers understand where patients and caregivers fall along this continuum to improve outcomes [32, 33].

Table 2. Models of medical decision making according to roles of the physician and patient or patient's surrogate during the three stages of the decision making process

Stages of decision making process	**Model of medical decision making**		
	Paternalistic	**Shared**	**Informed**
Information exchange	One-way flow of information from physician to patient/surrogate	Two-way flow of information to/from physician and patient/surrogate	One-way flow of information from physician to patient/ surrogate
Deliberation	Physician alone	Physician and patient/ surrogate	Patient/surrogate alone
Deciding on treatment to implement	Physician	Physician and patient/ surrogate	Patient/surrogate

Reproduced and modified from [27] with permission.

Studies of surrogate decision making preferences suggest that there is wide variability in terms of families' preferences in decision making roles [34], and that failure to identify preferences and tailor decision making accordingly may result in an increased risk of adverse consequences such as post-traumatic stress disorder among surrogates [35].

While patients in the outpatient setting with respiratory diseases are able to participate in conversations about medical decision making, many patients in the ICU lack the capacity to make decisions and are therefore unable to participate in discussions [36]. In this context, responsibility falls on a surrogate decision maker to engage in conversations on behalf of the patient. The surrogate decision maker should preferentially use a substituted judgement standard if possible, and if not, a best-interests standard should be used.

Use of a substituted judgement standard assumes that the surrogate has knowledge of the patient's values and preferences for or against certain medical interventions. These can be based either on explicit conversations with the patient, such as expressed in an advance directive, or by considering the patient's life goals and values, as expressed in words or by prior healthcare decisions. Best-interests standard refers to making decisions on the patient's behalf by comparing the benefits of an intervention against the burdens (pain, suffering, cost to patient and/or to patient's family) of that intervention and by proceeding with the intervention if its benefits outweigh its burdens, while forgoing the intervention if its burdens outweigh its benefits. Best-interests decision making should be used when the surrogate does not have knowledge of the patient's preferences or cannot infer such preferences as described above. A glossary of these and other terms related to bioethics and medical decision making are given in table 3.

Provision of palliative care

Advocates of palliative care argue that early palliative care may improve the quality of both life and death as well as decrease healthcare costs and utilisation. A 2014 US study of the Medicare hospice benefits suggested that those receiving hospice care for a cancer diagnosis had lower rates for hospitalisation and ICU admissions, fewer invasive procedures at the EOL and substantially lower healthcare costs in the last year of life [37]. Other studies have demonstrated that early integration of palliative care could result in increased survival [38, 39]. Still further, one study indicated that the place of death correlates with the EOL experience and caregiver mental health, with worse outcomes linked to the acute care and ICU setting and better outcomes associated with death at home with or without hospice care [40]. Other ancillary benefits associated with palliative care can include increased family satisfaction and comprehension [41], decreased conflict over goals of care [42] and better symptom assessment and patient comfort [43]. Thus, these findings support the assertion that providing palliative care assessments and treatments is beneficial to the experiences of both patients and families.

Consistent with this position, palliative care is increasingly being recognised as an important quality element in healthcare [44]. However, it should be recognised that the various cultures and societies around the world embrace differing viewpoints, in particular on death and dying, such as what constitutes a good quality of life or death and a meaningful existence, and whether it is ethically permissible to discontinue LST [45]. This lack of consensus complicates the standardisation of palliative and EOL practices globally.

Furthermore, many patients lack the ability to communicate preferences for care, in particular at the EOL when many decisions are required. Most have not previously articulated their values or preferences. This knowledge gap further challenges decision making and has resulted

Table 3. Glossary of terms related to bioethics and medical decision making

Term	Definition
Autonomy	Bioethical principle referring to the informed and competent adult patient's right to self-determination, respect for dignity and ability to refuse medical interventions and treatments
Beneficence	Bioethical principle referring to the goal of medicine to provide relief from pain and suffering and for the duty of physicians, nurses and other healthcare providers to promote the well-being of patients
Non-maleficence	Bioethical corollary to beneficence that healthcare providers have an ethical duty not to inflict harm on patients
Justice	Bioethical principle related to fairness, most commonly in the distribution of limited or scarce resources
Self-determination	The right of informed, competent adult patients to make choices based on their preferences for medical care
Informed consent	The legal and ethical concept related to self-determination in which a competent, adult patient agrees to undergo a specific medical intervention after being provided relevant information about that intervention: its indication, objectives, risks, benefits and alternatives, including the alternative of no intervention
Informed refusal	The legal and ethical concept related to self-determination in which a competent, adult patient refuses to undergo a specific medical intervention after being provided relevant information about that intervention: its indication, objectives, risks, benefits and alternatives, including the alternative of no intervention
Informed assent	The concept that reflects the willingness of a non-competent patient (*e.g.* a child or minor, or an adult who has lost or never had decision making capacity) to undergo a specific medical or research intervention
Substituted judgement	Bioethical principle referring to a surrogate decision maker making medical decisions for a patient who lacks sufficient capacity for decision making, based on knowledge of that patient's previously written or verbally expressed preferences for medical treatment or of the patient's values and life goals
Best-interests standard	Bioethical principle referring to a surrogate decision maker who lacks knowledge of a patient's preferences and who makes medical decisions for a patient who lacks sufficient capacity for decision making, based on a weighing of the benefits (*e.g.* life, quality of life, chances for survival) against the burdens (*e.g.* poor quality of life, financial costs, pain and suffering of patient and family) of a medical intervention and then making the decision on behalf of the patient after judging whether the benefits of the intervention outweigh its burdens (by choosing the intervention) or whether the burdens of the intervention outweigh the benefits (by forgoing the intervention)
Physician-assisted suicide	Medical act of a physician that assists a patient to commit suicide, *e.g.* prescribing a potentially lethal dose of a medication for the patient to administer to themselves at a later date with the objective being to cause cessation of the patient's life; this may be legal or illegal depending on state or country jurisdiction
Euthanasia	The act of administering an agent for the primary purpose of causing the patient's death
Surrogate decision maker	An individual either appointed or otherwise identified by a patient or legal authorised representative who has the legal and ethical authority to make healthcare decisions for a patient in the event that the patient is unable to make medical decisions for themselves, *i.e.* the patient lacks sufficient decision making capacity
Advance directive	Also known as a living will, this is a legal document in which a capable patient describes her or his preferences for medical care in advance of an illness that renders them incapable of making such decisions in the future

Continued

Table 3. Continued

Term	Definition
LST	A treatment that is required to sustain organ function and hence life; also referred to as "life support"
Paternalism	A traditional practice of physicians in which the physician makes medical decisions on behalf of the patient based on his or her expertise
Patient-/family-centred care	Healthcare that actively engages patients and families to participate in decision making processes and seeks to provide healthcare in accord with the values and preferences of the patient and family; the patient identifies their family members, *e.g.* may be blood- or legal-relatives or friends
Suffering	Physical or existential distress felt by patients and their families from illness or injury or in the process of medical care

in substantial variability in how medical decisions are made at the EOL [46, 47]. Furthermore, although technology may prolong life, it may not restore health or function to a quality of life consistent with that which the patient values. Moreover, technological interventions may not address the suffering, pain and distress that the patient and family must endure throughout the course of illness to achieve a meaningful quality of life.

These unanswered questions aggravate efforts to provide compassionate, patient-centred care. Communication and decision making in patients with respiratory diseases can be particularly challenging owing to the broad scope of diseases (*e.g.* obstructive, interstitial, pulmonary vascular, infectious, pleural and malignant) and the variability in outcomes, with some being chronic and slowly progressive, while others are more rapid or even acute, as in the case of acute respiratory distress syndrome. The type of disease impacts the timing and location of conversation, with some occurring in the outpatient setting, typically after strong physician–patient relationships have developed; still others occur in the ICU where trust is an ongoing process.

Models of providing palliative care

There are two broad models incorporating palliative care into clinical practice, including the ICU setting. The first is the consultative model where the primary healthcare provider is responsible for routine patient care, while palliative care is delivered on a consultative basis. Consulting specialists in hospice and palliative medicine assist with issues arising, including complex emotional distress, conflict between or among providers and patients/surrogates, challenging conversations, and difficult-to-control pain or suffering. One of the inherent advantages of the consultative model is that specialists in palliative care possess a unique skill set for addressing areas of concern that many other clinicians do not have. Additionally, palliative care teams often have robust interdisciplinary teams that include physicians, nurses, pharmacists, social workers and chaplains, allowing consultative teams to effectively and holistically address some of the key domains of palliative care (table 4). The latter were described in the Improving Palliative Care in the ICU (IPAL-ICU) project in 2010 [48] and were determined by the US National Consensus Project for Quality Palliative Care in 2013 [49]. Conversely, the consultative model is dependent on the primary team recognising the need for palliative care consultation, and necessitates suitable

Table 4. Domains of palliative care in clinical practice, including critical care

Patient- and family-centred values
Communication within the healthcare team and with patients and families
Continuity of care
Emotional and practical support for patients and families
Symptom management and comfort care
Spiritual support for patients and families
Emotional and organisational support for palliative care providers

Data from [48].

hospital resources to ensure that the consult team can provide their services as requested. Furthermore, it guarantees the need for additional consultations on patients who may already be receiving care from a large number of specialists, and could potentially duplicate or conflict with the efforts of the primary team [42].

An alternatively suggested model is the integrative model of palliative care where primary palliative care is provided directly by the practitioner caring for the patient. In this model, principles of palliative care are embedded into usual clinical practice, including ICU care. Accordingly, primary providers are expected to have basic competence with providing palliative care. Secondary palliative care can still be rendered on a consultative basis should additional assistance be needed. Integrated models have the benefit of expanding capacity to provide palliative care to all patients through the primary team without a need for consultation. However, it requires that healthcare providers receive suitable training in the basic principles and practices of palliative care in order to develop proficiency [48, 50].

No clear mandate or consensus opinion exists for either model, and data demonstrating greater efficacy for one *versus* the other is limited. As such, palliative care is commonly offered based on mechanisms and structures in place at individual institutions and is often dependent on the presence or absence of palliative care specialists, additional staffing resources, and the commitment of nonpalliative care specialists to engage with palliative care specialists for consultation and professional training in palliative care. It also remains uncertain which specific categories of patients are most likely to benefit from palliative care consultation, and the optimal time for such consultations. Nonetheless, it is hard to argue against the addition of systems that better address symptom management, communication concerning goals of care, and efforts to align values and preferences in patients suffering from advanced and terminal disease.

Global policy

Despite the deeply personal and private nature of PEOLC for individuals and families, many layers of health and social policy affect how, where, when, by whom and to whom PEOLC is rendered. Health and social policy, from the international level to the hospital ward or community agency level, influence the availability and accessibility of PEOLC across the globe. The WHO global atlas of palliative care outlines how policy serves as a conduit for PEOLC. Indeed, it is difficult for palliative care to become available, accessible and accepted without policies to support its provision. The WHO divides its discussion on policy into three vital elements: 1) policy in the form of laws, national standards, specialty or subspecialty recognition, acknowledgement of discrete knowledge of palliative care healthcare providers through granting of licensure, and national strategy to implement such care; 2) education policy to facilitate basic training provided in generalist education to all healthcare providers, intermediate or advanced training for those who frequently care for individuals with life-threatening illnesses, and specialty training in PEOLC; and 3) policies that shape availability of medication frequently used in PEOLC, as their access, especially opioids for relief of pain and breathlessness, is limited worldwide. Thus, the presence or absence of policies to guide these broad, yet integral aspects of PEOLC has wide-reaching effects [3].

Despite the wide acknowledgement of the value of PEOLC in minimising suffering in seriously ill individuals and their families and the recognition of PEOLC as a human right [3], there is great variability in the availability and accessibility of PEOLC services globally. The studies of Wright *et al.* [51] in 2008 and Lynch *et al.* [52] in 2013 provide an overview of this variability and how it has changed over time. The authors categorised countries into groups, based on the level of palliative care development, from group 1 nations, having no hospice or palliative care activity, to group 4b nations, in which hospice and palliative care services are well integrated into the general healthcare system. Lynch *et al.* [52] reported that nearly one-third of all countries had no known hospice or palliative care activity, more than half had limited but growing palliative care services, and only 20 countries had well-integrated PEOLC services in their general healthcare systems. While the availability of palliative care services increased globally by 9% from the 2008 study to the 2013 study, major increases are still required before PEOLC becomes generally accessible. The 2013 study by Lynch *et al.* [52] did find a "strong association" between availability of palliative care in a country and that country's score on the United Nations Human Development Index (UNHDI). For example, nearly 75% of countries in the most advanced groups (4a and 4b) had a high or very high level of development as measured by the UNHDI. The UNHDI is a summary measure of average achievement in three key dimensions of human development: 1) a long and healthy life (*i.e.* mean life-expectancy at birth); 2) being knowledgeable (*i.e.* mean years of schooling); and 3) having a decent standard of living (*i.e.* mean gross national income per capita) [53]. Conversely, over two-thirds of countries in group 1 (no hospice or palliative care services) had a low level of human development [52]. Taken together, one can appreciate how broad economic and sociopolitical forces can shape access to PEOLC services across the globe and why, in countries with low levels of human development as per their UNHDI, many patients who desire PEOLC are probably not receiving those services [5].

In addition to the variability in availability and accessibility of PEOLC, there is variability in EOL medical practices and the policies that guide these practices. Practices such as withholding or withdrawing LST vary according to cultural, regional, religious, statutory and healthcare provider factors [54, 55]. This is important, as the ICU and other hospital units are common places for the delivery of PEOLC for people with respiratory illnesses, especially those requiring technological support. The End-of-Life Practices in European Intensive Care Units (ETHICUS) [54], APPROPRICUS [56] and WELPICUS [45] studies illustrated principles and practices of PEOLC for critically ill individuals, as well as the impact of PEOLC on the healthcare providers that provide such care. Although withholding and withdrawing LSTs were generally accepted across ICUs in many European countries, there were regional differences in the rates of withdrawing *versus* withholding LSTs. These differences have been attributed to cultural, medicolegal and religious factors [54]. Active shortening of the dying process (defined as actions taken with the specific intent of hastening death) was uncommon and occurred in few countries [45, 54]. Such studies and consensus statements are important contributors to policy development because they can guide healthcare legislation, the establishment of infrastructure for PEOLC services, funding for research and healthcare provider training, and recognition of the particular needs of people with life-threatening illnesses, including those with advanced respiratory diseases.

While international efforts and frameworks guided by policy are important and helpful, such efforts must also keep in mind the context within which each nation provides PEOLC. An important aspect of this context is consideration of the leading causes of death and life-threatening illnesses in specific countries. The World Palliative Care Alliance highlights this regional variation. For example, adults mainly needed PEOLC for progressive, non-malignant diseases across the globe, but African and Southeast Asian regions had higher-than-average rates of death from HIV/AIDS, and the Americas and European and Western Pacific regions had a higher-than-average incidence of death from cancer [5].

Thus, policy can be both a barrier and a facilitator of PEOLC [57]. As a barrier, health policies in many nations do not provide an infrastructure for PEOLC as part of the overall healthcare system that could shape the provision of clinical services, training of the healthcare workforce, funding for research and access to opioid analgesics. In addition, health policies may be in place, but nations may have limited resources to enact such policies, or healthcare providers within the healthcare system and those receiving care may have mistaken perceptions about PEOLC. Finally, policy makers and the general public may be reluctant to talk about death and dying. PEOLC remains a relatively new concept, especially for low- to middle-income countries, and fear or lack of political or social will can shape which healthcare concerns are given time and attention by those in power. Without broad health and social policy support for PEOLC, growth may be confined to individual efforts to increase accessibility to PEOLC services.

On the other hand, health and social policy can serve as facilitators of PEOLC. Adoption of a broad, public health approach to PEOLC policy can guide the establishment of a palliative care infrastructure that fits the context of a particular country and meets the needs of its residents. Furthermore, this public health approach can shape healthcare provider training so that an adequate workforce is in place to provide the care and implement programmes created through a public health infrastructure. Finally, a public health approach to policy can intersect with medicolegal policy to further the discussion around patient and family involvement in PEOLC, appropriate use of LSTs, and access to necessary medications to limit pain and suffering near the EOL [5]. Table 5 highlights selected aspects of health and social policy affecting PEOLC across a number of representative countries.

Conclusion

Patients with advanced respiratory diseases often experience a significant burden of symptoms and other concerns that could benefit from palliative care. A problem-based approach to identifying when palliative care would be of benefit could prevent a delay in, or absence of, accessing such support. Palliative care seeks to improve quality of life, by focusing on comfort and quality of life rather than cure. To this end, palliative care emphasises patient- and family-centred care to mitigate physical, emotional, spiritual and moral distress not only during EOL care but also during many phases of illness (figure 1c). This is consistent with the basic bioethical principles of respect for autonomy and beneficence. Multiple professional healthcare organisations have recommended that medical decision making, including palliative care, be shared between providers and patients or

Table 5. PEOLC policies and practices in selected countries

Country	Classification of palliative care development [52]	Policy	Education	Medication availability[#]
Argentina	3b: Generalised provision (drop from approaching integration). In ALCP ranking (regional ranking): fourth highest of 18 nations.	No national palliative care programme. No statistically significant difference between ALCP nations with or without a palliative care programme [58].	Approximately one-fifth of medical schools offer undergraduate palliative care training[¶]. No data available for the number of nursing schools that offer undergraduate palliative care training. Four specialty programmes for postgraduate training of physicians[+]. Overall, 2.5 physicians accredited in palliative care per million inhabitants[§].	Consumption of strong opioids per capita: 12.88 mg of morphine[§]. Consumption of strong opioids per cancer death: 8665 mg of morphine per cancer death. Pharmacies that dispense strong opioids per million participants: no data available [58].
Belgium	4b: Advanced integration.	Law enacted in 2002 to preserve right of access to palliative care. Royal decrees outline minimum palliative care service provisions across various settings, and funding and free medical care for home palliative care and leave for informal caregivers. The National Cancer Plan outlines national and regional healthcare policy on palliative care. In Belgium, palliative care laws cover the definition of, right to and access to palliative care, its provision and quality assurance. Palliative care regulations cover the service provision, patient allowances, leave for informal caregivers and funding for services, while the National Cancer Plan provides national funding for palliative care services and provision. The general healthcare laws cover advance directives. A law legalising euthanasia, enacted in 2002, stipulates that the physician must offer options of palliative care to patients seeking euthanasia [59].	In Flanders (60% of population), there is no specialist accreditation in palliative care. Training is organised through Palliative Care Networks and the Federation Palliative Care Flanders, as well as through local universities. Training may be informed by the guidelines for symptom control and the Pathway for Palliative Care in Primary Care. This was commissioned by the Flemish Agency on Care and Health and the Federation Palliative Care Flanders. There are no national meetings in Belgium due to the organisation of the country [60]. As outlined in the Atlas of Palliative Care in Europe, the greatest palliative care issue facing the nation is capacity and workforce building, as well as retention. There is growth in undergraduate medical and nursing programmes for general training for pain and symptom management in EOL care. Similarly, there is postgraduate training in medical and nursing schools [60].	Belgian consumption of morphine: less than half of the European mean of 12.5917 mg per capita and consistent with the global mean of 5.9847 mg per capita. Opioids are generally available, with <25% of cost paid by patients (with cancer). No permits required for patients to receive opioids or for physicians to prescribe them. No barriers in forms used to prescribe (no need for duplicate and triplicate forms). Opioids are generally available at pharmacies, yet emergency prescription is prohibited to nurses and pharmacists, or over the telephone. Value-neutral language is used in opioid regulations [61].

Continued

Table 5. Continued

Country	Classification of palliative care development [52]	Policy	Education	Medication availability[#]
Israel	4a: Preliminary integration.	The National Health law guarantees care across the lifespan. The Ministry of Health recently published a paper defining the provision of palliative care across settings (hospital, community and nursing homes). The Law of the Dying stipulated that patients have the right to choose their preferred treatment for the end of their lives and the location of their death. A Directive of the Ministry of Health promotes broader awareness of PEOLC, creation of more inpatient palliative care beds, provision of palliative care in nursing homes and home-based palliative care. However, funding for palliative care development is at a standstill. The IPMS successfully led efforts against the passage of euthanasia legislation [60].	The IPMS led efforts to develop a national palliative care consensus and published guidelines. Palliative care nursing is recognised as a specialty, and palliative medicine is recognised as a subspecialty. The IPMS is leading efforts for specialty recognition in medicine. Palliative care is integrated in undergraduate nursing and medical education. There is postgraduate medical education in palliative care, whereas it is woven into postgraduate oncology training in nursing. The Israeli National Palliative Care Training is a national collaboration of physicians, nurses and social workers who provide basic palliative care training across the nation [60].	Access to essential medications is recognised as a legal and human right. A healthcare law makes opioids available by prescription. These prescriptions are more difficult to complete than general prescriptions. The 1996 prescription law allows for a 1-month supply of medication, removes maximum dosages and allows for as-needed dosing. No identified barriers to essential palliative care medications, including accessibility or affordability. Patients with cancer receive opioid prescriptions at no cost. Increased education efforts around prescription of opioids and decreasing fear [60].
Italy	4b: Advanced integration.	The National Law of Palliative Care (Law 38/2010) (2010) established palliative care as a basic right and stipulates that local healthcare services must implement regional palliative care networks to uphold this right. This law is both the general legislation and the national palliative care plan. The Italian National Health Service also describes palliative care throughout its plan for provision of cancer care. The Ministry of Health is the office to supervise the regional networks, measure its quality and evaluate opioid use. The Department of Health is responsible for overseeing the delivery of palliative care services. Law 38/2010 required that two palliative care networks be set up in each region (one for palliative care and one for pain), yet this can be hard to enact because each region has the right, provided by the Italian constitution, to autonomously organise its healthcare system. Law 38/2010 also requires that the Ministry of Health reports about the regional palliative care networks to the Italian parliament. A recent proposal for a law on advance directives received negative attention and assessment from the palliative care community and was never passed [60].	Law 38/2010 describes the standards for accreditation of services and professional requirements for physicians and nurses to work in palliative care. It also describes the national health organisation that defines and provides palliative care education for medicine, nursing and psychology. Law 38/2010 establishes the obligation to assess and treat pain of every terminally ill person. Integration of palliative care into undergraduate medical and nursing education is not clear. Of 40 medical schools, there are only two professors of palliative medicine. The Italian Society of Palliative Care plans training and conferences. They work with the Italian Federation of Palliative Care, an umbrella organisation of palliative care organisations, to produce consensus documents to move palliative care beyond cancer [60].	Italian consumption of morphine: approximately half of the global mean of 5.9847 mg per capita and approximately one-quarter of the European mean of 12.5917 mg per capita. Most opioids are available and free of charge to patients; several opioids are unavailable (propoxyphene, dihydrocodeine, pethidine injectable, hydromorphone immediate release). Law 38/2010 dictates that a particular kind of prescription is needed for injectable morphine or methadone, but no accommodations are needed for less potent opioids. Special forms are needed (duplicate and triplicate) to prescribe opioids and are freely available to physicians. Prescriptions are limited to 30 days. Opioids are generally available at any pharmacy. Prohibitions exist against emergency opioid prescribing over the telephone or by fax, or by nurses or pharmacists, and pharmacists cannot correct mistakes on opioid prescriptions (*e.g.* patient address). Value-neutral language found in regulations [61].

Continued

Table 5. Continued

Country	Classification of palliative care development [52]	Policy	Education	Medication availability#
Netherlands	4a: Preliminary integration.	No specific palliative care law, but the general healthcare law (the Dutch Act of Agreement on Medical Treatment) allocates patient allowances for payment of services and calls for advance directives in care. It also covers the role of palliative care volunteers. The "Termination of Life on Request and Assisted Suicide" was enacted in 2002. It stated that, for the law to be exercised, no reasonable alternative options can be available for the patient. Palliative care was not explicitly mentioned in the law [59]. The "Agreement Palliative Terminal Care" regulates funding and institutional regulation for specific palliative care settings. The national palliative care plan defines palliative care and covers the access to services, provision of services and quality assurance. The national and/or regional palliative care health policy "Plan van Aanpak Palliatieve Zorg" describes three elements of oversight: 1) organisation and finance of palliative care, such as the tasks, products and services of rural and regional palliative care organisations; 2) increased quality and transparency of palliative care services; and 3) education and competency in palliative care.	The "Plan van Aanpak Palliatieve Zorg", the national palliative care programme, was proposed in 2007. Among the three core elements is an emphasis on high-quality palliative care education and training. The palliative care plan covers palliative care training and research [59].	Dutch consumption of morphine: less than the European mean of 12.5917 mg per capita, yet higher than the global mean of 5.9847 mg per capita. Opioids are generally available, free of cost to patients (with cancer). No permits are required for patients to receive opioids or for physicians to prescribe them. No barriers in forms used to prescribe (no need for duplicate and triplicate forms). Opioids are generally available at pharmacies, yet emergency prescription is generally prohibited except for a fax sent in by a physician. Value-neutral language is used in opioid regulations [61].

Continued

Table 5. Continued

Country	Classification of palliative care development [52]	Policy	Education	Medication availability[#]
UK	4b: Advanced integration.	No specific laws or regulations concerning palliative care [59]. The general healthcare laws mention palliative care. Palliative care services are commissioned by local healthcare authorities [60]. A national palliative care plan covers quality assurance. National and/or regional healthcare policies about palliative care, such as the National Institute for Health and Care Excellence clinical guidance on supportive and palliative care, National Health Service cancer plan (2000), EOL care initiative (2003) and the EOL care strategy (2008) [59].	Limited information available about integration of palliative care into undergraduate or postgraduate medical and nursing training. There is an officially recognised certification for medicine (4–5 years of specialist training) and nursing (1–2 years of specialist training). The National Council on Palliative Care (1991) represents England, Wales and Northern Ireland. Palliative Care Scotland covers Scotland. Training is provided at the National Palliative Care Congress twice per year and through other interdisciplinary palliative care organisations. There is much research and many clinical collaborations within the UK and internationally [60].	UK consumption of morphine: over twice the European mean of 12.5917 mg per capita (~30 mg per capita) and nearly six times the global mean of 5.9847 mg per capita. Opioids are generally available, with <25% of cost paid by patients (with cancer). No permits required for patients to receive opioids or for physicians to prescribe them. No barriers in forms used to prescribe (no barriers for duplicate and triplicate forms). Prescriptions limited to 28–30 days. Opioids are generally available at pharmacies, and emergency prescriptions are allowed to be generated by nurses or pharmacists, and physicians can provide over-the-telephone prescriptions. Value-neutral language used in opioid regulations [61].

ALCP: Asociación Latinoamericana de Cuidados Paliativos (Latin American Association for Palliative Care); IPMS: Israel Palliative Medicine Society. #: ALCP indicator of opioid availability is measured in milligrammes of morphine per unit of interest; ¶: positive correlation between this parameter and availability of palliative care services per million inhabitants [58]; +: moderate correlation with palliative care service availability per million participants [58]; §: positive and significant correlation with palliative care service availability per million inhabitants [58].

their surrogates, *i.e.* using the shared decision making model (table 2). Nonetheless, because differences in national and local cultures impact the clinical practice of palliative care, such as acceptability to forgo life support, the decision making process should take into account the relevant cultural context. This is especially important when considering the creation and adaptation of global healthcare policy in providing PEOLC.

References

1. World Health Organization. WHO Definition of Palliative Care. www.who.int/cancer/palliative/definition/en/ Date last updated: 2016. Date last accessed: July 23, 2016.
2. Van Mechelen W, Aertgeerts B, De Ceulaer K, *et al.* Defining the palliative care patient: a systematic review. *Palliat Med* 2013; 27: 197–208.
3. Centers for Disease Control and Prevention. Deaths and Mortality. www.cdc.gov/nchs/fastats/deaths.htm Date last updated: February 25, 2016. Date last accessed: March 3, 2016.
4. Ecology Global Network. World Birth and Death Rates. www.ecology.com/birth-death-rates/ Date last updated: 2011. Date last accessed: March 3, 2016.
5. Worldwide Hospice Palliative Care Alliance. WHO Global Atlas on Palliative Care At the End of Life. Available from: www.thewhpca.org/resources/global-atlas-on-end-of-life-care Date last updated: July 10, 2014. Date last accessed: March 3, 2016.
6. World Health Organization. Chronic Respiratory Diseases: Burden of COPD. www.who.int/respiratory/copd/burden/en/ Date last updated: 2016. Date last accessed: June 6, 2016.
7. World Health Organization. Burden: mortality, morbidity and risk factors. *In:* Global Status Report on Noncommunicable Diseases 2010. Geneva, World Health Organization, 2011. www.who.int/nmh/publications/ncd_report_chapter1.pdf
8. Angus DC, Barnato AE, Linde-Zwirble WT, *et al.* Use of intensive care at the end of life in the United States: an epidemiologic study. *Crit Care Med* 2004; 32: 638–643.
9. Teno JM, Gozalo PL, Bynum JP, *et al.* Change in end-of-life care for Medicare beneficiaries: site of death, place of care, and health care transitions in 2000, 2005, and 2009. *JAMA* 2013; 309: 470–477.
10. Bekelman JE, Halpern SD, Blankart CR, *et al.* Comparison of site of death, health care utilization, and hospital expenditures for patients dying with cancer in 7 developed countries. *JAMA* 2016; 315: 272–283.
11. Bausewein C, Booth S, Gysels M, *et al.* Understanding breathlessness: cross-sectional comparison of symptom burden and palliative care needs in chronic obstructive pulmonary disease and cancer. *J Palliat Med* 2010; 32: 1109–1118.
12. Currow DC, Abernathy AP, Allcroft P, *et al.* The need to research refractory breathlessness. *Eur Respir J* 2016; 47: 342–343.
13. Canada.com. A Moral Force: The Story of Dr Balfour Mount. http://web.archive.org/web/20061215112019/http://www.canada.com/ottawacitizen/story.html?id=896d005a-fedd-4f50-a2d9-83a95fc56464 Date last updated: April 23, 2015. Date last accessed: July 22, 2016.
14. Lanken PN, Terry PB, Delisser HM, *et al.* An official American Thoracic Society clinical policy statement: palliative care for patients with respiratory diseases and critical illnesses. *Am J Respir Crit Care Med* 2008; 177: 912–927.
15. World Health Organization. Cancer Pain Relief and Palliative Care: Report of a WHO Expert Committee. Technical Report Series 804. Geneva, World Health Organization, 1990. http://apps.who.int/iris/bitstream/10665/39524/1/WHO_TRS_804.pdf
16. Meier DE, Isaacs SL, Hughes RG, eds. Palliative Care: Transforming the Care of Serious Illness. 1st Edn. San Francisco, Jossey-Bass, 2010.
17. Kübler-Ross E, ed. On Death and Dying: What the Dying Have to Teach Doctors, Nurses, Clergy and Their Own Families. New York, Simon & Schuster, 1969.
18. Saunders C, Baines M, Dunlop R, eds. Living with Dying: a Guide to Palliative Care. 3rd Edn. New York, Oxford University Press, 1995.
19. Davidson JE, Powers K, Hedayat KM, *et al.* Clinical practice guidelines for support of the family in the patient-centered intensive care unit: American College of Critical Care Medicine Task Force 2004–2005. *Crit Care Med* 2007; 35: 605–622.
20. American Academy of Hospice and Palliative Medicine. AAHPM Position Statements. http://aahpm.org/about/position-statements Date last updated: 2016. Date last accessed: March 19, 2016.
21. National Academies of Sciences, Engineering, and Medicine. Committee on Approaching Death: Addressing Key End of Life Issues. www.nationalacademies.org/hmd/Activities/Aging/TransformingEndOfLife.aspx Date last updated: October 15, 2015. Date last accessed: July 22, 2016.

22. Candy B, Elliott M, Moore K, *et al.* UK quality statements on end of life care in dementia: a systematic review of research evidence. *BMC Palliat Care* 2015; 14: 51.
23. Carlet J, Thijs LG, Antonelli M, *et al.* Challenges in end-of-life care in the ICU. Statement of the 5th International Consensus Conference in Critical Care: Brussels, Belgium, April 2003. *Intensive Care Med* 2004; 30: 770–784.
24. Thompson BT, Cox PN, Antonelli M, *et al.* Challenges in end-of-life care in the ICU: statement of the 5th International Consensus Conference in Critical Care: Brussels, Belgium, April 2003: executive summary. *Crit Care Med* 2004; 32: 1781–1784.
25. European Association for Palliative Care. www.eapcnet.eu/Home.aspx Date last updated: July 11, 2016. Date last accessed: July 22, 2016.
26. Charles C, Gafni A, Whelan T. Shared decision-making in the medical encounter: what does it mean? (or it takes at least two to tango). *Soc Sci Med* 1997; 44: 681–692.
27. Charles C, Gafni A, Whelan T. Decision-making in the physician-patient encounter: revisiting the shared treatment decision-making model. *Soc Sci Med* 1999; 49: 651–661.
28. Murray E, Charles C, Gafni A. Shared decision-making in primary care: tailoring the Charles *et al.* model to fit the context of general practice. *Patient Educ Couns* 2006; 62: 205–211.
29. The American Heritage Dictionary of the English Language. 5th Edn. New York, Houghton Mifflin Harcourt Publishing Company, 2011.
30. Gillon R. Philosophical Medical Ethics. 1st Edn. Chichester, John Wiley & Sons Ltd, 1986.
31. Fiester A. Viewpoint: why the clinical ethics we teach fails patients. *Acad Med* 2007; 82: 684–689.
32. Curtis JR, White DB. Practical guidance for evidence-based ICU family conferences. *Chest* 2008; 134: 835–843.
33. Curtis JR, Vincent JL. Ethics and end-of-life care for adults in the intensive care unit. *Lancet* 2010; 376: 1347–1353.
34. Heyland DK, Cook DJ, Rocker GM, *et al.* Decision-making in the ICU: perspectives of the substitute decision-maker. *Intensive Care Med* 2003; 29: 75–82.
35. Gries CJ, Engelberg RA, Kross EK, *et al.* Predictors of symptoms of posttraumatic stress and depression in family members after patient death in the ICU. *Chest* 2010; 137: 280–287.
36. Prendergast TJ, Luce JM. Increasing incidence of withholding and withdrawal of life support from the critically ill. *Am J Respir Crit Care Med* 1997; 155: 15–20.
37. Obermeyer Z, Makar M, Abujaber S, *et al.* Association between the Medicare hospice benefit and health care utilization and costs for patients with poor-prognosis cancer. *JAMA* 2014; 312: 1888–1896.
38. Temel JS, Greer JA, Muzikansky A, *et al.* Early palliative care for patients with metastatic non-small-cell lung cancer. *N Engl J Med* 2010; 363: 733–742.
39. Higginson IJ, Bausewein C, Reilly CC, *et al.* An integrated palliative and respiratory care service for patients with advanced disease and refractory breathlessness: a randomized controlled trial. *Lancet Respir Med* 2014; 2: 978–987.
40. Wright AA, Keating NL, Balboni TA, *et al.* Place of death: correlations with quality of life of patients with cancer and predictors of bereaved caregivers' mental health. *J Clin Oncol* 2010; 28: 4457–4464.
41. Azoulay E, Pochard F, Chevret S, *et al.* Impact of a family information leaflet on effectiveness of information provided to family members of intensive care unit patients: a multicenter, prospective, randomized, controlled trial. *Am J Respir Crit Care Med* 2002; 165: 438–442.
42. Lilly CM, De Meo DL, Sonna LA, *et al.* An intensive communication intervention for the critically ill. *Am J Med* 2000; 109: 469–475.
43. Erdek MA, Pronovost PJ. Improving assessment and treatment of pain in the critically ill. *Int J Qual Health Care* 2004; 16: 59–64.
44. Aslakson RA, Curtis JR, Nelson JE. The changing role of palliative care in the ICU. *Crit Care Med* 2014; 42: 2418–2428.
45. Sprung CL, Truog RD, Curtis JR, *et al.* Seeking worldwide professional consensus on the principles of end-of-life care for the critically ill. The Consensus for Worldwide End-of-Life Practice for Patients in Intensive Care Units (WELPICUS) study. *Am J Respir Crit Care Med* 2014; 190: 855–866.
46. Prendergast TJ, Claessens MT, Luce JM. A national survey of end-of-life care for critically ill patients. *Am J Respir Crit Care Med* 1998; 158: 1163–1167.
47. Cohen S, Sprung C, Sjokvist P, *et al.* Communication of end-of-life decisions in European intensive care units. *Intensive Care Med* 2005; 31: 1215–1221.
48. Nelson JE, Bassett R, Boss RD, *et al.* Models for structuring a clinical initiative to enhance palliative care in the intensive care unit: a report from the IPAL-ICU Project (Improving Palliative Care in the ICU). *Crit Care Med* 2010; 38: 1765–1772.
49. National Consenus Project Task Force. Clinical Practice Guidelines for Quality Palliative Care, 3rd Edn. Pittsburgh, National Consenus Project for Quality Palliative Care, 2013.
50. Quill TE, Abernethy AP. Generalist plus specialist palliative care – creating a more sustainable model. *N Engl J Med* 2013; 368: 1173–1175.
51. Wright M, Wood J, Lynch T, *et al.* Mapping levels of palliative care development: a global view. *J Pain Symptom Manage* 2008; 35: 469–485.

52. Lynch T, Connor S, Clark D. Mapping levels of palliative care development: a global update. *J Pain Symptom Manage* 2013; 45: 1094–1106.
53. United Nations Development Programme. Human Development Index (HDI). http://hdr.undp.org/en/content/human-development-index-hdi Date last updated: 2015. Date last accessed: April 29, 2016.
54. Sprung CL, Cohen SL, Sjokvist P, *et al.* End-of-life practices in European intensive care units: the Ethicus Study. *JAMA* 2003; 290: 790–797.
55. Mark NM, Rayner SG, Lee NJ, *et al.* Global variability in withholding and withdrawal of life-sustaining treatment in the intensive care unit: a systematic review. *Intensive Care Med* 2015; 41: 1572–1585.
56. Piers RD, Azoulay E, Ricou B, *et al.* Perceptions of appropriateness of care among European and Israeli intensive care unit nurses and physicians. *JAMA* 2011; 306: 2694–2703.
57. World Health Organization. Strengthening of palliative care as a component of integrated treatment throughout the life course. *J Pain Palliat Care Pharmacother* 2014; 28: 130–134.
58. Pastrana T, Torres-Vigil I, De Lima L. Palliative care development in Latin America: an analysis using macro indicators. *Palliat Med* 2014; 28: 1231–1238.
59. Van Beek K, Woitha K, Ahmed N, *et al.* Comparison of legislation, regulations and national health strategies for palliative care in seven European countries (results from the Europall Research Group): a descriptive study. *BMC Health Serv Res* 2013; 13: 275.
60. Centeno C, Lynch T, Donea O, *et al.* EAPC Atlas of Palliative Care in Europe 2013 – Full Edition. Milan, EAPC Press, 2013. Available from: www.eapcnet.eu/Themes/Organisation/DevelopmentinEurope/EAPCAtlas2013.aspx
61. Cherny NI, Baselga J, de Conno F, *et al.* Formulary availability and regulatory barriers to accessibility of opioids for cancer pain in Europe: a report from the ESMO/EAPC Opioid Policy Initiative. *Ann Oncol* 2010; 21: 615–626.

Acknowledgements: The authors would like to thank the anonymous reviewers for their thoughtful comments.

Disclosures: None declared.

Chapter 2

The need for palliative care

Sabrina Bajwah[1], Eve Namisango[1], Daisy J.A. Janssen[2,3], Deborah Dudgeon[4,5], Anna-Marie Stevens[6] and Jayne Wood[6]

Patients with life-limiting respiratory diseases, such as lung cancer, COPD, IPF and cystic fibrosis, have physical, psychological, social and spiritual needs. Palliative care can help meet these needs, and improve the quality of life of these patients and their families.

Palliative care aims to prevent and relieve suffering by controlling symptoms and providing support to patients and families in order to maintain and improve their quality of life (QoL) [1]. COPD is the most common CRD that requires palliation, but other progressive respiratory diseases such as IPF are coming to the forefront, with recent studies showing the scale of suffering for both patients and carers [2, 3]. In delivering effective palliative care to large numbers of patients with respiratory disease, the epidemiology of advanced respiratory disease needs to be considered, including the challenges of delivering palliative care in a resource-challenged setting. In addition, there must be a focus on improving the physical, psychosocial and spiritual needs of those living with non-malignant lung diseases (including COPD and IPF), cancer and cystic fibrosis (CF). This chapter will highlight the palliative care needs of each of these individual disease groups.

Epidemiology of advanced respiratory diseases

Incidence and prevalence

23 million people in countries of the European Union suffer from moderate to very severe COPD, resulting in 1.1 million hospital admissions and 150 000 deaths a year [4]. The prevalence of COPD is estimated to range from 4% to up to 20% in adults over 40 years of age [5–8], with a considerable increase by age, particularly among smokers. Large differences exist among countries. These are attributable to differences in diagnostic methods, year of study, age of the population and prevalence of the main risk factors, such as tobacco smoking [9]. Limited data are available for resource-limited settings, but with a prevalence of 6.3%, a total of 56.6 million moderate to severe COPD cases is estimated in 12 countries in Asia [9]. COPD prevalence has always been higher in the older age groups in resource-limited settings

[1]Dept of Palliative Care, Policy and Rehabilitation, Cicely Saunders Institute, King's College London, London, UK. [2]Dept of Research and Education, CIRO, Horn, The Netherlands. [3]Centre of Expertise for Palliative Care, Maastricht University Medical Centre+ (MUMC+), Maastricht, The Netherlands. [4]Dept of Medicine, Queen's University, Kingston, ON, Canada. [5]Canadian Partnership Against Cancer, Person-Centred Perspective, Toronto, ON, Canada. [6]Royal Marsden Hospital NHS Foundation Trust, London, UK.

Correspondence: S. Bajwah, Cicely Saunders Institute of Palliative Care and Rehabilitation, Bessemer Rd, London SE5 9PJ, UK. E-mail: sabrina.bajwah@kcl.ac.uk

 Print ISBN: 978-1-84984-071-2. Online ISBN: 978-1-84984-072-9. Print ISSN: 2312-508X. Online ISSN: 2312-5098.

but is now increasing in the 20–44 years age bracket due to the increase in tobacco consumption in this group [10].

Lung cancer is the most common cancer worldwide, with nearly 1.83 million new cases of lung cancer diagnosed in 2012 [11]. In Europe alone, more than 410 000 new cases of lung cancer were estimated to have been diagnosed in 2012 [11]. The UK incidence rate is the seventh lowest in Europe for males and the seventh highest for females [11].

The prevalence of IPF in the USA varies, with estimates of between 14 and 27.9 cases per 100 000 population using narrow case definitions, and between 42.7 and 63 per 100 000 population using broad case definitions [12]. In Europe, IPF prevalence ranges from 1.25 to 23.4 cases per 100 000 population [12]. The annual incidence of IPF in the USA is estimated at 6.8–8.8 per 100 000 population using narrow case definitions and at 16.3–17.4 per 100 000 population using broad case definitions [12]. In Europe, the annual incidence ranges between 0.22 and 7.4 per 100 000 population [12]. IPF prevalence and incidence increase with age, are higher among males and appear to have been on the increase in recent years [12].

Mortality

Respiratory diseases are among the leading causes of death worldwide (table 1) [13, 14]. Lung infections (mostly pneumonia and tuberculosis), lung cancer and COPD together accounted for 9.5 million deaths worldwide during 2008, one-sixth of the global total [13]. More than 3 million people died of COPD in 2012, which was equal to ~6% of all deaths globally that year [13]. Over 90% of these COPD deaths occurred in low- and middle-income countries [15]. This trend is largely attributed to poverty-associated problems, which are associated with poor health outcomes [15]. In the 28 countries of the European Union, respiratory diseases account for one in eight deaths [15]. In the next two decades, the proportion of deaths caused by respiratory disease in Europe is likely to remain stable, with a decrease in deaths from lung infections balanced by a rise in lung cancer and COPD mortality [13].

Lung cancer is the most common cause of death from cancer worldwide, estimated to be responsible for nearly one in five (1.4 million) deaths [16]. Because of its high fatality (the

Table 1. The 10 most common causes of death in 2008

Deaths attributed to	Worldwide	WHO European Region
Ischaemic heart disease	7.3 million (12.8%)	2.40 million (24.7%)
Cerebrovascular disease	6.2 million (10.8%)	1.40 million (14.0%)
Lower respiratory infections	3.5 million (6.1%)	0.23 million (2.3%)
COPD	3.3 million (5.8%)	0.25 million (2.5%)
Diarrhoeal diseases	2.5 million (4.3%)	0.03 million (0.3%)
HIV/AIDS	1.8 million (3.1%)	0.08 million (0.8%)
Trachea/bronchus/lung cancer	1.4 million (2.4%)	0.38 million (3.9%)
Tuberculosis	1.3 million (2.4%)	0.08 million (0.8%)
Diabetes mellitus	1.3 million (2.2%)	0.17 million (1.7%)
Road traffic accidents	1.2 million (2.1%)	0.12 million (1.2%)

WHO: World Health Organization. Reproduced from [13] with permission. Data from [14].

overall ratio of mortality to incidence is 0.87) and the relative lack of variability in survival in different world regions, the geographical patterns in mortality closely follow those of incidence [16].

Morbidity

Globally, respiratory diseases present a serious public health problem and are associated with high morbidity, mortality, economic burden and impact on patient QoL, as well as that of their families. COPD is a major cause of chronic morbidity worldwide [17, 18]. COPD severely impacts QoL [19, 20]. Exacerbations lead to substantial reductions in health-related QoL (HRQoL), in both physical and other areas [21]. In the European Union, among respiratory diseases, COPD is the leading cause of work days lost [13]. In addition, recent qualitative research shows that other respiratory diseases such as IPF have a much greater impact than previously thought, with far-reaching implications of the disease on every aspect of patient and carers' lives [2, 3].

The paucity of data on respiratory diseases in resource-limited settings is attributed to the limited diagnostic capacity, weak surveillance systems that do not include respiratory diseases in the national health management information systems for national level tracking, and a lack of vital statistics. However, it is likely that the burden of respiratory diseases is underreported.

The World Health Organization (WHO) estimated that respiratory diseases accounted for one-tenth of the DALYs lost worldwide in 2008 (table 2) [13, 14].

Health service burden

In 2013, there were approximately 6.5 million in-patients with diseases of the respiratory system discharged from hospitals in the European Union [22]. Almost half of respiratory admissions in Europe are attributable to acute infections (including pneumonia), and episodes of infection are often a cause of exacerbations of asthma and COPD. More than one-quarter of respiratory admissions are due to lung cancer and COPD, diseases that are strongly related to smoking [13]. Other respiratory diseases such as IPF also experience

Table 2. The 10 most common causes of DALYs lost worldwide in 2008

DALYs lost to	Worldwide	WHO European Region
Lower respiratory infections	79 million (5.4%)	2.2 million (1.5%)
HIV/AIDS	65 million (4.4%)	2.6 million (1.8%)
Ischaemic heart disease	64 million (4.4%)	16.0 million (11.3%)
Diarrhoeal diseases	56 million (3.8%)	1.1 million (0.7%)
Cerebrovascular disease	48 million (3.3%)	9.3 million (6.4%)
Road traffic accidents	45 million (3.1%)	3.4 million (2.4%)
COPD	33 million (2.3%)	2.9 million (2.0%)
Tuberculosis	29 million (2.0%)	1.7 million (1.2%)
Diabetes mellitus	22 million (1.5%)	2.6 million (1.8%)
Trachea/bronchus/lung cancer	13 million (0.9%)	3.2 million (2.2%)

WHO: World Health Organization. Reproduced from [13] with permission. Data from [14].

increased healthcare resource utilisation and direct medical costs [23]. This is important, because, as the population gets older, we can expect the burden on healthcare to increase [23].

Future projections

By 2030, the WHO estimates that the four major potentially fatal respiratory diseases (pneumonia, tuberculosis, lung cancer and COPD) will account for about one in five deaths worldwide, compared with one-sixth of all deaths globally in 2008. Within the WHO European Region, the proportion is expected to remain stable at about one-tenth of all deaths, with an increase in COPD and lung cancer deaths balancing a decline in deaths from lower respiratory infections and tuberculosis. IPF is predominately a disease of later life, with two-thirds of patients being over 60 years of age at presentation [24]. This demographic profile is important, as the incidence of IPF is set to double by 2030 as populations age [25]. Therefore, we can expect that the burden on healthcare will increase [23].

In developing countries, the WHO's objectives for improving the management of respiratory diseases include decreasing the burden of illness, preventing avoidable deaths and increasing the QoL of patients [26]. The critical need for palliative care in respiratory diseases requires building capacity for healthcare professionals to provide palliative care to an array of patients with respiratory symptoms and increased access to appropriate medicines to improve care outcomes with only a modest investment of additional resources into the health system.

Palliative care needs in people with non-malignant lung disease

The probability of patients with COPD receiving palliative care is much lower than for patients with cancer. Moreover, if patients are referred to palliative care services, referral occurs late in the course of the disease (about 10 days before death). Patients with COPD who are not referred to palliative care are more likely to receive life-prolonging treatment than palliative treatment [27]. Patients with IPF are also unlikely to be referred to palliative care. A recent study showed that only 14% of deceased patients with IPF were referred for a palliative care consultation, and the majority of these were within 1 month of death [28]. Barriers to palliative care provision in patients with non-malignant lung disease include: 1) the variable disease trajectory, leading to difficulty in predicting prognosis and identifying patients appropriate for palliative care; 2) reluctance among clinicians and patients to discuss palliative care; and 3) health-system issues, including reimbursement structures [29].

Symptom distress

Symptom burden is high in patients with advanced chronic lung diseases [30, 31]. Dyspnoea is the most reported symptom [32, 33] and, according to bereaved relatives, 94% of patients with COPD suffered from dyspnoea in their last year of life [34]. Moreover, patients with a noncancer diagnosis experience more severe dyspnoea over a longer period of time than lung cancer patients [35]. Some patients even have dyspnoea at rest; it increases with exertion and can also increase during exacerbations of the disease [36]. Episodes of acute dyspnoea may occur several times a day and are described by patients as extremely frightening [37–39]. Patients also suffer from other symptoms; for example, fatigue, coughing, muscle weakness, sleeplessness, pain, and symptoms of anxiety and depression are frequently reported [31, 32, 40]. Symptoms are often poorly addressed; for example, in one study, only a minority of outpatients with advanced COPD reported receiving treatment for fatigue, muscle weakness, low mood or sleeplessness [30]. Moreover, if the patients received treatment for their symptoms, they were only moderately satisfied with its effect [30].

Impaired HRQoL

HRQoL is impaired in patients with advanced non-malignant lung disease. Gore *et al.* [41], in a study in 2000, showed that patients with advanced COPD had worse HRQoL than patients with advanced cancer. A more recent study in 2015 confirmed that these findings are still true [42]. Symptom distress correlates with impairment in HRQoL [31, 43]. In fact, patients with higher depression scores or an increase in dyspnoea severity are more likely to experience a decline in HRQoL [44].

Functional and social limitations

Living with advanced non-malignant lung disease has major consequences for patients, as well as for their loved ones. Patients experience symptoms such as dyspnoea during normal daily activities, and this naturally leads to the avoidance of exertion. However, this is a harmful response to dyspnoea and results in functional impairment. Functional impairment results in care dependency [45]. Care dependency is frequently reported by patients with advanced lung disease and is associated with impairment in HRQoL and increased mortality risk [43, 46]. Functional impairment and care dependency limit the ability to engage in social activities and therefore result in a change in social role [45]. Loved ones may also need to adapt their life and often change their role towards being a family caregiver [47]. The QoL and emotional well-being of family caregivers can be impaired [48]. In fact, family caregivers experience disruption of daily tasks and financial, family and health burdens [49]. Nevertheless, family caregivers also experience positive aspects of caregiving and may value their role as a caregiver [47].

Disease trajectory and advance care planning

Patients with non-malignant lung diseases often live for many years with their chronic disease, and loved ones often describe the end of their life as unanticipated [50]. The disease trajectories of non-malignant lung diseases are characterised by uncertainty, and progression of COPD or IPF is very heterogeneous [51–53]. Every exacerbation can be life threatening [54]. Indeed, mortality following a hospital admission due to an exacerbation of COPD is about 10% [54] and increases to about one-quarter for patients in need of invasive mechanical ventilation [55]. Moreover, patients with non-malignant lung disease may also die from other diseases. Patients often suffer from comorbidities, which also compromise survival as well as QoL [56–60].

The uncertain disease trajectory creates a challenge for clinicians. On the one hand, the likelihood of sudden deterioration and sudden death increases the need for timely advance care planning [61]. Indeed, advance care planning interventions increase the occurrence and quality of discussions about EOL care and improve concordance between preferences for care and delivered care [62]. On the other hand, the uncertain disease trajectory is mentioned as a barrier towards advance care planning [61, 63]. Therefore, advance care planning is often poorly done in patients with advanced non-malignant lung disease [64]. Clinicians rarely discuss LST preferences with their patients with COPD, despite the fact that patients are able to indicate their preferences [65]. Moreover, EOL fears, such as concerns about dying and fear of breathlessness, are highly prevalent among patients but are barely addressed by professional caregivers [66]. Most patients will wait for caregivers or health professionals to initiate a discussion about the EOL [67]. Topics that are important for patients to address during advance care planning conversations include diagnosis and the expected disease process, treatment options (including LSTs), prognosis and what dying might be like [67, 68].

Benefits of palliative care interventions

Patients often live for a long time with their chronic disease and deliberating symptoms, impaired daily functioning, care dependency and impaired HRQoL. Moreover, loved ones are also confronted with the disease of the patients and a changed role as the family caregiver. Finally, advance care planning, including communication about EOL care, is of major importance. These complex needs require a multidimensional palliative care approach. Recent studies have shown the benefits of palliative care interventions for patients with advanced non-malignant lung disease. Higginson *et al.* [69] showed that a breathlessness support service, integrating palliative care, respiratory medicine, physiotherapy and occupational therapy, resulted in improvements in breathlessness mastery, as well as in survival in patients with refractory dyspnoea and advanced disease. Furthermore, Bajwah *et al.* [70] showed that a palliative intervention, including a case conference and care plan, improved symptoms and QoL in patients with IPF.

Palliative care needs in people with cancer

In 2012, there were 14.1 million cases of cancer in the world with an expected increase to 24 million by 2035 [71]. Lung cancer is the most common cancer worldwide and contributed 13% of the total number of new cancer cases in 2012 [71]. Pulmonary metastases, the second most common site for spread, are seen in 20–54% of extrathoracic malignancies, with prevalence depending on primary cancer type [72]. Mesothelioma rates are rising in Europe [73]. However, there is much geographical variation in the risk, with annual rates ranging from around 8 per 100 000 population in Scotland, England and The Netherlands to lower than 1 per 100 000 population in Spain [73].

People with a diagnosis of cancer suffer from a number of physical, psychological, social and existential/spiritual needs throughout the course of their illness. Numerous studies have demonstrated that early integration of palliative care can improve not only satisfaction, symptoms, depression, anxiety, QoL and length of life but also health services utilisation and costs [74–77].

Psychological needs

A diagnosis of cancer can lead to normal feelings of vulnerability, sadness and fears that can become disabling, with depression, anxiety, panic, social isolation and spiritual crisis. A qualitative study found that patients with lung cancer perceive that they are particularly stigmatised because others associate their disease with smoking and dirt, and because patients with lung cancer are portrayed as dying in an unpleasant way [76]. Lung cancer patients report significant distress [79]. In a study of patients starting chemotherapy or radiation therapy, one-third of patients had high levels of distress, and most reported physical (84%) or emotional (56%) problems [80]. In a cross-sectional study that compared the prevalence and intensity of needs expressed by cancer patients at the time of first recurrence with those at the time of disease progression, the recurrent group expressed more symptom-related problems, but there were no differences in reported psychological problems, responses to recurrence or their greatest concern [81].

Physical needs

In a cohort of over 45 000 cancer patients who completed a screening Edmonton Symptom Assessment System as part of standardised symptom screening in Ontario, Canada, fatigue was the most prevalent (75%) symptom with over one-half of patients reporting pain or shortness of breath and about half of those in the moderate to severe range [82]. Lung cancer patients had the worst burden of symptoms, with the intensity of shortness of breath, depression, anxiety and a poor sense of well-being being highest in this group. In a subgroup of this cohort who died, shortness of breath, drowsiness, well-being, lack of appetite and tiredness increased in severity over time, particularly in the month before death [83]. In a study of 5386 cancer patients, Currow *et al.* [84] showed that intensity of breathlessness and the prevalence of severe breathlessness increased as death approached, with a significant increase in the rate of change between 3 and 10 days before death. Other studies of patients with lung cancer have shown that 97% had decreased their activities and 80% had socially isolated themselves from friends and family [85], 36% were housebound and 10% were largely chairbound because of their breathlessness [41]. Screening for distress is the first step and should lead to a comprehensive assessment followed by timely and appropriate interventions. Recent trials of holistic breathlessness interventions [86, 87] have shown promising effects on physical and psychological symptoms.

It is important that the underlying aetiology of the identified needs is determined, as it may be treatment related, secondary to a comorbid condition, indirectly related to the cancer or due to the underlying cancer itself. In a study of terminally ill cancer patients who were short of breath, patients had a median of five different abnormalities that could have contributed to their dyspnoea, some of which were potentially correctable such as hypoxia, anaemia and bronchospasm [88]. Another study of 923 cancer outpatients found that the intensity of shortness of breath was significantly associated with the presence of hilar, mediastinal and rib metastases, and, surprisingly, the presence of mediastinal or hilar metastases was associated with a higher intensity of dyspnoea than the presence of lung metastases [89]. Patients with advanced cancers can develop malignant pleural effusions, pericardial effusions, superior vena cava or airway obstructions, phrenic nerve paralysis, and multiple tumour or pulmonary emboli. Treatments with surgery, systemic therapies and radiation, alone or in combination, can result in significant shortness of breath, emphasising the need for thorough assessment.

In a study of 289 patients with NSCLC, cough was the most common (>60%) and most severe symptom at presentation, with 80% having a cough before death. In this group of patients, cough and breathlessness were not as well controlled as other symptoms [90]. A cough can be very distressing [91]; it may cause pain, fractured ribs, heaving or retching, and can cause many patients to restrict their social lives [92].

Haemoptysis can result from bleeding in the respiratory tract anywhere from the nose to the lungs. It varies from blood streaking of sputum to coughing up massive amounts of blood. In patients with lung cancer, haemoptysis is the presenting symptom 7–10% of the time, it occurs in 20% of patients during their clinical course and 3% of people with lung cancer will die of massive haemoptysis [93].

Cachexia is another serious and often unrecognised and undertreated consequence of cancer, occurring secondary to a systemic inflammatory response [94]. It has traditionally been understood as weight loss but more recently has been defined as loss of muscle with or without loss of fat. In a study of 441 patients with NSCLC, 46.8% had computed tomography imaging evidence of severe muscle wasting. These patients had muscularity levels known to be associated with increased mortality and functional disability, which could have potential implications for systemic therapy dosing [95].

Palliative care needs in people with CF

Emergent research is highlighting the potentially valuable place of a specialist palliative care team in CF, either through direct working with the patient and family or indirectly by offering specialist palliative care guidance to specialist professionals working within the field of CF [96, 97]. Based on this and in consideration of the WHO definition of palliative care [1], the implementation of palliative care early in the illness of patients with CF should be supported.

Introducing palliative care to CF patients and their families

Research has indicated that early referral to palliative care for patients with CF and their families should be considered to support their needs. It is important to recognise that patients with CF will have known the teams caring for them and will have close relationships with them. Research by Lowton [98] explored the meaning of place of death for adults with CF. This research involved in-depth interviews over a 4-year period and analysis of letters received from families of patients who had died from CF. While the focus of this study related to EOL care, interesting information was made available on the way in which palliative care was introduced to some families. In one instance, a mother recounted how, 2 h before the death of her adult daughter, she was asked to meet the palliative care nurse for the first time [98]. In this example, the opportunity to be reviewed by the palliative care nurse was declined by the participant, as she chose not to meet a stranger at that time. This illustrates that introducing palliative care at this stage is too late for families, and may be the same for patients.

Unpublished data from a recent doctoral study indicated that, for patients, building a relationship with professionals is important [99]. Sixteen patients with CF who were interviewed alluded to the importance of having a therapeutic relationship with the teams looking after them and the need for more information determining what palliative care services could offer [99]. They actively stated that they would not want to be seen by a team who was unknown to them when they were dying. Tomison and MacDowell [100] also established that patients with non-malignant conditions are much less likely to be referred early to palliative care, and that the first meeting of the patient and family is usually at a crisis point when patients are distressed and families are frightened. Patients with CF often have long established relationships with most of the core multidisciplinary team, and it is understandable that they would prefer earlier establishment of palliative care relationships.

Symptom management and models of palliative care for patients with CF

CF is a chronic disease with a substantial symptom burden that is not always comparable with the severity of the pulmonary disease. The impact that specialist palliative care services can offer towards the control of patients' symptoms has been illustrated previously [101, 102], but referral patterns to specialist palliative care teams remain unclear [103]. An integrated approach involving the specialist knowledge of the CF team together with the guidance of the symptom management expertise of a palliative care team is optimal for delivery of holistic care and can support patients at different stages of the illness, including transplant. A multidisciplinary approach is essential, as all aspects of social, spiritual and psychological concerns can have an effect on the patient's experience of symptoms. While there is limited evidence on other supportive interventions such as distraction, relaxation and complementary therapies in patients with CF, it has been shown previously in other groups that techniques such as distraction therapy and relaxation should be considered to support symptom control, especially related to breathlessness [98].

Symptom control includes the management of headache and gastrointestinal discomfort. Upper body pain, particularly of the chest and rib areas, is frequent. This is predominantly related to either coughing and/or infection. Optimising pain management will not only allow the patient to feel better but will also help support the recommended physiotherapy plan. The management of pain invariably consists of a combination of pharmacological interventions and massage, physical activities, rest, heat therapies and distraction activities [99]. Alongside the symptom of pain, patients' needs continue with the management of breathlessness, cough, anxiety and distress, nausea and vomiting. CF patients also have psychological palliative care needs. They can experience unresolved symptoms of confusion, fear and anxiety, which can, for some, lead to increasing terminal restlessness as death approaches. The opportunity to explore some of these issues with the patient's consent should be considered prior to the introduction of medications. It is also important to acknowledge the spiritual needs of the patient. More recently, an attempt has been made to broaden the description of spirituality. For some patients, their religion as the ability to worship is central to their spirituality, while for others it is the search for meaning [104]. Organisations can offer spiritual care in various ways, including physical resources such as quiet rooms for reflection or prayer rooms, and can also provide support from other support services, such as volunteers or chaplains. Effective communication between staff and patients while facilitating patients to discover meaning, and staff supporting them through this, can add to creating a spiritual environment.

Palliative care in CF is poorly understood [96, 97]. A study undertaken by Braithwaite *et al.* [97] involved interviewing staff, patients and families, with the focus being on determining unmet needs in EOL care. Within this study, it was recognised that patients lacked knowledge about palliative care services, and therefore offering patients with CF information regarding what palliative services can offer may help in introducing it early within the patient's disease journey. The management of such symptoms is addressed elsewhere in this *Monograph*; however, the issue in terms of need is in recognising when specialist help from palliative care should be initiated and when integrated care should begin. Patients with CF may benefit symptomatically either from support received directly from a palliative care team or indirectly through support and advice given to CF professionals. The exact model of care should be individualised for each patient and clinical scenario.

Advance care planning

Many adults with CF have thought about their future care and may well have already addressed this with their family and friends [105]. Interestingly, although patients may have discussed this with family and friends, fewer than one-third of patients have discussed this with the teams delivering their care [106]. Some clinicians may have concerns about broaching discussions with patients and families relating to advance care planning; however, for some, the opportunity to address such issues, including preferences around care and death, is welcomed. Palliative care services, integrated with CF specialists, are in an optimum position to support these discussions and facilitate patient preference.

EOL care

Discussion and decisions concerning the ceiling of care and outlining the treatment plan can at times be difficult to address due to the uncertainty of the disease and the response to proposed treatments. Integrating palliative care services early in the patient's illness to support symptoms can be advantageous in establishing relationships with patients and families while patients are still relatively well, and, when appropriate, enabling discussions about EOL preferences and wishes.

Conclusion

Respiratory diseases are among the leading causes of death worldwide with high levels of morbidity and health service burden. In addition, patients with respiratory diseases have numerous physical, psychological, social and existential/spiritual needs throughout the course of their illness. Both the prevention and treatment of lung diseases will need to be improved if their impact on longevity and QoL of individuals, and their economic burden on society, are to be reduced in Europe and worldwide. Appropriate skills are required to determine the underlying aetiology and access to individuals skilled in delivering the appropriate palliative care interventions needed. Early integration of palliative care (where possible) can help ensure that complex needs are addressed. However, achieving this in resource-limited settings is a challenge.

References

1. World Health Organization. WHO Definition of Palliative Care. www.who.int/cancer/palliative/definition/en/ Date last updated: 2016. Date last accessed: July 2016.
2. Bajwah S, Koffman J, Higginson IJ, *et al.* "I wish I knew more…" the end-of-life planning and information needs for end-stage fibrotic interstitial lung disease: views of patients, carers and health professionals. *BMJ Support Palliat Care* 2013; 3: 84–90.
3. Bajwah S, Higginson IJ, Ross JR, *et al.* The palliative care needs for fibrotic interstitial lung disease: a qualitative study of patients, informal caregivers and health professionals. *Palliat Med* 2013; 27: 869–876.
4. Lunardi W, Lopes EA, Kehde E, *et al.* Pneumonite e fibrose pulmonar por amiodarona: relato de dois casos com microscopia óptica e eletrônica [Pneumonitis and pulmonary fibrosis due to amiodarone: report of two cases with optic and electronic microscopy]. *Arq Bras Cardiol* 1986; 46: 415–419.
5. Viegi G, Pedreschi M, Pistelli F, *et al.* Prevalence of airways obstruction in a general population: European Respiratory Society vs American Thoracic Society definition. *Chest* 2000; 117: Suppl. 2, 339S–345S.
6. Halbert RJ, Isonaka S, George D, *et al.* Interpreting COPD prevalence estimates: what is the true burden of disease? *Chest* 2003; 123: 1684–1692.
7. Celli BR, Halbert RJ, Isonaka S, *et al.* Population impact of different definitions of airway obstruction. *Eur Respir J* 2003; 22: 268–273.
8. Viegi G, Matteelli G, Angino A, *et al.* The proportional Venn diagram of obstructive lung disease in the Italian general population. *Chest* 2004; 126: 1093–1101.
9. Cruz AA, Bousquet J, Khaltaev N. Global Surveillance, Prevention and Control of Chronic Respiratory Diseases: A Comprehensive Approach. Geneva, World Health Organization, 2007.
10. de Marco R, Accordini S, Cerveri I, *et al.* An international survey of chronic obstructive pulmonary disease in young adults according to GOLD stages. *Thorax* 2004; 59: 120–125.
11. Cancer Research UK. Lung Cancer Incidence Statistics. www.cancerresearchuk.org/health-professional/cancer-statistics/statistics-by-cancer-type/lung-cancer/incidence Date last accessed: March 3, 2016.

12. Nalysnyk L, Cid-Ruzafa J, Rotella P, *et al.* Incidence and prevalence of idiopathic pulmonary fibrosis: review of the literature. *Eur Respir Rev* 2012; 21: 355–361.
13. Strachan D, Gupta RA, Limb E, *et al.* The burden of lung disease. *In:* Gibson JG, Loddenkemper R, Sibille Y, *et al.* eds. European Lung White Book. Sheffield, European Respiratory Society, 2013; pp. 2–15.
14. World Health Organization. World Health Statistics 2011. Available from: www.who.int/whosis/whostat/2011/en/
15. World Health Organization. Global Status Report on Non-communicable Diseases 2010. Description of the Global Burden of NCDs, their Risk Factors and Determinant. Geneva, World Health Organization, 2011.
16. World Health Organization. GLOBOCAN 2012: Estimated Cancer Incidence, Mortality and Prevalence Worldwide in 2012. http://globocan.iarc.fr/Pages/fact_sheets_cancer.aspx Date last updated: July 12, 2012. Date last accessed: February 25, 2016.
17. Pauwels RA, Buist AS, Calverley PM, *et al.* Global strategy for the diagnosis, management, and prevention of chronic obstructive pulmonary disease. NHLBI/WHO Global Initiative for Chronic Obstructive Lung Disease (GOLD) Workshop summary. *Am J Respir Crit Care Med* 2001; 163: 1256–1276.
18. American Thoracic Society. Standards for the diagnosis and care of patients with chronic obstructive pulmonary disease. *Am J Respir Crit Care Med* 1995; 152: S77–S121.
19. Jones P, Lareau S, Mahler DA. Measuring the effects of COPD on the patient. *Respir Med* 2005; 99: Suppl. B, S11–S18.
20. ZuWallack RL, Haggerty MC, Jones P. Clinically meaningful outcomes in patients with chronic obstructive pulmonary disease. *Am J Med* 2004; 117: Suppl. 12A, 49–59.
21. Schmier JK, Halpern MT, Higashi MK, *et al.* The quality of life impact of acute exacerbations of chronic bronchitis (AECB): a literature review. *Qual Life Res* 2005; 14: 329–347.
22. Eurostat. Respiratory Diseases Statistics 2015. http://ec.europa.eu/eurostat/statistics-explained/index.php/Respiratory_diseases_statistics Date last updated: October, 2015. Date last accessed: February 25, 2016.
23. Collard HR, Ward AJ, Lanes S, *et al.* Burden of illness in idiopathic pulmonary fibrosis. *J Med Econ* 2012; 15: 829–835.
24. Kim DS, Collard HR, King TE Jr. Classification and natural history of the idiopathic interstitial pneumonias. *Proc Am Thorac Soc* 2006; 3: 285–292.
25. Fernandez Perez ER, Daniels CE, Schroeder DR, *et al.* Incidence, prevalence, and clinical course of idiopathic pulmonary fibrosis: a population-based study. *Chest* 2010; 137: 129–137.
26. Ait-Khaled N, Enarson DA, Bissell K, *et al.* Access to inhaled corticosteroids is key to improving quality of care for asthma in developing countries. *Allergy* 2007; 62: 230–236.
27. Beernaert K, Cohen J, Deliens L, *et al.* Referral to palliative care in COPD and other chronic diseases: a population-based study. *Respir Med* 2013; 107: 1731–1739.
28. Lindell KO, Liang Z, Hoffman LA, *et al.* Palliative care and location of death in decedents with idiopathic pulmonary fibrosis. *Chest* 2015; 147: 423–429.
29. Vermylen JH, Szmuilowicz E, Kalhan R. Palliative care in COPD: an unmet area for quality improvement. *Int J Chron Obstruct Pulmon Dis* 2015; 10: 1543–1551.
30. Janssen DJ, Spruit MA, Uszko-Lencer NH, *et al.* Symptoms, comorbidities, and health care in advanced chronic obstructive pulmonary disease or chronic heart failure. *J Palliat Med* 2011; 14: 735–743.
31. Blinderman CD, Homel P, Billings JA, *et al.* Symptom distress and quality of life in patients with advanced chronic obstructive pulmonary disease. *J Pain Symptom Manage* 2009; 38: 115–123.
32. Janssen DJ, Spruit MA, Wouters EF, *et al.* Daily symptom burden in end-stage chronic organ failure: a systematic review. *Palliat Med* 2008; 22: 938–948.
33. Lee AS, Mira-Avendano I, Ryu JH, *et al.* The burden of idiopathic pulmonary fibrosis: an unmet public health need. *Respir Med* 2014; 108: 955–967.
34. Edmonds P, Karlsen S, Khan S, *et al.* A comparison of the palliative care needs of patients dying from chronic respiratory diseases and lung cancer. *Palliat Med* 2001; 15: 287–295.
35. Weingaertner V, Scheve C, Gerdes V, *et al.* Breathlessness, functional status, distress, and palliative care needs over time in patients with advanced chronic obstructive pulmonary disease or lung cancer: a cohort study. *J Pain Symptom Manage* 2014; 48: 569–581.
36. Parshall MB, Schwartzstein RM, Adams L, *et al.* An official American Thoracic Society statement: update on the mechanisms, assessment, and management of dyspnea. *Am J Respir Crit Care Med* 2012; 185: 435–452.
37. Disler RT, Green A, Luckett T, *et al.* Experience of advanced chronic obstructive pulmonary disease: metasynthesis of qualitative research. *J Pain Symptom Manage* 2014; 48: 1182–1199.
38. Dunger C, Higginson IJ, Gysels M, *et al.* Breathlessness and crises in the context of advanced illness: a comparison between COPD and lung cancer patients. *Palliat Support Care* 2015; 13: 229–237.
39. Simon ST, Weingartner V, Higginson IJ, *et al.* Definition, categorization, and terminology of episodic breathlessness: consensus by an international Delphi survey. *J Pain Symptom Manage* 2014; 47: 828–838.
40. Russell AM, Ripamonti E, Vancheri C. Qualitative European survey of patients with idiopathic pulmonary fibrosis: patients' perspectives of the disease and treatment. *BMC Pulm Med* 2016; 16: 10.

41. Gore JM, Brophy CJ, Greenstone MA. How well do we care for patients with end stage chronic obstructive pulmonary disease (COPD)? A comparison of palliative care and quality of life in COPD and lung cancer. *Thorax* 2000; 55: 1000–1006.
42. Javadzadeh S, Chowienczyk S, Booth S, *et al.* Comparison of respiratory health-related quality of life in patients with intractable breathlessness due to advanced cancer or advanced COPD. *BMJ Support Palliat Care* 2015; 6: 105–108.
43. Janssen DJ, Franssen FM, Wouters EF, *et al.* Impaired health status and care dependency in patients with advanced COPD or chronic heart failure. *Qual Life Res* 2011; 20: 1679–1688.
44. Wilke S, Spruit MA, Wouters EF, *et al.* Determinants of 1-year changes in disease-specific health status in patients with advanced chronic obstructive pulmonary disease: a 1-year observational study. *Int J Nurs Pract* 2015; 21: 239–248.
45. Janssen DJ, Wouters EF, Spruit MA. Psychosocial consequences of living with breathlessness due to advanced disease. *Curr Opin Support Palliat Care* 2015; 9: 232–237.
46. Janssen DJ, Wouters EF, Schols JM, *et al.* Care dependency independently predicts two-year survival in outpatients with advanced chronic organ failure. *J Am Med Dir Assoc* 2013; 14: 194–198.
47. Janssen DJ, Spruit MA, Wouters EF, *et al.* Family caregiving in advanced chronic organ failure. *J Am Med Dir Assoc* 2012; 15: 447–456.
48. Pinto RA, Holanda MA, Medeiros MM, *et al.* Assessment of the burden of caregiving for patients with chronic obstructive pulmonary disease. *Respir Med* 2007; 101: 2402–2408.
49. Sautter JM, Tulsky JA, Johnson KS, *et al.* Caregiver experience during advanced chronic illness and last year of life. *J Am Geriatr Soc* 2014; 62: 1082–1090.
50. Pinnock H, Kendall M, Murray SA, *et al.* Living and dying with severe chronic obstructive pulmonary disease: multi-perspective longitudinal qualitative study. *BMJ* 2011; 342: d142.
51. Murray SA, Kendall M, Boyd K, *et al.* Illness trajectories and palliative care. *BMJ* 2005; 330: 1007–1011.
52. Casanova C, de Torres JP, Aguirre-Jaime A, *et al.* The progression of chronic obstructive pulmonary disease is heterogeneous: the experience of the BODE cohort. *Am J Respir Crit Care Med* 2011; 184: 1015–1021.
53. Martinez FJ, Safrin S, Weycker D, *et al.* The clinical course of patients with idiopathic pulmonary fibrosis. *Ann Intern Med* 2005; 142: 963–967.
54. Steer J, Gibson J, Bourke SC. The DECAF Score: predicting hospital mortality in exacerbations of chronic obstructive pulmonary disease. *Thorax* 2012; 67: 970–976.
55. Hajizadeh N, Goldfeld K, Crothers K. What happens to patients with COPD with long-term oxygen treatment who receive mechanical ventilation for COPD exacerbation? A 1-year retrospective follow-up study. *Thorax* 2015; 70: 294–296.
56. Frei A, Muggensturm P, Putcha N, *et al.* Five comorbidities reflected the health status in patients with chronic obstructive pulmonary disease: the newly developed COMCOLD index. *J Clin Epidemiol* 2014; 67: 904–911.
57. Vanfleteren LE, Spruit MA, Groenen M, *et al.* Clusters of comorbidities based on validated objective measurements and systemic inflammation in patients with chronic obstructive pulmonary disease. *Am J Respir Crit Care Med* 2013; 187: 728–735.
58. Hartl S, Lopez-Campos JL, Pozo-Rodriguez F, *et al.* Risk of death and readmission of hospital-admitted COPD exacerbations: European COPD Audit. *Eur Respir J* 2016; 47: 113–121.
59. Divo M, Cote C, de Torres JP, *et al.* Comorbidities and risk of mortality in patients with chronic obstructive pulmonary disease. *Am J Respir Crit Care Med* 2012; 186: 155–161.
60. Barnes P, Celli B. Systemic manifestations and comorbidities of COPD. *Eur Respir J* 2009; 33: 1165–1185.
61. Curtis JR. Palliative and end-of-life care for patients with severe COPD. *Eur Respir J* 2008; 32: 796–803.
62. Houben CH, Spruit MA, Wouters EF, *et al.* A randomised controlled trial on the efficacy of advance care planning on the quality of end-of-life care and communication in patients with COPD: the research protocol. *BMJ Open* 2014; 4: e004465.
63. Gott M, Gardiner C, Small N, *et al.* Barriers to advance care planning in chronic obstructive pulmonary disease. *Palliat Med* 2009; 23: 642–648.
64. Knauft E, Nielsen EL, Engelberg RA, *et al.* Barriers and facilitators to end-of-life care communication for patients with COPD. *Chest* 2005; 127: 2188–2196.
65. Janssen DJ, Spruit MA, Schols JM, *et al.* A call for high-quality advance care planning in outpatients with severe COPD or chronic heart failure. *Chest* 2011; 139: 1081–1088.
66. Gardiner C, Gott M, Small N, *et al.* Living with advanced chronic obstructive pulmonary disease: patients concerns regarding death and dying. *Palliat Med* 2009; 23: 691–697.
67. Heffner JE, Fahy B, Hilling L, *et al.* Attitudes regarding advance directives among patients in pulmonary rehabilitation. *Am J Respir Crit Care Med* 1996; 154: 1735–1740.
68. Curtis JR, Wenrich MD, Carline JD, *et al.* Patients' perspectives on physician skill in end-of-life care: differences between patients with COPD, cancer, and AIDS. *Chest* 2002; 122: 356–362.
69. Higginson IJ, Bausewein C, Reilly CC, *et al.* An integrated palliative and respiratory care service for patients with advanced disease and refractory breathlessness: a randomised controlled trial. *Lancet Respir Med* 2014; 2: 979–987.

70. Bajwah S, Ross JR, Wells AU, *et al.* Palliative care for patients with advanced fibrotic lung disease: a randomised controlled phase II and feasibility trial of a community case conference intervention. *Thorax* 2015; 70: 830–839.
71. World Cancer Research Fund International. Worldwide data. www.wcrf.org/int/cancer-facts-figures/worldwide-data
72. Cheng S, Mohammed TL. Metastatic disease to the lungs and pleura: an overview. *Semin Roentgenol* 2003; 48: 335–343.
73. Montanaro F, Bray F, Gennaro V, *et al.* Pleural mesothelioma incidence in Europe: evidence of some deceleration in the increasing trends. *Cancer Causes Control* 2003; 14: 791–803.
74. Temel JS, Greer JA, Muzikansky A, *et al.* Early palliative care for patients with metastatic non-small-cell lung cancer. *N Engl J Med* 2010; 363: 733–742.
75. Zimmermann C, Swami N, Krzyzanowska M, *et al.* Early palliative care for patients with advanced cancer: a cluster-randomised controlled trial. *Lancet* 2014; 383: 1721–1730.
76. Bakitas M, Lyons KD, Hegel MT, *et al.* Effects of a palliative care intervention on clinical outcomes in patients with advanced cancer: the Project ENABLE II randomized controlled trial. *JAMA* 2009; 302: 741–749.
77. Ferrell B, Sun V, Hurria A, *et al.* Interdisciplinary palliative care for patients with lung cancer. *J Pain Symptom Manage* 2015; 50: 758–767.
78. Chapple A, Ziebland S, McPherson A. Stigma, shame, and blame experienced by patients with lung cancer: qualitative study. *BMJ* 2004; 328: 1470.
79. Carlson LE, Waller A, Mitchell AJ. Screening for distress and unmet needs in patients with cancer: review and recommendations. *J Clin Oncol* 2012; 30: 1160–1177.
80. Hollingworth W, Metcalfe C, Mancero S, *et al.* Are needs assessments cost effective in reducing distress among patients with cancer? A randomized controlled trial using the Distress Thermometer and Problem List. *J Clin Oncol* 2013; 31: 3631–3638.
81. Dudgeon DJ, Raubertas RF, Doerner K, *et al.* When does palliative care begin? A needs assessment of cancer patients with recurrent disease. *J Palliat Care* 1995; 11: 5–9.
82. Barbera L, Seow H, Howell D, *et al.* Symptom burden and performance status in a population-based cohort of ambulatory cancer patients. *Cancer* 2010; 116: 5767–5776.
83. Seow H, Barbera L, Sutradhar R, *et al.* Trajectory of performance status and symptom scores for patients with cancer during the last six months of life. *J Clin Oncol* 2011; 29: 1151–1158.
84. Currow DC, Smith J, Davidson PM, *et al.* Do the trajectories of dyspnea differ in prevalence and intensity by diagnosis at the end of life? A consecutive cohort study. *J Pain Symptom Manage* 2010; 39: 680–690.
85. Brown ML, Carrieri V, Janson B, *et al.* Lung cancer and dyspnea: the patient's perception. *Oncol Nurs Forum* 1986; 13: 19–24.
86. Farquhar MC, Prevost AT, McCrone P, *et al.* The clinical and cost effectiveness of a Breathlessness Intervention Service for patients with advanced non-malignant disease and their informal carers: mixed findings of a mixed method randomised controlled trial. *Trials* 2016; 17: 185.
87. Higginson IJ, Bausewein C, Reilly CC, *et al.* An integrated palliative and respiratory care service for patients with advanced disease and refractory breathlessness: a randomised controlled trial. *Lancet Respir Med* 2014; 2: 979–987.
88. Dudgeon DJ, Lertzman M. Dyspnea in the advanced cancer patient. *J Pain Symptom Manage* 1998; 16: 212–219.
89. Dudgeon DJ, Kristjanson L, Sloan JA, *et al.* Dyspnea in cancer patients: prevalence and associated factors. *J Pain Symptom Manage* 2001; 21: 95–102.
90. Muers MF, Round CE. Palliation of symptoms in non-small cell lung cancer: a study by the Yorkshire Regional Cancer Organisation Thoracic Group. *Thorax* 1993; 48: 339–343.
91. Harle AS, Blackhall FH, Smith JA, *et al.* Understanding cough and its management in lung cancer. *Current Opin Support Palliat Care* 2012; 6: 153–162.
92. Molassiotis A, Lowe M, Ellis J, *et al.* The experience of cough in patients diagnosed with lung cancer. *Support Care Cancer* 2011; 19: 1997–2004.
93. Kvale PA, Simoff M, Prakash UB, *et al.* Lung cancer. Palliative care. *Chest* 2003; 123: Suppl., 284S–311S.
94. Scott HR, McMillan DC, Forrest LM, *et al.* The systemic inflammatory response, weight loss, performance status and survival in patients with inoperable non-small cell lung cancer. *Br J Cancer* 2002; 87: 264–267.
95. Baracos VE, Reiman T, Mourtzakis M, *et al.* Body composition in patients with non-small cell lung cancer: a contemporary view of cancer cachexia with the use of computed tomography image analysis. *Am J Clin Nutr* 2010; 91: 1133S–1137S.
96. Bourke S, Doe S, Gascoigne A, *et al.* An integrated model of provision of palliative care to patients with cystic fibrosis. *Palliat Med* 2009; 23: 512–517.
97. Braithwaite M, Philip J, Tranberg H, *et al.* End of life care in CF: patients, families and staff experiences and unmet needs. *J Cyst Fibros* 2011; 10: 253–257.
98. Lowton K. "A bed in the middle of nowhere": parents' meanings of place of death for adults with cystic fibrosis. *Soc Sci Med* 2009; 69: 1056–1062.
99. Stevens AM. An exploration of early palliative care in adult patients with cystic fibrosis. PhD thesis. Guildford, University of Surrey, 2015.

100. Tomison G, McDowell JR. Nurses' needs in delivering palliative care for long-term conditions. *Br J Commun Nurs* 2011; 16: 274–281.
101. Edmonds PM, Stuttaford JM, Penny J, *et al.* Do hospital palliative care teams improve symptom control? Use of a modified STAS as an evaluation tool. *Palliat Med* 1998; 12: 345–351.
102. Stevens AM, Gwilliam B, A'hern R, *et al.* Experience in the use of the palliative care outcome scale. *Support Care Cancer* 2005; 13: 1027–1034.
103. Fadul N, Elsayem A, Palmer JL, *et al.* Predictors of access to palliative care services among patients who died at a Comprehensive Cancer Center. *J Palliat Med* 2007; 10: 1146–1152.
104. Bluebond-Langner M. In the Shadow of Illness: Parents and Siblings of the Chronically Ill Child. Princeton, Princeton University Press, 2000.
105. Dellon EP, Shores MD, Nelson KI, *et al.* Family caregiver perspectives on symptoms and treatments for patients dying from complications of cystic fibrosis. *J Pain Symptom Manage* 2010; 40: 829–837.
106. Sawicki GS, Sellers DE, Robinson WM. Self-reported physical and psychological symptom burden in adults with cystic fibrosis. *J Pain Symptom Manage* 2008; 35: 372–380.

Disclosures: None declared.

Chapter 3

Access to palliative care

Tim Peel[1], Lynn F. Reinke[2] and Claudia Bausewein[3]

Various (integrated) service models of palliative care for both inpatient and community settings have been developed around the world. The importance of collaboration between palliative and respiratory medicine has been recognised in recent national and international guidance. However, specialist palliative care support for patients is still variable, with higher acceptance for patients with malignant lung disease and more sporadic access for patients with chronic, non-malignant lung disease. Barriers to access are related to disease trajectories, service configuration and delivery, and lack of training for both generalist and specialist palliative care. Access to palliative care is facilitated by systematic needs assessment and recognition of both disease- and symptom-related triggers to initiate palliative care.

Palliative care services have been established widely around the world. Also, the need for palliative care involvement for people with advanced malignant and non-malignant disease has been recognised and supported by evidence. However, this does not necessarily mean that patients with advanced lung disease have sufficient access to palliative care in both generalist and specialist settings. Ways for respiratory medicine and specialist palliative care to cooperate need to be established because for many patients with chronic, non-malignant lung disease the respiratory physician will be the primary contact for a long time. Access to specialist palliative care should then be based on needs rather than diagnosis and prognosis.

Hospice and palliative care service models

Palliative care has developed around the world with various service models for both inpatient and community settings. In many countries, palliative care provision is differentiated between generalist/primary and specialist palliative care. Generalist or primary palliative care is seen as the task of healthcare providers, such as GPs, hospital doctors and nurses, and district nurses. It seeks to integrate palliative approaches within the regular care plan to address unmet needs in the advanced stages of illness [1]. Specialist palliative care services are those where the main activity is the provision of palliative care and clinicians have had additional training [2]. These services generally care for patients with complex and difficult clinical problems. Specialist palliative care therefore requires a

[1]Retired Consultant in Respiratory and Palliative Medicine, Northumbria Palliative Care Unit, North Tyneside General Hospital, Northumbria Healthcare NHS Foundation Trust, North Shields, UK. [2]Health Services R&D, VA Puget Sound Health Care System, Seattle, WA, USA. [3]Dept of Palliative Medicine, LMU Munich, Munich University Hospital, Munich, Germany.

Correspondence: Claudia Bausewein, LMU Munich, Dept of Palliative Medicine, Munich University Hospital, Marchioninistraße 15, 81377 Munich, Germany. E-mail: Claudia.bausewein@med.uni-muenchen.de

 Print ISBN: 978-1-84984-071-2. Online ISBN: 978-1-84984-072-9. Print ISSN: 2312-508X. Online ISSN: 2312-5098.

high level of palliative care education, appropriate staff, and other resources and is provided by multiprofessional teams [3].

Differences in service models mainly relate to local structures and national healthcare systems with some components being similar and others being different although bearing the same name. This is particularly apparent in the USA where "hospice" tends to refer to EOL services, often community-based, and "palliative care" often refers to hospital-based advisory teams that may allow potentially more integrated care depending on local service funding models. An overview of specialist palliative care services as defined by the European Association for Palliative Care (EAPC) is provided in table 1. Some forms of specialist services, such as inpatient hospices or palliative care units, take over the care of the patients completely whereas other types of services provide specialist support to general services and aim to improve general palliative care in the setting where the patient is found [2]. This latter model reaches far more patients than specialist units can care for.

Palliative care is provided by a multiprofessional team of specially trained physicians, nurses, social workers, chaplains, and other specialists with advanced training in palliative care who work with each patient's other clinicians to provide an extra layer of support [4]. Clinicians who are specifically trained in palliative care can provide in-depth pain and symptom management, communication regarding goals of care, and care coordination across settings and over time.

Hospice and palliative medicine is now recognised as a medical specialty in England, Ireland, Australia and New Zealand, and as subspecialty by the American Board of Medical Specialties (ABMS), as well as in many European countries (*e.g.* France, Germany, Norway) [5]. Many other European countries are also in the process of developing certification for palliative care [6]. Specialty and subspecialty palliative care services are mainly available in high-income countries; in low-income countries, the availability of subspecialty palliative care services is generally quite limited.

Healthcare specialties and professions

The importance of collaboration between palliative and respiratory medicine has been recognised in recent national and international guidance [7–10]. Patients with respiratory diseases will usually be under the care of the primary healthcare team after the diagnosis has been established in the respiratory clinic. As the complexity of their illness increases, it is likely that they will be referred to secondary care, usually to a respiratory physician. At this stage, management will focus on disease modification, aimed at reversing or at least halting the progression of the disease process. In patients with lung cancer, other clinicians such as surgeons and oncologists will also be involved.

Within each specialty there are different professionals who fulfil different roles in each patient's care. For example, in COPD, apart from respiratory physicians, there are important roles for CNSs, physiotherapists, pharmacists, clinical psychologists, and dieticians.

The GP will usually know the patient and their family better than the secondary care professionals. From this point of view, the GP is in a good position for recognising the overall disease trajectory and advance care planning, and can help the patient make decisions about

Table 1. Services providing specialist palliative care

Organisational unit	Structure	Goal of treatment	Comment
Inpatient palliative care unit	Ward within or adjacent to a hospital, but also as a stand-alone service	Crisis intervention for patients with complex symptoms and problems or providing EOL care for patients where home care is no longer possible Alleviate disease- and therapy-related discomfort; if possible, stabilise functional status and offer patient and carers psychological and social support allowing for discharge or transfer to another care setting	In many countries, the function of an inpatient hospice is similar to that of a palliative care unit, whereas, in other countries, a clear distinction can be observed
Inpatient hospices	Autonomous organisational unit with its own team	Patients in their last phase of life, when treatment in a hospital is not necessary and care at home or in a nursing home is not possible	
Hospital palliative care support teams	Specialist palliative care advice and support to other clinical staff, patients and their families and carers in the hospital environment	Alleviation of multiple symptoms of patients on different hospital wards Mentoring the attending staff and supporting patients and relatives	Countries with high proportion of hospital palliative care support teams: Belgium, France, Ireland and the UK
Home palliative care teams	Multiprofessional team supporting people at home or in a nursing home	Specialist palliative care to patients at home and support to families and carers at the patient's home Specialist advice to GPs, family doctors and nurses caring for the patient at home	
Day hospices	Day hospices or day-care centres are spaces in hospitals, hospices, palliative care units or the community	Patients usually spend part of the day in the day-care centre, either each day or once weekly Promote recreational and therapeutic activities among palliative care patients	
Palliative outpatient clinics	Consultation for patients living at home who can visit the clinic	Usually affiliated to specialist palliative care units or inpatient hospices	

Data from [3].

their future. A GP will not have as much in-depth knowledge about the specific disease processes as secondary care professionals, or about difficult symptom control, as specialist palliative care clinicians.

Respiratory physicians have expertise in the pathophysiology of lung diseases and in the treatments aimed at disease modification. Communication skills and general palliative care should be an integral part of respiratory medicine higher training, forming the basis for any management of respiratory patients. However, presently this is not generally the case.

Some respiratory physicians who wish to have more in-depth knowledge about palliative care take modules or diplomas in specialist palliative care during their training. This is more popular in some countries than others. Alternatively, a rotation to a palliative care service during respiratory medicine specialist training might provide a good insight and further expertise in palliative care. On a less formal level, training opportunities already exist within hospitals, and at regional, national and international levels at specialist society meetings.

Specialist palliative care physicians and CNSs are well trained in symptom control, communication skills, and ethical issues but have less experience of managing the reversible elements of respiratory diseases and of acute conditions that may occur during the course of a chronic illness.

In most respiratory diseases there will not be a precise point at which the management switches from treatment of the underlying condition to palliation of the symptoms. Rather, a palliative approach should be considered early in the disease in addition to disease modification. The American Thoracic Society (ATS) therefore suggests that when patients become symptomatic, palliative care should be made available at all times during the natural history of a progressive or CRD or critical illness [10]. Generally, palliative care should be made available when curative/restorative care begins and while it continues, after life-prolonging treatments are withheld or withdrawn, and, for the benefit of the patient's family, after the patient has died [10].

Collaboration and innovation

As the specialist expertise from both respiratory medicine and palliative care is most beneficial for patients, collaboration between the two disciplines fosters optimal care. A number of different models for collaboration have evolved over recent years based on local structures, personal engagement, or research with evidence supporting the newly developed models. A few are introduced here.

Multidisciplinary team meetings and collaborative services

The concept of a multidisciplinary team for the management of most respiratory diseases is now well established, particularly for cancer and for some rarer diseases, where local expertise may be limited.

Multidisciplinary teams are well established in lung cancer care and usually include a specialist palliative care presence. Multidisciplinary teams can be used to access specialist palliative care [11]. Most general hospitals in the UK, but also in other countries, have a weekly lung cancer multidisciplinary team meeting. Apart from respiratory physicians and CNSs, team members include oncologists, thoracic surgeons, radiologists, pathologists, and usually specialist palliative care professionals (either consultants or CNSs).

In England, regional ILD multidisciplinary teams exist throughout the country [12]. They tend to concentrate on diagnostic issues and disease modification. Palliative patients are often not discussed. Once ILD patients have completed any disease-modifying treatment, they will be followed up in the respiratory clinic. If housebound and oxygen-dependent, they tend to return to the care of their primary healthcare team.

There are documented examples of specialist palliative care input into adult cystic fibrosis (CF) multidisciplinary teams with success [13], although the overall care will continue with the respiratory physician. In CF, specific challenges occur with the integration of palliative care with the high burden of daily symptoms in CF, especially pain and depression, on the one hand, and more invasive EOL care, partly because of changes in the demographics of death in CF and partly because of the wider pursuit of lung transplantation, on the other hand [14].

The integration of specialist palliative care with COPD remains challenging. The large number of patients and the unpredictability of the disease trajectory mean that COPD multidisciplinary teams have not become commonplace [15]. "Red flag" events, such as the need for NIV, might be used as triggers for consideration of future care needs (*e.g.* to introduce educational or self-management strategies) or finally involvement of palliative care and, if available, specialist palliative care. However, there are initiatives that integrate palliative principles into COPD care within the existing resources [16, 17].

Joint clinics

In lung cancer, parallel respiratory, oncology, and nurse-led clinics are commonplace with palliative medicine increasingly involved in the manner of an extended team rather than taking over care. Because of the high prevalence of symptoms in lung cancer patients, this may be an appropriate use of a scarce resource and clinical trials of early integration of palliative care in lung cancer have shown benefit [18]. This is not the case in general respiratory clinics [19].

There is no single model of care for the palliative needs of respiratory patients. Those providing their regular care need to be alert to when they need help from specialist palliative care. Those working in specialist palliative care need to be readily accessible to provide advice and education, but also to be directly involved in the care if necessary.

Breathlessness services

Over recent years, a number of breathlessness services have been developed; these are mainly based on research following the Medical Research Council Framework [20]. These short-term services focus on refractory breathlessness as the most dominant and disabling symptom of patients with respiratory disease, while also taking into account other symptoms and concerns about the life-limiting disease. Originally, nurse-led clinics were further developed into a multiprofessional Breathlessness Intervention Service with predominantly palliative medicine and physiotherapy input [21]. In another model, medical input was extended with close collaboration of respiratory and palliative medicine professionals seeing the patient jointly [22]. These services also play a major role in the early integration of palliative care into the disease trajectory of patients with advanced, non-malignant respiratory disease [22]. However, there is still little evidence to show which service model or delivery is needed for which patients. A recent RCT of people with lung cancer investigated whether a single breathlessness management session provided the same benefit as three sessions, with less breathlessness-related distress [23]. Researchers found no evidence that three sessions conferred additional benefits over one. Thus, a single session seemed appropriate, minimised patient burden, and was more cost-effective. It is important to monitor the benefit–harm balance of interventions even when the interventions do not involve a drug, device or surgical intervention. Breathlessness services are still relatively new to the respiratory community. Pulmonary rehabilitation is a much more familiar concept to respiratory physicians. However, patients with a more advanced disease might not be fit enough to attend several weeks of pulmonary rehabilitation but suffer increasingly from intractable breathlessness. This is the gap that breathlessness services intend to fill.

Integrated care models for patients with respiratory disease

With increasing numbers of patients suffering from respiratory disease, the need for integrated care models is constantly rising [24]. Also, care for patients with advanced lung disease has been criticised for being fragmented and often complex. Adding another element, such as specialist palliative care, can thus be a challenge [1]. Therefore, the ATS favours an individualised integrated model of palliative care in which a patient receives palliative care at the onset of symptoms from a progressive respiratory disease and then concurrently with curative/restorative care [10]. Thus, several care models have been developed around the world that integrate assessment, education, optimisation of management and self-management, and improved access to services.

The National Institute for Health and Care Excellence (NICE) has included palliative care in its COPD guidance and related pathway as an example for embedding access to palliative care into policy [25]. Breathing Space is a community service for people with COPD and other respiratory conditions and their carers provided by the Rotherham NHS Foundation Trust in the UK [26]. It provides inpatient care for people with exacerbations, pulmonary rehabilitation, oxygen services, education and lifestyle support, a residential 7-day programme targeting breathlessness, and respite and hospice care for those who need it. These services are all tailored to the needs of patients rather than the anticipated prognosis [26].

The Western Australian COPD model of care names care and EOL support explicitly as a Chronic Respiratory Disease Service Improvement Framework [8]. The BREATHE programme provides nursing, physiotherapy, occupational therapy, clinical psychology, pharmacy and community care aid services in a client's home at a flexible level according to their level of fitness and complexity of healthcare needs [27]. The COPD-Home model is an integrated model for patients with severe and very severe COPD. It includes education for patients and involves nurses, improved coordination of levels of care with joint visits and telephone checks, improved accessibility through a call centre for GP support, and an individualised management plan [28]. INSPIRED (Implementing a Novel and Supportive Program of Individualized care for patients and families living with Respiratory Disease) is a home-based model to support COPD patients in Canada. It includes education according to patients' and carers' needs, a COPD Action Plan to help manage COPD and acute exacerbations, support with navigating the healthcare system and gaining access to programmes/services, and the opportunity to discuss advance care planning [1, 16].

Barriers to access

Trajectories

The disease trajectory of chronic lung diseases, such as COPD and pulmonary fibrosis, is variable and characterised by considerable uncertainty [15]. While patients typically have a phase of gradual decline, the trajectory can change abruptly because of exacerbations of the underlying lung disease or events caused by a comorbid disease.

Patients with advanced COPD usually experience a gradual but progressive decline in exercise tolerance and the development of oxygen dependence that is typically punctuated by acute exacerbations [29]. Patients with COPD are frequently hospitalised at the EOL, often in the ICU, although this will vary from country to country with patients being more frequently admitted to ICUs in the USA compared to Europe. However, there is some evidence that over time, fewer patients are dying in acute care hospitals. One retrospective cohort study examined fee-for-service Medicare beneficiaries who died in 2000, 2005 or 2008 with a diagnosis of cancer, COPD or dementia [30]. In the cohort with COPD, between 2000 and 2009, more patients died at home in 2009 than in 2000 (28 *versus* 24%), fewer died in acute care hospitals (32 *versus* 44%), and more patients were under hospice care at the time of their death (39 *versus* 20%).

Every COPD exacerbation can be life-threatening and is associated with an increased risk of dying. Approximately 10% of patients hospitalised with an acute exacerbation of COPD die during hospital admission [31]. This proportion increases to about a quarter for patients who need invasive mechanical ventilation because of respiratory failure [32]. About half of the patients admitted for an exacerbation do not survive 4 years after discharge [33].

Importantly, not all patients follow this hypothetical disease trajectory of a gradual decline interspersed with acute exacerbations. In fact, the progression of COPD is very heterogeneous [34], and the end of the patient's life is often unanticipated by their loved ones [15]. Despite the heterogeneity in clinical course in patients with COPD, certain parameters predict a greater likelihood of death within 12 months: decrease in 6-min walk distance of 50 m; change towards a very sedentary lifestyle based on a single question; change towards feeling upset or downhearted; an increase in arterial carbon dioxide tension of <5 mmHg; or a decrease in arterial oxygen tension >3 mmHg [35].

IPF is usually characterised by a gradual and inexorable decline in respiratory capacity. However, patients may remain stable for a longer period of time or may be confronted with frequent hospital admissions because of acute worsening of respiratory symptoms [36]. The median survival for IPF is 2–3 years, although some patients live much longer [37]. Most patients experience a subacute worsening over one or more months, while a minority have an acute deterioration <1 month. The majority of patients with IPF die in a hospital setting, and in contrast to the data for COPD, there is no evidence that this number has declined over time or that hospice enrolment has increased [38]. In one study of adult patients with IPF living in the USA, only 14% were referred to palliative care and most referrals occurred in the last month of life [38].

The trajectory of lung cancer is more clearly defined than chronic lung diseases. For patients diagnosed with NSCLC, the greatest impact on prognosis is the tumour–node–metastasis staging. On average, median survival is 59 months for patients diagnosed with stage 1A disease and only 4 months for patients with stage IV disease [39].

The most important prognostic factor in patients with SCLC is the extent of disease (stage) at presentation. For patients with limited-stage disease, median survival ranges from 15 to 20 months, and the reported 5-year survival rate is 10–13%. In contrast, for patients with extended-stage disease, median survival is 8–13 months, and the 5-year survival rate is 1–2% [40].

These prognostic data support oncology guidelines recommending the integration of palliative into oncological care for patients with advanced metastatic lung cancer [41]. A clinical opinion from the American Society of Clinical Oncology (ASCO) advises combining standard oncological care and palliative care early on in the course of illness for all patients with metastatic cancer and/or a high symptom burden [42]. Despite these recommendations, few integrative practice models exist [18, 43, 44].

Attitudes towards palliative care

Despite the benefits, palliative care remains an unmet need for many patients with chronic lung disease. Barriers to accessing palliative care services include patients' lack of understanding of the progressive nature of their disease and possibility they could die from COPD [45], and clinicians not broaching the topic, also in the belief that palliative care is only for dying people. Unfortunately, this misconception about palliative care as care for the dying is not only held by patients but also by professionals and the public, which makes it even more challenging to integrate palliative care earlier on in the disease trajectory.

Lack of communication

In a study of patients with oxygen-dependent COPD in the USA, only 32% of patients reported having discussed with their clinician the care they would want if they were too sick to speak for themselves [46]. A Dutch study confirmed that clinicians rarely discuss LST preferences with their patients with COPD, despite the fact that patients can indicate their preferences regarding LSTs [47]. In a cross-sectional study, outpatients were asked to complete a quality of communication questionnaire. Patients with severe COPD rated their clinicians' general communication skills, such as listening and answering questions, highly. Conversely, patients rated their clinicians' skills at discussing EOL topics as poor. In fact, topics such as prognosis, what dying might be like, and spiritual issues were not discussed at all [48]. These findings underscore the need for improving the communication skills of professionals caring for patients with advanced lung disease. Training in communication skills must be an integral part of any specialist training. Palliative care clinicians have the necessary communication skills and by working with other clinicians they can often support them in developing these skills. The World Health Organization lists COPD as one of the most common conditions for which palliative care is an appropriate, yet underutilised service [49].

Service configuration/delivery

Since the formal recognition of palliative care as a medical (sub)specialty nearly a decade ago in the USA and almost 30 years ago the in the UK, there has been an increase in the number of programmes throughout the USA and Europe [22, 50, 51].

The number of hospital-based palliative care programmes has increased rapidly and, as of 2013, programmes were in place at more than 67% of US hospitals with more than 50 beds [50].

The EAPC reported that the number of palliative care beds per million inhabitants ranged between 45 and 75 beds in most advanced European countries [52]. Studies have demonstrated significant cost reductions in care as a result of palliative care consults helping patient and families align their treatment preferences with the care they receive [53]. Concordance of patient goals and treatments results in less invasive care and a reduction in the length of stay [53, 54].

Models of hospital-based palliative care services include palliative care consultation services that provide recommendations to the requesting provider or service, palliative care units, and integrated palliative care models. Inpatient palliative care units and palliative care providers either have primary responsibility for patients or provide a consulting role. Inpatient palliative care units are most appropriate for patients with symptoms that cannot be easily controlled; when medical needs cannot be optimally managed in another setting; when distressed families need a higher level of support; when there is a need for transferring out of a critical care setting; and for patients who are close to dying. In one study, a dedicated palliative care unit reduced daily costs by 74% compared to usual care patients [55]. Integrated palliative care models that enhance palliative care within different settings are being developed; successful models include ICUs [56] and more recently EDs [57, 58]. ICU-based palliative care is growing because evidence shows that this model saves costs by appropriating care that aligns with patient and family members' preferences [59, 60]. Palliative care in critical care settings can be delivered by intensivists, nurses, social workers, or palliative care specialists depending on the ICU model. Evidence suggests that the quality of palliative care in the ICU varies depending on factors such as staffing, stakeholder interaction, and eligibility ascertainment. The use of electronic health record triggers based on a combination of patient criteria (*e.g.* days on mechanical ventilation, poor outcomes and needs assessment) holds promise to improve the quality of palliative care [60].

Outpatient or community palliative care services provide continuity of care for patients who are discharged from the hospital or referred by a primary care or subspecialty provider. Community palliative care teams provide pain and symptom management, psychosocial support, and coordination of home care needs. Community-based programmes are less common than inpatient consultation programmes; however, a growing number of studies support the benefits of community-based and telemedicine palliative care services. These benefits include improved patient satisfaction, symptom control, quality of life, and reduced healthcare use [18, 61–63].

Barriers to palliative care referrals exist for patients, families, and providers [64, 65]. These barriers include the unawareness of palliative care services in patients and their families and the tendency of clinicians to equate palliative care with EOL care [66]. This misunderstanding calls for clear definitions in lay terms on the meaning of palliative care [4]. One study found the term "supportive care" more acceptable to patients and families [65]. Providers may be more amenable to consulting palliative care for supportive care or symptom management services. In addition to misperceptions of palliative care, issues related to reimbursement and the shortage of palliative care clinicians and services are very important and need to be addressed by policymakers, insurers, and medical and nursing school educational models.

Lack of training

For the large number of patients with an advanced and life-threatening illness to benefit from palliative care, it is important that supportive services be provided not only by specialists but also incorporated into the practices of all clinicians who are caring for persons with serious and complex illnesses such as chronic lung disease. Some term this primary palliative care, to distinguish it from subspecialty palliative care. This encompasses any type of supportive care that is delivered by all healthcare professionals caring for patients with a life-threatening illness. Optimal palliative care for patients with respiratory diseases should ideally incorporate both primary and subspecialty palliative care. However, clinicians caring for these patients need to attain competence in providing comprehensive supportive care. The lack of palliative care training is frequently cited by clinicians as the reason why they do not incorporate palliative care into their practice. Training all clinicians on the basic tenets of palliative care and on how to conduct goals of care conversations is becoming more available and is offered in various teaching formats, *e.g.* mobile apps, videos, case-based role playing, in addition to traditional classroom settings (table 2). Furthermore, this specialist training should be made systematic by incorporating it into all clinician training.

Facilitators to access

Systematic needs assessment: recognition and triage

Systematic assessment of symptoms and functional ability should be standardised in routine clinical practice to facilitate the recognition of patients' problems and changes over time. The use of simple, valid measurement tools for common respiratory symptoms, such as dyspnoea, fatigue and cough, and functional status may improve earlier referral to palliative care specialists. Examples of measurement tools include the Edmonton Symptom Assessment System and the Palliative Performance Scale version 2, a modification of the Karnofsky Performance Status Scale [68].

Identification of patient palliative care needs can be divided into three distinct levels of care based on data such as diagnosis, age, hospitalisations and ED visits over the past 12 months. The first level recognises that all patients need education about the importance of advance care planning and identifies a surrogate decision-maker. The second level targets at-risk patients diagnosed with one or more serious illnesses that may result in distressing symptoms, psychological or spiritual needs, or that may progress to a terminal phase. These patients would benefit from routine screening and more specific advance care planning. The third level includes high-need patients with a shorter prognosis (<2 years), those with a higher symptom burden, or more significant psychosocial or spiritual needs [69].

Trigger tools, including electronic forms, have been developed using palliative care indicators. These tools improve the recognition of palliative care needs for patients with non-malignant diagnoses and unmet needs that may benefit from an earlier needs assessment, a review of care goals, and anticipatory care planning [70].

The use of specific criteria or triggers to prompt proactive referrals for palliative care consultation in ICUs reduces the use of ICU resources and increases involvement of palliative care specialists for critically ill patients and families in need. Criteria should be tailored and implemented in ICUs depending on the identified process and outcome measures [59, 71].

Early integration and triggers/transitions to palliative care (chronic progressive, generalist *versus* specialist palliative care)

For patients with an advanced and life-threatening illness, such as chronic lung disease, palliative care should be offered early in the disease process and should be available

Table 2. Examples of primary palliative care educational opportunities

Educational opportunity	Description	Website
NHS Health Education England	The e-learning programme End of Life Care for All aims to enhance the training and education of the health and social care workforce	www.e-lfh.org.uk/programmes/end-of-life-care/
Center to Advance Palliative Care	A national membership-based organisation offering tools, training and technical assistance to front-line clinicians	www.capc.org
VitalTalk	An online resource that teaches clinicians EOL communication skills	www.vitaltalk.org
End-of-Life Nursing Education Consortium	Offers worldwide training to nurses of all levels; classroom courses and online-modules are available on basic palliative care and specialty topics	www.aacn.nche.edu/elnec
Palliative Care Education and Practice	Training for nurse educators and physicians	http://www.hms.harvard.edu/pallcare/PCEP/PCEP.htm
MJHS Institute for Innovation in Palliative Care	Online palliative care webinars for healthcare professionals	www.mjhspalliativeinstitute.org/e-learning/
Professional societies		
American Academy of Hospice and Palliative Medicine		www.aahpm.org
Hospice and Palliative Nurses Association		
National Hospice and Palliative Care Organization		www.nhpco.org/eol
European Association for Palliative Care	Identifies 10 core competencies for health and social care professionals delivering basic palliative care	www.eapc.eu (general); www.eapcnet.eu/LinkClick.aspx?fileticket=xc-tl28Ttfk=&tabid=194 (Core competencies in palliative care: an EAPC White Paper on palliative care education – part 1)

Reproduced and modified from [67] with permission.

throughout the patient's course if needed to address difficult-to-control symptoms, goals of care, or coordination across sites of care. The ideal setting and time to introduce palliative care and engage in early goals of care conversations is the outpatient setting when the patient is in a stable disease state thus enabling shared decision-making [45]. If palliative care cannot be introduced during an outpatient visit, several studies have demonstrated the benefits of inpatient palliative care consultation during hospitalisation, including patients with multimorbidities such as COPD, heart failure, and IPF [61]. Patient-centred outcomes of palliative care consultation include communication, access to home services, emotional and spiritual support, well-being and dignity, and care around the time of death [72].

Indications for a palliative care consultation

Ideally, clinicians caring for patients with chronic lung disease should be able to manage most of their patients' palliative care issues. However, there are many situations where a consultation with a palliative care specialist may be beneficial. The initiation of a palliative care consultation should be led by patient or family need rather than by the clinical or physiological stage of the underlying disease. As some individuals will cope with advanced disease, and indeed symptoms, more independently than others, it is not possible to generalise for any one person or condition. There may, however, be triggers that can be identified for making such a referral, such as: if the burden of physical symptoms is felt to be unacceptable by the individual, carer or clinician involved in regular care; when the emotional needs (related to the illness) are unmet; to help with decision-making about treatment options; or when there is concern (from any of the above parties) about EOL and the need for advance care planning.

There may also be disease-specific triggers for patients not previously seen by palliative care. For example, in COPD, a referral might follow an admission involving invasive ventilation or NIV; a number of patients say "never again", and this may be an indication for a more detailed exploration of future care preferences, although they may change their mind with the next exacerbation. In the case of lung cancer and mesothelioma, when the oncologist feels that they are unfit for further oncological intervention, this can be a devastating blow to the patient; therefore, integrating palliative care at the onset of lung cancer can improve symptom burden and quality of life. In CF and IPF, if patients are ineligible for a transplant, this may trigger a referral to a palliative care specialist.

Several transition points in chronic lung disease and lung cancer have been identified by patients, carers and clinicians, and confirmed by studies, that should serve to prompt a discussion about goals of care and palliative care: the start of new or different treatments, *e.g.* initiation of oxygen therapy; a lack of further life-prolonging treatment options; functional decline associated with increased severity of breathlessness and fatigue; frequent exacerbations, *e.g.* >2 per year; frequent hospitalisations/ED visits, *e.g.* >2 every 6 months; and progressive breathlessness over time.

While disease-specific criteria, *e.g.* COPD GOLD stage IV or a decline in FVC for patients with IPF, serve as markers for many clinicians to consult palliative care, earlier integration of palliative care may lessen symptom burden by incorporating self-management skills into daily care regimens.

An initial palliative care assessment should include the aspects outlined in table 3 [67, 73, 74].

Table 3. Primary palliative care assessment of patients with chronic lung disease

Understanding of illness/prognosis and treatment options

Does the patient/family/surrogate understand the current illness, their prognosis for quantity and quality of life, expected disease trajectory/uncertainty about disease trajectory, and treatment options?

Symptom management

Does the patient have uncontrolled/distressing symptoms? In particular, does the patient have any of the following: pulmonary symptoms (cough, dyspnoea) with daily activities; pain; fatigue and sleep disturbance; distressing psychological symptoms (depression and anxiety); or constitutional symptoms (anorexia and weight loss)?

Social/spiritual assessment

Are there significant social or spiritual concerns affecting the patient's daily life?

Decision-making

Is the patient comfortable making healthcare decisions or does the patient rely on family members, friends or healthcare professionals to make decisions?

Has the patient identified a surrogate decision-maker and talked with this person about their goals and values?

Would the patient/family/surrogate like help with treatment decision-making?

Identification of patient-centred goals of care

What are the goals of care, as identified by the patient/family/surrogate?

Are treatment options matched to informed patient-centred goals?

Has the patient participated in an advance care planning process?

Has the patient completed an advance care planning document?

Coping with life-threatening illness

How is the patient coping with their illness?

How are the family/caregivers coping with the illness?

Coordination of care

Are there barriers to safe and sustainable transitions from one setting to another (*e.g.* transport to appointments)?

Are systems in place to enable good communication between multiple providers?

Reproduced and modified from [67] with permission. Data from [73] and [74].

Conclusions

Access to palliative care for patients with chronic malignant and non-malignant lung disease has improved over recent years, with specialist palliative care services available in an increasing number of countries. Collaboration of respiratory and palliative care professionals is paramount for providing the best care for these patients. Various service models have been developed, especially for patients with non-malignant lung disease, but wide coverage of such concepts is still missing. More systematic assessment and identification of those in need of (specialist) palliative care as well as systematic inclusion of palliative care principles in medical and nursing training is still needed.

References

1. Rocker GM, Simpson AC, Horton R. Palliative care in advanced lung disease: the challenge of integrating palliation into everyday care. *Chest* 2015; 148: 801–809.
2. Radbruch L, Payne S, on behalf of the EAPC Board of Directors. White Paper on standards and norms for hospice and palliative care in Europe: part 1. *Eur J Palliat Care* 2009; 16: 278–289.

3. Radbruch L, Payne S, on behalf of the EAPC Board of Directors. White Paper on standards and norms for hospice and palliative care in Europe: part 2. *Eur J Palliat Care* 2010; 17: 22–33.
4. Center to Advance Palliative Care. www.capc.org Date last accessed: March 20, 2016.
5. Bolognesi D, Centeno C, Biasco G. Specialisation in Palliative Medicine for Physicians in Europe 2014. A supplement of the EAPC Atlas of Palliative Care in Europe. Milan, EAPC Press, 2014. www.eapcnet.eu/Portals/0/Organization/Development%20in%20Europe%20TF/Specialisation/2014_SpecialisationPMPhysicianInEurope.pdf
6. Shipman C, Gysels M, White P, *et al.* Improving generalist end of life care: national consultation with practitioners, commissioners, academics, and service user groups. *BMJ* 2008; 337: a1720.
7. National Institute for Health and Care Excellence (NICE). Idiopathic pulmonary fibrosis in adults. Quality Standard (QS79). www.nice.org.uk/guidance/qs79 Date last accessed: June 9, 2016. Date last updated: January, 2015.
8. Dept of Health Western Australia. Chronic Obstructive Pulmonary Disease Model of Care. Subiaco, Dept of Health, Government of Western Australia, 2012.
9. Siouta N, van Beek K, Preston N, *et al.* Towards integration of palliative care in patients with chronic heart failure and chronic obstructive pulmonary disease: a systematic literature review of European guidelines and pathways. *BMC Palliat Care* 2016; 15: 18.
10. Lanken PN, Terry PB, Delisser HM, *et al.* An official American Thoracic Society clinical policy statement: palliative care for patients with respiratory diseases and critical illnesses. *Am J Respir Crit Care Med* 2008; 177: 912–927.
11. Connors S, Graham S, Peel T. An evaluation of a physiotherapy led non-pharmacological breathlessness programme for patients with intrathoracic malignancy. *Palliat Med* 2007; 21: 285–287.
12. Bradley B, Branley HM, Egan JJ, *et al.* Interstitial lung disease guideline: the British Thoracic Society in collaboration with the Thoracic Society of Australia and New Zealand and the Irish Thoracic Society. *Thorax* 2008; 63: Suppl. 5, 1–58.
13. Bourke SJ, Doe SJ, Gascoigne AD, *et al.* An integrated model of provision of palliative care to patients with cystic fibrosis. *Palliat Med* 2009; 23: 512–517.
14. Robinson WM. Palliative and end-of-life care in cystic fibrosis: what we know and what we need to know. *Curr Opin Pulm Med* 2009; 15: 621–625.
15. Pinnock H, Kendall M, Murray SA, *et al.* Living and dying with severe chronic obstructive pulmonary disease: multi-perspective longitudinal qualitative study. *BMJ* 2011; 342: d142.
16. Rocker GM, Cook D. 'INSPIRED' approaches to better care for patients with advanced COPD. *Clin Invest Med* 2013; 36: E114–E120.
17. Boland J, Owen J, Ainscough R, *et al.* Developing a service for patients with very severe chronic obstructive pulmonary disease (COPD) within resources. *BMJ Support Palliat Care* 2014; 4: 196–201.
18. Temel JS, Greer JA, Muzikansky A, *et al.* Early palliative care for patients with metastatic non-small-cell lung cancer. *N Engl J Med* 2010; 363: 733–742.
19. Curtis C, Challand S, Harrison S, *et al.* Integrated palliative care/advanced respiratory disease (ARDS) clinics: a multi-centre pilot project. *BMJ Support Palliat Care* 2014; 4: A94–A95.
20. Booth S, Moffat C, Farquhar M, *et al.* Developing a breathlessness intervention service for patients with palliative and supportive care needs, irrespective of diagnosis. *J Palliat Care* 2011; 27: 28–36.
21. Farquhar MC, Prevost AT, McCrone P, *et al.* Is a specialist breathlessness service more effective and cost-effective for patients with advanced cancer and their carers than standard care? Findings of a mixed-method randomised controlled trial. *BMC Med* 2014; 12: 194.
22. Higginson IJ, Bausewein C, Reilly CC, *et al.* An integrated palliative and respiratory care service for patients with advanced disease and refractory breathlessness: a randomised controlled trial. *Lancet Respir Med* 2014; 2: 979–987.
23. Johnson MJ, Kanaan M, Richardson G, *et al.* A randomised controlled trial of three or one breathing technique training sessions for breathlessness in people with malignant lung disease. *BMC Med* 2015; 13: 213.
24. Partridge MR. Integrated care: delivering better outcomes for patients with respiratory disease. *Br J Health Care Manage* 2015; 21: 7–9.
25. National Institute for Health and Care Excellence (NICE). Chronic Obstructive Pulmonary Disease in Over 16s: Diagnosis and Management (CG101). Available from www.nice.org.uk/guidance/cg101/ Date last accessed: June 9, 2016. Date last updated: June 2010.
26. Rotherham NHS Foundation Trust. BreathingSpace. www.therotherhamft.nhs.uk/breathing_space/ Date last accessed: June 9, 2016.
27. Taylor R, Marley A. An integrated model for community COPD care. *Aust J Prim Health* 2006; 12: 45–50.
28. Sunde S, Walstad RA, Bentsen SB, *et al.* The development of an integrated care model for patients with severe or very severe chronic obstructive pulmonary disease (COPD): the COPD-Home model. *Scand J Caring Sci* 2014; 28: 469–477.
29. Murray SA, Kendall M, Boyd K, *et al.* Illness trajectories and palliative care. *BMJ* 2005; 330: 1007–1011.
30. Teno JM, Gozalo PL, Bynum JP, *et al.* Change in end-of-life care for Medicare beneficiaries: site of death, place of care, and health care transitions in 2000, 2005, and 2009. *JAMA* 2013; 309: 470–477.

31. Steer J, Gibson J, Bourke SC. The DECAF score: predicting hospital mortality in exacerbations of chronic obstructive pulmonary disease. *Thorax* 2012; 67: 970–976.
32. Hajizadeh N, Goldfeld K, Crothers K. What happens to patients with COPD with long-term oxygen treatment who receive mechanical ventilation for COPD exacerbation? A 1-year retrospective follow-up study. *Thorax* 2015; 70: 294–296.
33. Piquet J, Chavaillon JM, David P, *et al.* High-risk patients following hospitalisation for an acute exacerbation of COPD. *Eur Respir J* 2013; 42: 946–955.
34. Casanova C, de Torres JP, Aguirre-Jaíme A, *et al.* The progression of chronic obstructive pulmonary disease is heterogeneous: the experience of the BODE cohort. *Am J Respir Crit Care Med* 2011; 184: 1015–1021.
35. Benzo R, Siemion W, Novotny P, *et al.* Factors to inform clinicians about the end of life in severe chronic obstructive pulmonary disease. *J Pain Symptom Manage* 2013; 46: 491–499. e4.
36. Martinez FJ, Safrin S, Weycker D, *et al.* The clinical course of patients with idiopathic pulmonary fibrosis. *Ann Intern Med* 2005; 142: 963–967.
37. Ley B, Collard HR, King TE Jr. Clinical course and prediction of survival in idiopathic pulmonary fibrosis. *Am J Respir Crit Care Med* 2011; 183: 431–440.
38. Lindell KO, Liang Z, Hoffman LA, *et al.* Palliative care and location of death in decedents with idiopathic pulmonary fibrosis. *Chest* 2015; 147: 423–429.
39. Siegel RL, Miller KD, Jemal A. Cancer statistics, 2016. *CA Cancer J Clin* 2016; 66: 7–30.
40. Silvestri GA, Tanoue LT, Margolis ML, *et al.* The noninvasive staging of non-small cell lung cancer: the guidelines. *Chest* 2003; 123: Suppl. 1, 147–156.
41. Griffin JP, Koch KA, Nelson JE, *et al.* Palliative care consultation, quality-of-life measurements, and bereavement for end-of-life care in patients with lung cancer: ACCP evidence-based clinical practice guidelines (2nd edition). *Chest* 2007; 132: Suppl. 3, 404–422.
42. Smith TJ, Temin S, Alesi ER, *et al.* American Society of Clinical Oncology provisional clinical opinion: the integration of palliative care into standard oncology care. *J Clin Oncol* 2012; 30: 880–887.
43. King JD, Eickhoff J, Traynor A, *et al.* Integrated onco-palliative care associated with prolonged survival compared to standard care for patients with advanced lung cancer: a retrospective review. *J Pain Symptom Manage* 2016; 51: 1027–1032.
44. Ferrell B, Sun V, Hurria A, *et al.* Interdisciplinary palliative care for patients with lung cancer. *J Pain Symptom Manage* 2015; 50: 758–767.
45. Curtis JR, Engelberg RA, Nielsen EL, *et al.* Patient-physician communication about end-of-life care for patients with severe COPD. *Eur Respir J* 2004; 24: 200–205.
46. Knauft E, Nielsen EL, Engelberg RA, *et al.* Barriers and facilitators to end-of-life care communication for patients with COPD. *Chest* 2005; 127: 2188–2196.
47. Janssen DJ, Curtis JR, Au DH, *et al.* Patient-clinician communication about end-of-life care for Dutch and US patients with COPD. *Eur Respir J* 2011; 38: 268–276.
48. Reinke LF, Slatore CG, Uman J, *et al.* Patient-clinician communication about end-of-life care topics: is anyone talking to patients with chronic obstructive pulmonary disease? *J Palliat Med* 2011; 14: 923–928.
49. Connor SR, Sepulveda Bermedo MC, eds. Global Atlas of Palliative Care at the End-of-Life. London, Worldwide Palliative Care Alliance, 2014. www.who.int/nmh/Global_Atlas_of_Palliative_Care.pdf
50. Dumanovsky T, Augustin R, Rogers M, *et al.* The growth of palliative care in U.S. hospitals: a status report. *J Palliat Med* 2016; 19: 8–15.
51. Gomes B, Calanzani N, Curiale V, *et al.* Effectiveness and cost-effectiveness of home palliative care services for adults with advanced illness and their caregivers. *Cochrane Database Syst Rev* 2013; 6: CD007760.
52. Centeno C, Clark D, Lynch T, *et al.* Facts and indicators on palliative care development in 52 countries of the WHO European region: results of an EAPC Task Force. *Palliat Med* 2007; 21: 463–471.
53. May P, Garrido MM, Cassel JB, *et al.* Palliative care teams' cost-saving effect is larger for cancer patients with higher numbers of comorbidities. *Health Aff* 2016; 35: 44–53.
54. May P, Normand C, Morrison RS. Economic impact of hospital inpatient palliative care consultation: review of current evidence and directions for future research. *J Palliat Med* 2014; 17: 1054–1063.
55. Smith TJ, Coyne P, Cassel B, *et al.* A high-volume specialist palliative care unit and team may reduce in-hospital end-of-life care costs. *J Palliat Med* 2003; 6: 699–705.
56. Curtis JR, Treece PD, Nielsen EL, *et al.* Integrating palliative and critical care: evaluation of a quality-improvement intervention. *Am J Respir Crit Care Med* 2008; 178: 269–275.
57. Grudzen CR, Richardson LD, Johnson PN, *et al.* Emergency department-initiated palliative care in advanced cancer: a randomized clinical trial. *JAMA Oncol* 2016; 2: 591–598.
58. Lamba S, Quest TE, Weissman DE. Palliative care consultation in the emergency department #298. *J Palliat Med* 2016; 19: 108–109.
59. Frontera JA, Curtis JR, Nelson JE, *et al.* Integrating palliative care into the care of neurocritically ill patients: a report from the Improving Palliative Care in the ICU Project Advisory Board and the Center to Advance Palliative Care. *Crit Care Med* 2015; 43: 1964–1977.

60. Cox CE, Curtis JR. Using technology to create a more humanistic approach to integrating palliative care into the intensive care unit. *Am J Respir Crit Care Med* 2016; 193: 242–250.
61. Enguidanos SM, Cherin D, Brumley R. Home-based palliative care study: site of death, and costs of medical care for patients with congestive heart failure, chronic obstructive pulmonary disease, and cancer. *J Soc Work End Life Palliat Care* 2005; 1: 37–56.
62. Rabow M, Kvale E, Barbour L, *et al.* Moving upstream: a review of the evidence of the impact of outpatient palliative care. *J Palliat Med* 2013; 16: 1540–1549.
63. Bakitas MA, Tosteson TD, Li Z, *et al.* Early *versus* delayed initiation of concurrent palliative oncology care: patient outcomes in the ENABLE III randomized controlled trial. *J Clin Oncol* 2015; 33: 1438–1445.
64. Schenker Y, Park SY, Maciasz R, *et al.* Do patients with advanced cancer and unmet palliative care needs have an interest in receiving palliative care services? *J Palliat Med* 2014; 17: 667–672.
65. Maciasz RM, Arnold RM, Chu E, *et al.* Does it matter what you call it? A randomized trial of language used to describe palliative care services. *Support Care Cancer* 2013; 21: 3411–3419.
66. Mason B, Buckingham S, Finucane A, *et al.* Improving primary palliative care in Scotland: lessons from a mixed methods study. *BMC Fam Pract* 2015; 16: 176.
67. Reinke LF, Janssen D, Curtis JR. Palliative care for adults with nonmalignant chronic lung disease. *In*: Post TW, ed. UpToDate. Waltham, UpToDate, 2016. Available from: www.uptodate.com Date last accessed: May 13, 2016.
68. National Program of Cancer Registries. Monitoring and Evaluation Tools. www.npcrc.org/content/25/Measurement-and-Evaluation-Tools.aspx
69. Parrish M, Kinderman A, Rabow M. Weaving Palliative Care into Primary Care: A Guide for Community Health Centers. Available from: www.chcf.org/publications/2015/08/weaving-palliative-care Date last accessed: June 9, 2016. Date last updated: August 2015.
70. Highet G, Crawford D, Murray SA, *et al.* Development and evaluation of the Supportive and Palliative Care Indicators Tool (SPICT): a mixed-methods study. *BMJ Support Palliat Care* 2014; 4: 285–290.
71. Nelson JE, Curtis JR, Mulkerin C, *et al.* Choosing and using screening criteria for palliative care consultation in the ICU: a report from the Improving Palliative Care in the ICU (IPAL-ICU) Advisory Board. *Crit Care Med* 2013; 41: 2318–2327.
72. Casarett D, Pickard A, Bailey FA, *et al.* Do palliative consultations improve patient outcomes? *J Am Geriatr Soc* 2008; 56: 593–599.
73. Jacobsen J, Jackson V, Dahlin C, *et al.* Components of early outpatient palliative care consultation in patients with metastatic nonsmall cell lung cancer. *J Palliat Med* 2011; 14: 459–464.
74. Weissman DE, Meier DE. Identifying patients in need of a palliative care assessment in the hospital setting: a consensus report from the Center to Advance Palliative Care. *J Palliat Med* 2011; 14: 17–23.

Disclosures: None declared.

Chapter 4

Supporting informal carers

Morag Farquhar

Carers play a vital role in supportive, palliative and EOL care for patients with advanced respiratory conditions. They enable patients to be cared for, and even die, in their place of choice. However, this caring role comes at a cost in terms of psychosocial distress, physical and psychological health impacts (including carer mortality), and pressure on finances. Ensuring that carers are supported can ameliorate these effects. Healthcare professionals must respond to policy rhetoric and be dramatically better at identifying carers, working with them to assess and prioritise their support needs, and responding to and reviewing those needs. Evidence-based tools and approaches exist and can help, but are not a one-off exercise. Carers' needs may change as the patient's condition (or location of care) changes, or as carer health or systems change. Carers' needs may also exist beyond the patient's death. Clinical and academic researchers need to robustly develop and evaluate interventions for carers and include appropriate carer outcomes in evaluations of patient-targeted interventions.

Advanced respiratory disease has a high symptom burden that causes physical disability, anxiety and depression, and loss of independence and dignity, and often occurs alongside other patient comorbidities. It places a huge burden not only on patients and health systems, but also on informal carers (families and friends who support them at home). These carers can experience isolation due to the restrictions placed on their lives, role change, and a range of emotions including anxiety and anger. Carers play a crucial role, but a considerable care burden falls on them, with well-established impacts. There is substantial evidence that carers are largely unsupported. This chapter aims to increase awareness of carers and their important role, the impact of caring, carers' support needs, ways to support active and bereaved carers, and implications for research.

The profile and importance of carers

Informal carers are "lay people in a close supportive role who share in the illness experience of the patient and who undertake vital care work and emotion management" [1]; they are also known as "family carers", "caregivers", "supporters" or simply "carers". While at least half of carers provide care in the same household [2], care can be provided by a complex and diffuse network of both families and friends [3].

Primary Care Unit, Dept of Public Health and Primary Care, University of Cambridge, Institute of Public Health, Cambridge, UK.

Correspondence: Morag Farquhar, Primary Care Unit, Dept of Public Health and Primary Care, University of Cambridge, Institute of Public Health, Robinson Way, Cambridge, CB2 0SR. E-mail: mcf22@medschl.cam.ac.uk

 Print ISBN: 978-1-84984-071-2. Online ISBN: 978-1-84984-072-9. Print ISSN: 2312-508X. Online ISSN: 2312-5098.

In the USA, 34.2 million people (14.3% of the population) provided unpaid care to an adult aged ⩾50 years in 2015 [4]. One in 10 patients on any UK GP practice list are carers [5] and 1.4 million people provide ⩾50 h unpaid care per week [2]. By 2030, 10.9 million people will be providing informal care across the EU for at least 35 h a week, with 21.5 million providing care for at least 20 h a week [6]. Carers play a crucial role in providing supportive care to relatives [7], reducing formal care costs [8–10], and contributing to the social care economy [11]. It is well established that carers enable patients to be cared for, and even to die, in their place of choice [12].

There is a vast generic literature on carers, and on carers of patients with advanced disease [13–16], but there is also more discrete literature on carers supporting patients with breathlessness in advanced disease, or patients with advanced conditions causing breathlessness. This small but growing literature relates predominantly to COPD but also to cancer.

Data on the number of carers supporting patients with breathlessness in advanced disease are scarce. An RCT of a UK breathlessness intervention service reported that at least 60% of recruited patients with advanced, cancer-related breathlessness [17] and 66% of those with breathlessness due to advanced, non-malignant disease (predominantly COPD) had a carer [18]. A retrospective Norwegian survey of next of kin of COPD patients by Gautun *et al.* [19] reported that >70% of patients had one or more carers, and a UK prospective observational study of a well-defined, population-based cohort of patients with advanced COPD found that 77% of patients had a carer [20].

Analysis by Currow *et al.* [21] of retrospective carer data from the South Australian Health Omnibus found that the mean±SD age of carers of patients with end-stage lung disease was 51.2±16.5 years (range 17–85 years) and one in five was a spouse. One in five of these carers provided physical care (20.8%), either on a daily basis or as intermittent hands-on care, for a mean±SD period of 40.1±56.9 months [21]. Miravitlles *et al.* [22] reported data from the 2008 Survey on Disabilities, Personal Autonomy, and Dependency Situations (Encuesta de Discapacidad, Autonomía personal y situaciones de Dependencia (EDAD)) on the characteristics of Spanish patients disabled by COPD and their carers: the mean±SD age of carers was 56.5±14.9 years and 76% were female.

Farquhar *et al.* [20] reported on an older cohort of carers. In their UK prospective, population-based sample of 115 carers of patients with advanced COPD, the median age of carers was 68 years (interquartile range (IQR) 59–75 years), 73% were female, and 80% were spouses. Most of these carers (87%) lived with the patient, nearly a third reported having other caring responsibilities (32%), and they reported having been in their caring role for a median of 7 years (IQR 3–12 years). This was a changing role. Three-quarters (73%) reported that the amount of caring they gave had changed over that time, and two-thirds (66%) that the type of care they gave had changed. Most gave help every day (90%) and a third gave help for >50 h per week (33%). These carers were not just caring for someone with COPD; they also identified other comorbidities patients had that had an impact on their caring role, a factor noted by others [23].

Carers of patients with advanced respiratory disease carry out a range of often complex personal care tasks including washing, dressing, managing symptoms, administering medicines, or managing home oxygen. As well as this practical help, they also provide emotional support. This is an aspect of caring that is probably not captured in the data about caring hours noted earlier. Thus, carers' roles are multiple [20], often including overnight vigilance [24, 25]. Booth *et al.* [25] described carers providing support and care at night, lying awake to make sure their patient was breathing, or helping their patient be comfortable.

Carers have been shown to have a positive impact on the well-being of patients with COPD: having a carer is associated with better adherence to treatment, reduced rate of smoking, and less frequent emergency visits [26–28]. A qualitative study by Hynes *et al.* [29] found that caring involved continually assessing the state of play by drawing on intimate and nuanced knowledge of the patient's expression of symptoms. While these carers lacked understanding of COPD and reported feeling out of their depth, Hynes *et al.* [29] found that carers built up expertise, skill, and tacit knowledge which came into play in decision-making during symptom exacerbations and which healthcare professionals should acknowledge; McPherson *et al.* [30] similarly reported on the need for health and social care to recognise carer expertise.

Impact of the caring role

The caring role comes at a cost. Negative effects on carers' physical and psychological health (including premature mortality) are well established in the generic caring literature [7, 31–35], and these effects have been shown to be worse for those living in the same household [36] (the most common scenario in respiratory conditions). Using qualitative and quantitative methods, a number of studies have reported the experiences and impacts of the caring role for carers of people with end-stage lung disease [21]. The predominant finding is of a negative impact, but some have also noted some positive aspects of the caring role [24, 37–39].

Most of the carers in the study of advanced COPD by Farquhar *et al.* [20] were older with chronic health problems of their own, reporting a range of self-identified physical and mental health problems that had an impact on their ability to care, *e.g.* back pain (20%), arthritis (19%), heart problems (14%), and mental health problems (14%). The mean Hospital Anxiety and Depression Scale scores for anxiety and depression of these carers were higher than population norms: 27% had probable clinical anxiety and 11% had probable clinical depression [20]. Similarly, Miravitlles *et al.* [22] reported that up to 35% of carers had health-related problems: feeling tired was the most frequent problem, followed by feeling depressed. Health effects and existing health problems in carers have implications for healthcare professionals in meeting carers' support needs [40].

Impacts extend beyond health. Caring is a highly individual experience; carer appraisal of the situation, as opposed to the symptoms they are required to manage, may determine how they cope [41, 42]. Carers of patients with advanced respiratory disease have reported strain, isolation, fear, anxiety, emotional distress, uncertainty, powerlessness, helplessness, depression, uncertainty about the future, restrictions, social isolation and loss [19, 22, 24, 25, 37, 43–54]. Hynes *et al.* [29] found losses related to a previous life, independence, a hoped-for future, financial security and earning capacity. The economic or occupation-related impact of supporting someone with COPD among younger carers has been noted by others [22, 53].

A qualitative study by Simpson *et al.* [55] reported that carers and patients with COPD can have different expectations of the carer and some spousal carers perceived the patient to have child-like needs or attitudes. Others [49, 50] noted that a couple's identity may change over time. An exploratory study by Leidy and Traver [56] found that family members perceived patients with COPD to have disquieting behaviours and there was discrepancy between family and patient views of social behaviour that suggested sources of distress. Furthermore, a small quantitative study by PINTO *et al.* [57] reported that one of the most important predictors of carer burden was the relationship between carers and patients (in addition to carers' mental health scores). The impact of these changed carer–patient relationships can be compounded by isolation. As patients deteriorate, carers can find themselves incrementally providing more care and becoming detached from others; they can feel that the patient is their responsibility alone and no one else's [37]. Social isolation can lead to emotional strain, and can be deepened by a poor understanding of COPD and worry that exacerbations can be fatal [25].

Disease stage may influence a range of impacts. MALIK *et al.* [58] performed a survey of carers of breathlessness patients with lung cancer or heart failure and identified fewer positive caring experiences for carers of patients with more severe breathlessness. FIGUEIREDO *et al.* [54] demonstrated that those caring for people with advanced COPD reported higher subjective burden, more depression, and poorer self-rated mental health than did those caring for people with early COPD. Similarly, MIRAVITLLES *et al.* [22] found that the probability of a problem arising in a carer was positively associated with the degree of dependence of the COPD patient. Furthermore, the likelihood of developing health problems was higher among carers of patients with great, severe, or moderate dependence than among those caring for non-dependent patients. With regard to leisure and social problems, the degree of dependence was also associated with the probability of not being able to go on holiday, not having time for friends and for self-care, and having conflict with a partner (only in the highest level of dependence). Disease stage has also been shown to have an impact on the coping styles adopted by carers of patients with COPD. The cross-sectional interview study by FIGUEIREDO *et al.* [59] reported that those caring for patients with advanced disease used three types of coping: problem-solving, emotion-cognitive and managing stress coping. By contrast, those caring for patients with early disease were more likely to use just problem-solving to cope. This suggests that patient decline in functioning leads to increased dependence on the carer, requiring the carer to adjust to their demanding caregiving role [59].

Little is known about whether different disease trajectories and inequitable access to palliative care and social support have a differential impact on carer outcomes [60], but longitudinal and qualitative studies have demonstrated how the course of non-malignant disease, such as COPD, is lengthy and beset with uncertainty [21, 61]. This unpredictable trajectory is associated with challenges for healthcare professionals in providing a prognosis, even in end-stage disease, leaving patients and carers with significant gaps in information on the disease course [47, 62–64]. This uncertainty, combined with living in the shadow of fear of breathlessness [52], can further exacerbate the already heavy burden for patients and carers. This literature resonates with the objective and subjective stressors and situational context of the caring process identified in broad theoretical models of caring [65–68].

Despite this, carers can still remain unnoticed or invisible [3, 69]. This is in part because carers can be reluctant to ask for support, only seeking help at a time of crisis [25, 37, 70]. Healthcare professionals need a better understanding of the barriers to seeking and accepting proactive support [71]. Many carers do not consider themselves "carers"; rather, they see themselves as a spouse, child or other relative [72], a role for which they may not feel they should, or could, ask for help. They can feel guilty about "not coping" and can have difficulty in acknowledging how serious the patient's illness is [16, 73]. Some value self-reliance and independence [74] but are also often reluctant to request help for fear of diverting resources from patient care [14]. Health services are mostly geared towards the patient's medical needs, mainly acute needs and symptom management [25], thus healthcare professionals predominantly focus on the patient and can neglect to identify who carers are and how they are managing. Further, despite being patients themselves [75], carers can be ambivalent about their own health needs, and the reality of caring often means putting their own health second [24, 76, 77]; it can be difficult to access care for their own health where they are unable (or reluctant) to leave the patient. Currow *et al.* [78] suggested a range of potential carer, patient and healthcare professional reasons for help not being given or asked for, including: embarrassment in asking for help; upskilling of carers over time; lack of consensus between patients and carers about the help needed or wanted; patient and carer hoping that the patient will recover to the previous level; recalibration or response shift to a new "normal"; slow and unpredictable disease progression making it difficult to determine stages; disease-specific factors (*e.g.* surreptitious onset, stigma, discreditation by healthcare professionals, acceptance that breathlessness is a normal symptom); lack of appreciation by healthcare professionals about the help needed; and lack of knowledge or signposting to services by healthcare professionals.

Whatever the reasons for not accessing help, carers lack rudimentary support or assistance [24, 25, 37]. Farquhar *et al.* [20] reported that two-thirds of advanced COPD carers could not identify a healthcare professional for their caring role. When they did identify someone, this was often couched in terms of who they would contact for help in an emergency, rather than someone who was giving them direct ongoing support. Data from healthcare professional interviews within the same study resonated with this: they rarely reported assessing carers' health or support needs, or knowing who their patient's carer was [79].

Carer support needs

The evidence base for carer needs in relation to caring for someone with advanced respiratory disease, or with breathlessness as a result of an advanced disease, is growing. Unmet needs include knowledge and strategies to support the patient and manage their caring role, and feelings of helplessness and powerlessness [25, 37, 43]. Analysis by Currow *et al.* [21] of survey responses of bereaved carers to the South Australian Health Omnibus reported that over a third of carers of someone with end-stage lung disease indicated that they had unmet needs (109 (38%) out of 290), including for support with physical care (17%) or symptom control (11%), for information about the future course of the illness (11%) or service availability (11%), and for emotional support for their patient (11%). Similarly, the prospective study by Farquhar *et al.* [20] found that more than half of carers of patients with advanced COPD wanted more support with knowing what to expect in the future, and more than a third with understanding the illness, knowing who to contact when concerned, having time for themselves in the day, and dealing with their feelings and worries. Around 20% wanted more support with practical help in the home, equipment to help care for their relative, looking after their own health, and talking with their relative about their condition.

Farquhar *et al.* [20] also found that carers were unprepared for many aspects of the caring role despite, or perhaps because of, the longevity of their caring role (median duration 7 years): more than half felt unprepared for finding out about and setting up services, and more than a third felt unprepared for getting help and information from the health system, and for responding to and handling breathlessness. This feeling of being ill-prepared and lacking confidence in caring tasks and situations has been identified by others [21, 25, 37, 43, 80–85]. It is a source of anxiety and has an impact on carers' ability to ask for help [85, 86], leading to crises. Carers lack information about, and access to, professional services and only use help in acute situations [87], *e.g.* SPENCE *et al.* [37] found little carer awareness of the potential of palliative care.

Carers want support to better manage symptoms such as breathlessness [21, 25], *e.g.* having a response plan is important to them [61]. There is a fear associated with acute exacerbations [43]; fear of breathlessness drives demand for emergency healthcare, which in itself is distressing [88], costly [89], and may sometimes be unwarranted [88, 90]. Older carers describe significantly lower COPD-related knowledge than younger carers and may require more education on the use of drugs and symptom management [91]. Healthcare professionals receive appropriate training on managing patient needs, but many carers receive no such guidance and feel ill-prepared to care [80, 81]. Educating carers about breathlessness, evidence-based, non-pharmacological interventions for breathlessness, and relevant breathlessness management (*e.g.* what patients can be expected to do, what a carer can do in a breathlessness episode) may meet both patient and carer needs.

PENFOLD *et al.* [92] interviewed 25 patient–carer dyads living with breathlessness due to advanced cancer or advanced COPD to identify what these carers wanted to learn about. They found that carers wanted an educational intervention that was "for carers" and identified six interrelated topics that carers of patients with breathlessness wanted to learn about; these are shown in table 1.

PENFOLD *et al.* [92] found that most carers wanted to learn "with" the patient, but not for every topic. There was a tension for carers with regard to wanting to know what to expect in the future but also not wanting to upset the patient. This reflects the findings of PHILIP *et al.* [61] that some carers believe the information they need may differ from the information the patient needs. Carers want information about the disease trajectory [21, 37, 61, 87]; they experience feelings of uncertainty about patient deterioration and what the future holds [43]. They also have a need for medical staff to introduce the idea of future planning or need for additional help so carers do not have to do this themselves [61].

Table 1. Six topics that carers of patients with breathlessness due to advanced disease want to learn about

Topic	Aspects of topic
Understanding breathlessness	The causes of breathlessness and the experience of breathlessness (*i.e.* how it feels)
Responding to breathlessness, anxiety and panic	How to manage breathlessness, how to recognise and respond confidently to panic
Managing infections	How to avoid infections and how to respond to them
Supporting activity, exercise and rest	What is helpful and what is safe to encourage
Living positively with breathlessness	How to maintain a reasonable quality of life, overcoming isolation and restrictions
Knowing what to expect in the future	How to enable carers to be proactive rather than reactive as the illness progresses

Data from [92].

Supporting carers

Improved life expectancy for people with long-term conditions means more informal care will be required for longer periods. Carers of patients with advanced chronic non-malignant diseases face particular challenges given the longevity of their caring role [7, 93], coupled with uncertainty and complexity [16]. Demands on carers will increase further as policies to increase the number of home deaths become effective (*e.g.* see the UK Dept of Health strategy from 2008 [94]). In addition, home-based care and early discharge of very ill patients, who may also be dependent on technology such as NIV, raise questions about how both patients and their carers should be supported in the home [29].

There is some evidence that effective management of the patient's condition can impact positively on carers, but carers also need direct support for themselves. In this context, "support" covers a range of activities enabling carers to manage life with advanced disease. It might include the provision of tangibles such as information, education or services [95], but could also include the provision of comfort (sharing emotional burden, sympathy, encouragement), strengthening (bolstering the individual's ability to sustain functioning by conveying understanding and demonstrating kindness, concern and competence) and advocacy (demonstrating having the individual's interest foremost) [96].

There is policy rhetoric that carers should be supported, but little guidance on how this should be achieved in clinical practice [97]. Kamal and Dionne-Odom [98] noted that definitions of palliative care consider the "unit of care" to be the patient and family and that palliative care seeks, as a speciality, to address the distress of both. They suggest that palliative care should meet "societal need and take on the family caregivers as a new focus of its specialised care" [98]. However, carer support is not just the remit of specialists; generalists have the skills to provide carer support, or to be the vehicles for provision of carer support (*i.e.* to identify carers and identify need). Furthermore, evidence-based resources have been developed to train support workers or volunteers to deliver carer support [99]. Healthcare professionals need to be better at working with carers, supporting them in their role, and helping them identify and manage changes in the patient and in their own needs. Table 2 summarises six steps to consider in order to achieve this, with more detail given in the following sections.

Identifying and acknowledging carers

Identifying carers is the first step in offering them support, but carers are rarely acknowledged or supported by healthcare systems [61, 73, 100]. A recent UK population-based, primary care cohort study by Sampson *et al.* [70] found that recording of carers of people dying from cancer, lung disease, or dementia was suboptimal. Healthcare professionals lack protocols for the identification of carers in primary care. In the UK, GPs can be remunerated *via* the Quality and Outcomes Framework for holding dementia carer registers and conducting annual carer health and support needs assessments (DEM002 indicator) [101], but not in other chronic conditions. In addition, greater acknowledgement and recognition of carer expertise is needed [29, 30].

Identifying and prioritising support needs

There is a key distinction between professionally defined and user-defined need. Bradshaw [102] argued that professionally defined or "normative needs" relate to need as determined by "experts", whereas user-defined need can be conceptualised either as "expressed need" in terms

Table 2. Six steps to consider in order to achieve carer support

Steps	Key considerations
1. Identify the carer	Ask the patient: "Who gives you help and support at home?" Be aware that both patients and/or carers may not identify carers as "carers" (they are a husband, wife, son or daughter, or friend first) There may be more than one carer (and this in itself can be a source of tension) The carer may be aged <18 years The carer may not be who you think they are The carer may not be geographically close The carer may change Record who the carer is Record who the carer's GP is
2. Acknowledge their role	Acknowledge the carer and their role Acknowledge their insight and expertise Reassure them about what they are doing well: many will have developed their own strategies over time
3. Identify need for (more) support	Identify their need for more support using an evidence-based tool Identify their desire for more support (presence of a need may not translate into a desire for intervention) Sometimes needs just need acknowledging (that in itself is an intervention; it legitimises need) Record their needs and desire for more support
4. Prioritise needs	Prioritise needs with the carer The greatest need may not be their highest priority Record the priority need
5. Respond to priority need	Identify how to address that priority need with the carer; this may involve providing information, signposting or referring on Record how the need was addressed
6. Reassess need	Consider when to reassess need for more support Record the reassessment

of demand for particular services, or "felt need" relating to a person's experiences. Policy initiatives have begun to emphasise the integration of user involvement into the need identification process to address the extent to which professionally defined needs have dominated clinical encounters and the shaping of user-defined need by their expectations [103].

Carer need is different to carer burden; knowing how burdened a carer is might indicate or suggest what their support needs are, but it does not directly identify support needs. Ewing and Grande [97] highlighted the important distinction between measurement tools that are indicators of carer need (aspects of an individual's experience, such as burden, that suggest a need for support) and tools that can be used to directly identify carer support needs (areas needing assistance). This resonates with the work of Bradshaw [102], in which the former are useful within a normative definition of need whereas the latter facilitate expression of felt need. Despite the plethora of research tools for identifying carer experiences, such as burden, there is a distinct lack of tools for identifying carer need in clinical practice [60]. Two recent exceptions are the Carers' Alert Thermometer [104, 105] and Carer Support Needs Assessment Tool [97, 106–108].

The Carers' Alert Thermometer is a tool to alert practitioners to carers who are at risk and in need of a formal needs assessment [104]. It is professionally led and comprises 10 questions that fall into two domains within the current caring situation, including exploring the needs of carers in their caring role and carers' own health and well-being. The Carers' Alert Thermometer uses a traffic light system to score the risk of the alerts (green=low; amber=intermediate; and red=high) and provides a set of generic support responses in relation to each of the alert areas [104]. Further information about the Carers' Alert Thermometer, and on how to register to use it, is available on the Carers' Alert Thermometer website [109].

The Carer Support Needs Assessment Tool is an evidence-based, carer-completed tool designed for use in clinical practice that focuses on supporting carers to identify unmet support needs, *i.e.* areas where they need help or require further assessment [97]. The Carer Support Needs Assessment Tool is a direct measure of support need integrated into a person-centred approach to practice. It consists of 14 questions (support domains), seven relating to support the carer may need for themselves (direct support needs), and seven relating to support the carer may need to enable them to care (enabling needs). Carers complete the tool to identify areas where they feel they need more support. It enables carers to consider, express, and discuss these needs with a practitioner. This conversation (which includes carer prioritisation of identified unmet needs) forms the basis for developing a plan of action and to tailor appropriate support for the carer. Importantly, the process of using the tool is practitioner-facilitated but carer-led, with carers themselves determining their support needs and supportive actions [107]. Inspection copies of the Carer Support Needs Assessment Tool and information about training in using the tool are available *via* its website [110].

Clinicians can worry that using such tools could open a floodgate of needs they cannot respond to, and this is sometimes given as a reason for not engaging with carers in the first place. However, a needs assessment, particularly where it is carer-led, is an intervention in itself. Carers completing tools such as the Carer Support Needs Assessment Tool, in part, addresses need. The process legitimises need and flags up potential future need. It opens up the conversation between clinicians and carers, and sometimes that is all that is required for carers to feel better supported. However, there are ways of addressing need if further support is required.

Responding to support needs and reassessment

Responses to need take the form of either preventive support or of repairing problems [60, 111], depending on their timing; however, interventions often come too late [28]. There are two broad types of carer interventions: 1) existing patient and carer resources; and 2) carer-specific educational, training or psychosocial interventions. Despite the evidence base for carer needs, the evidence base for the effectiveness of the latter interventions is limited: few educational, training or psychosocial interventions for carers are supported by rigorous research [14, 60, 112–114]. There is a particular lack of robustly developed and evaluated interventions to enhance caregiving capacity at the EOL [112, 115], in cancer [81], in chronic disease [116] and, more specifically, in COPD [117–119], and in relation to breathlessness in advanced disease [120].

A range of existing patient and carer resources can be harnessed to meet aspects of carer need. These resources vary by locality but can be broadly categorised by area of support, as shown in table 3. Many are resources that are for "patients"; however, carers are "just" patients who happen to be looking after someone else in a supportive role.

Table 3. Existing resources for carers

Area of support	Examples of resources
Physical	Services such as generalist community care, community respiratory care, hospital-at-home, hospice-at-home, statutory or voluntary care services, out-of-hours and night support, respite care (sitters may be preferable to admissions [13]) Addressing carer's physical health needs (back injuries and fatigue are common [111]), *e.g.* directly or through referral to GP or onwards (with consent) Medical equipment and aids [13]
Emotional/psychological	Relaxation and complementary therapies or carer sessions offered by hospice day care or cancer support centres (attendance can be difficult if the carer cannot leave the patient [14] but this could be facilitated through care services or respite care, or by harnessing existing support from wider family/friends) Peer support groups, such as those related to a patient's diagnosis that target patients and carers, or groups specifically for carer support Addressing carer's mental health needs through referral to GP/counselling, or onwards (with consent) Anxiety management interventions Opportunities to talk and be listened to by healthcare professionals with an understanding of breathlessness (there are neurophysiological explanations for why empathy is helpful in the management of breathlessness [121]) Acknowledgement of carers' needs in their own right
Social	Identify activities that are important to the carer and enable continued engagement even if in a limited way, *e.g.* through care services or respite care, or harnessing existing support from wider family/friends Referral to activities (*e.g.* golf, choir, *etc.*) with co-provision of respite if required Identify activities the patient and carer could access together (this may require facilitating patient access through mobility aids, portable oxygen, *etc.* [56]) Carer support groups/services, *e.g.* hospice-provided carer sessions Online carer support Services such as statutory or voluntary care services, respite care Social services carer's assessment
Financial	Supporting ability to carry on working if wished, *e.g.* through care services or respite care, or harnessing existing support from wider family/friends Social services Citizens Advice State welfare provision Charitable funds
Spiritual	Referral to a faith practitioner or group Supporting ability to attend faith group, *e.g.* through care services or respite care, or harnessing existing support from wider family/friends Carer support groups
Holistic	Specialist palliative care: palliative care is a speciality that seeks to address the needs of both patients and carers [98], and many "carer interventions" are part of everyday palliative care provision [14]

Continued

Table 3. Continued

Area of support	Examples of resources
Indirect	Patient-targeted interventions may have an impact on carers (either positively or negatively) [28, 112] How patient healthcare is organised can impact on carers (positively or negatively), particularly in long-term conditions [28, 30] Clinical interventions aimed at improving patient understanding and management of breathlessness may ameliorate some carer needs, *e.g. via* specialist respiratory services, pulmonary rehabilitation (carers have benefitted from inclusion in single pulmonary rehabilitation sessions) [122], and specialist palliative care breathlessness intervention services [17–18] (which may include online resources, *e.g.* [123]) Information on local patient (and carer) support groups, *e.g.* in the UK the British Lung Foundation provides Breath Easy support groups [124]

Specialist palliative care services, including specialist breathlessness services, can play a role in meeting carer needs in advanced respiratory disease. Both patients and their carers using the Cambridge Breathlessness Intervention Service liked the time it provided to talk about breathlessness with experts who understood life with breathlessness; it legitimised the symptom through expert acknowledgement [17, 18]. They gained knowledge about breathlessness and strategies to manage it. This increased confidence in living with it, and patients and carers no longer felt alone [17, 18]. The attention given to carers was unexpected and some carers noted an indirect effect through upskilling of the patient, reporting receiving fewer phone calls from their patient [17]. Similarly, the RCT of a breathlessness support service by Higginson *et al.* [125] found that earlier integration of palliative care was beneficial for patients and carers living with breathlessness due to either cancer or non-malignant conditions. The benefits of early integration of palliative care have been noted by others [126–132].

Information and education is a response to many unmet carer needs. It can be delivered *ad hoc* or by carer-specific educational, training or psychosocial interventions. However, carers do not need to be taught everything. Penfold *et al.* [92] found that carers' educational needs varied; any response to their educational needs should fit their need and be personalised. Tools such as the Carers' Alert Thermometer or Carer Support Needs Assessment Tool may help identify what carers want to learn about. Information and educational needs may be specific to respiratory disease (such as those identified by Penfold *et al.* [92], reported in table 1) or relate to generic carer skills, some of which are outlined in table 4.

Carers form part of a dyad; thus there are additional considerations in responding to carers' needs that relate to the patient. Carers' needs may differ from, and may even be incompatible with, patients' needs, and clinicians need to discern whose needs take priority. Carers' needs may also be disproportionate to patients' needs, *i.e.* they may be quantitatively, as well as qualitatively, different. These considerations raise ethical and clinical questions. Ethically, a patient's autonomy must be respected and this may mean that their carer's needs cannot be met, *e.g.* where a patient refuses respite admissions. Outside of the dyad there is also the issue of refuted need, where a clinician identifies a carer's need that the carer denies or is unaware of, *e.g.* where the carer believes they are doing the right thing for breathlessness management by preventing the patient from doing anything physical.

Table 4. Generic knowledge and skills for carers

Generic knowledge and skills	Examples
Accessing care and support in their locality	Mapping of local services, including voluntary provision, for patients and carers (as service provision varies widely by locality) How to access health and social services, for both patients and carers How to access out-of-hours care, *e.g.* strategies to deal with queries and forward planning to avoid crisis situations and unwanted or unnecessary admissions
Emergency plan	Holding a locatable emergency plan Checking understanding of the emergency plan Ensuring the emergency plan is reviewed regularly Reviewing the effectiveness of the emergency plan after use
Practical caring/nursing skills	Skills to minimise the carer's physical burden, *e.g.* lifting or transferring Skills to facilitate the patient's adherence to a treatment plan (which may have positive knock-on effects on carer well-being and coping), *e.g.* how and when to take medication
New life skills	New life skills may be required where the carer is taking on roles or tasks previously performed by the patient [55, 118], *e.g.* cooking, laundry, managing finances, basic DIY or house maintenance, IT skills
Communication and negotiation skills	Skills to interact with a range of people (*e.g.* healthcare professionals across a range of settings, social care professionals, healthcare and social care administrative staff, wider family members and friends) to obtain the help they need, to act as an advocate for the patient [13], and (potentially) to share bad news with others [133]

Regardless of how carers' support needs are met, both the identified needs and the agreed means of addressing them should be communicated and reviewed. Good practice includes communication with the carer and with other relevant care professionals (such as the carer's GP), *e.g.* a letter detailing the outcome of an assessment and an agreed plan. In reviewing the outcome, the carer and healthcare professional should consider whether the intervention met the need or whether needs have changed (either in relation to changes in carer experience, patient need or service provision). Identifying and responding to carers' needs is not a one-off exercise; reassessment is important.

When the caring changes or comes to an end

Transition in care setting

Temporary or permanent transitions in care settings, such as hospital admission or a patient moving into long-term care, can result in the caring role changing. This can be a source of respite for carers, but also a source of additional stress. Hynes *et al.* [29] described how carers of patients with advanced COPD can feel hospital staff do not appreciate their knowledge about the patient and that failure to actively engage with carers may compound carer burden. Hospitalisation has an added physical burden for carers in terms of journeying to and from visits, and an emotional burden in terms of the watchfulness over care and decision-making deemed essential for the carer's advocacy role and implications for care following discharge. Some may also experience guilt [134].

Patient death

Carers may have very practical needs immediately after the patient's death, such as for information about the arrangements they need to make [13], but at a time when they are also grieving. Bereavement is emotionally stressful [135] and carers can experience negative after-effects [136]. A significant proportion develops complicated grief, depression and anxiety [135], and there is evidence of experience of guilt [38, 137]. There is also evidence of new and increased psychotropic drug prescription in the year after bereavement [70, 138].

Where the patient and carer were spouses who attended the same primary care practice, staff are likely to be aware of the bereavement and may offer support. However, not all carers are spouses and not all spouses are registered at same practice. Bereavement support can be provided through individual support or bereavement support groups [13], and there are many carer (and patient) organisations offering online or written resources providing advice and information (*e.g.* [139–141]). Bereavement may relate to the loss of the person cared for, but also the loss of the caring role itself [38, 137], so some carers may need support in re-establishing themselves after the caring role has ended. There may also be economic concerns [137].

This chapter has advocated the assessment of carer support needs to provide person-centred carer support while the patient is living. Such attention and resulting support may better facilitate transitions to widowhood [142]. However, the same can be said for carer support in bereavement: effective assessment of need for support is required [143]. Bereavement risk assessment measures with acceptable psychometric properties do exist, but their suitability for use in clinical practice varies widely [143].

Implications for research

Research should address the mechanisms for identifying carers, use appropriate measures of need where this is the concept of interest (as opposed to burden), and robustly develop and evaluate carer interventions. In addition, Al-Janabi *et al.* [28] have called for the collection of more data on the effect of patient interventions on carers and routine use of these data to inform reviews, meta-analyses and economic evaluations. This may be motivated by a need to ensure carers are effective in their caring role and can facilitate patient compliance with interventions and therapies (referred to as "enabling needs" by Ewing and Grande [97]), but may also concern the direct support needs of carers themselves. Al-Janabi *et al.* [28] note that the UK's National Institute for Health and Care Excellence (NICE) already stipulates that economic evaluations of new interventions should consider carers' health outcomes as well as patients' [144], but that this is rarely done [28, 145].

Conclusion

Carers play a vital role in supportive, palliative and EOL care, enabling care and, ultimately, death in the patients' place of choice. They are "an absolutely essential component of high-quality healthcare delivery" [98]. However, this caring role comes at a cost in terms of psychosocial distress, physical and psychological health impacts (including carer mortality), and pressure on finances. Ensuring carer support can ameliorate these effects. Healthcare professionals need to respond to policy rhetoric and be dramatically better at supporting carers. They need to identify carers, work with them to assess and prioritise their support needs, and respond to and review those needs. Evidence-based tools and approaches exist and can help, but are not a one-off exercise: there may be changes in carers' needs as the patient's condition (or location of care) changes, carer health changes and systems change. Carers' needs may also exist beyond the patient's death. Finally, clinical and academic researchers need to robustly develop and evaluate interventions for carers supporting patients living with breathlessness in advanced disease and include appropriate carer outcomes in evaluations of patient-targeted interventions.

References

1. National Institute for Clinical Excellence (NICE). Guidance on Cancer Services: Improving Supportive and Palliative Care for Adults with Cancer. The Manual. London, NICE, 2004. www.nice.org.uk/guidance/csg4/resources/improving-supportive-and-palliative-care-for-adults-with-cancer-773375005
2. Carers UK. Facts About Carers 2014. London, Carers UK, 2014. Available from: www.carersuk.org/for-professionals/policy/policy-library/facts-about-carers-2014
3. Burns CM, Abernethy AP, Dal Grande E, *et al.* Uncovering an invisible network of direct caregivers at the end of life: a population study. *Palliat Med* 2013; 27: 608–615.
4. National Alliance for Caregiving, Public Policy Institute. Caregiving in the United States 2015. www.aarp.org/ppi/info-2015/caregiving-in-the-united-states-2015/ Date last accessed: June 12, 2016. Date last updated: June 4, 2015.
5. The Princess Royal Trust for Carers, Royal College of General Practitioners. Supporting Carers: an Action Guide for General Practitioners and Their Teams. 2nd Edn. Woodford Green, The Princess Royal Trust for Carers, 2011. http://static.carers.org/files/supporting-carers-an-action-guide-for-general-practitioners-and-their-teams-second-edition-5877.pdf
6. Grammenos S. Implications of Demographic Ageing in the Enlarged EU in the Domains of Quality of Life, Health Promotion and Health Care. Various Studies on Policy Implications of Demographic Changes in National and Community Policies. Lot 5. Contract VC/2004/0076. No. SI2.396079. Brussels, Centre for European Social and Economic Policy, 2005. http://ec.europa.eu/employment_social/social_situation/docs/lot5_health_summary_en.pdf
7. Morris SM, King C, Turner M, *et al.* Family carers providing support to a person dying in the home setting: a narrative literature review. *Palliat Med* 2015; 29: 487–495.
8. Higginson IJ, Jarman B, Astin P, *et al.* Do social factors affect where patients die: an analysis of 10 years of cancer deaths in England. *J Public Health Med* 1999; 21: 22–28.
9. Aoun SM, Kristjanson LJ, Currow DC, *et al.* Caregiving for the terminally ill: at what cost? *Palliat Med* 2005; 19: 551–555.
10. Rolls L, Seymour JE, Froggatt KA, *et al.* Older people living alone at the end of life in the U.K.: research and policy challenges. *Palliat Med* 2011; 25: 650–657.
11. Buckner L, Yeandle S. Valuing Carers 2015: The Rising Value of Carers' Support. London, Carers UK, 2015. Available from: www.carersuk.org/for-professionals/policy/policy-library/valuing-carers-2015
12. Gomes B, Higginson IJ. Factors influencing death at home in terminally ill patients with cancer: systematic review. *BMJ* 2006; 332: 515–521.
13. Payne S, Hudson P, Grande G, *et al.* White Paper on improving support for family carers in palliative care: part 1. *Eur J Palliat Care* 2010; 17: 238–245.
14. Payne S, Hudson P, Grande G, *et al.* White Paper on improving support for family carers in palliative care: part 2. *Eur J Palliat Care* 2010; 17: 286–290.
15. Stajduhar K, Funk L, Toye C, *et al.* Part 1: Home-based family caregiving at the end of life: a comprehensive review of published quantitative research (1998–2008). *Palliat Med* 2010; 24: 573–593.
16. Funk L, Stajduhar K, Toye C, *et al.* Part 2: Home-based family caregiving at the end of life: a comprehensive review of published qualitative research (1998–2008). *Palliat Med* 2010; 24: 594–607.
17. Farquhar MC, Prevost AT, McCrone P, *et al.* Is a specialist breathlessness service more effective and cost-effective for patients with advanced cancer and their carers than standard care? Findings of a mixed-method randomised controlled trial. *BMC Med* 2014; 12: 194.
18. Farquhar MC, Prevost AT, McCrone P, *et al.* The clinical and cost effectiveness of a Breathlessness Intervention Service for patients with advanced non-malignant disease and their informal carers – mixed findings of a mixed method randomised controlled trial. *Trials* 2016; 17: 185.

19. Gautun H, Werner A, Lurås H. Care challenges for informal caregivers of chronically ill lung patients: results from a questionnaire survey. *Scand J Public Health* 2012; 40: 18–24.
20. Farquhar M, Ewing G, Moore C, *et al.* Preparedness to care in advanced COPD: how prepared are informal carers and what are their support needs? Baseline data from an ongoing longitudinal study. *BMJ Support Palliat Care* 2014; 4: Suppl. 1, A8–A9.
21. Currow DC, Ward A, Clark K, *et al.* Caregivers for people with end-stage lung disease: characteristics and unmet needs in the whole population. *Int J Chron Obstruct Pulmon Dis* 2008; 3: 753–762.
22. Miravitlles M, Peña-Longobardo LM, Oliva-Moreno J, *et al.* Caregivers' burden in patients with COPD. *Int J Chron Obstruct Pulmon Dis* 2015; 10: 347–356.
23. Barnes PJ, Celli BR. Systemic manifestations and comorbidities of COPD. *Eur Respir J* 2009; 33: 1165–1185.
24. Bergs D. "The Hidden Client" – women caring for husbands with COPD: their experience of quality of life. *J Clin Nurs* 2002; 11: 613–621.
25. Booth S, Silvester S, Todd C. Breathlessness in cancer and chronic obstructive pulmonary disease: using a qualitative approach to describe the experience of patients and carers. *Palliat Support Care* 2003; 1: 337–344.
26. Trivedi RB, Bryson CL, Udris E, *et al.* The influence of informal caregivers on adherence in COPD patients. *Ann Behav Med* 2012; 44: 66–72.
27. Wakabayashi R, Motegi T, Yamada K, *et al.* Presence of in-home caregiver and health outcomes of older adults with chronic obstructive pulmonary disease. *J Am Geriatr Soc* 2011; 59: 44–49.
28. Al-Janabi H, Nicholls J, Oyebode J. The need to "carer proof" healthcare decisions. *BMJ* 2016; 352: i1651.
29. Hynes G, Stokes A, McCarron M. Informal care-giving in advanced chronic obstructive pulmonary disease: lay knowledge and experience. *J Clin Nurs* 2012; 21: 1068–1077.
30. McPherson KM, Kayes NK, Moloczij N, *et al.* Improving the interface between informal carers and formal health and social services: a qualitative study. *Int J Nurs Stud* 2014; 51: 418–429.
31. Dept of Health. Carers at the Heart of 21st-century Families and Communities. "A Caring System on Your Side. A Life of Your Own." London, Dept of Health, 2008. www.gov.uk/government/uploads/system/uploads/attachment_data/file/136492/carers_at_the_heart_of_21_century_families.pdf
32. Dept of Health. Care Act 2014. London, Dept of Health, 2014. Available from: www.legislation.gov.uk/ukpga/2014/23/contents/enacted
33. Schulz R, O'Brien AT, Bookwala J, *et al.* Psychiatric and physical morbidity effects of dementia caregiving: prevalence, correlates, and causes. *Gerontologist* 1995; 35: 771–791.
34. Schulz R, Beach SR. Caregiving as a risk factor for mortality: the Caregiver Health Effects Study. *JAMA* 1999; 282: 2215–2219.
35. Pinquart M, Sörensen S. Associations of stressors and uplifts of caregiving with caregiver burden and depressive mood: a meta-analysis. *J Gerontol B Psychol Sci Soc Sci* 2003; 58: 112–128.
36. Pinquart M, Sörensen S. Correlates of physical health of informal caregivers: a meta-analysis. *J Gerontol B Psychol Sci Soc Sci* 2007; 62: 126–137.
37. Spence A, Hasson F, Waldron M, *et al.* Active carers: living with chronic obstructive pulmonary disease. *Int J Palliat Nurs* 2008; 14: 368–372.
38. Hasson F, Spence A, Waldron M, *et al.* Experiences and needs of bereaved carers during palliative and end-of-life care for people with chronic obstructive pulmonary disease. *J Palliat Care* 2009; 25: 157–163.
39. Gabriel R, Figueiredo D, Jácome C, *et al.* Day-to-day living with severe chronic obstructive pulmonary disease: towards a family-based approach to the illness impacts. *Psychol Health* 2014; 29: 967–983.
40. De Korte-Verhoef MC, Pasman HR, Schweitzer BP, *et al.* Burden for family carers at the end of life; a mixed-method study of the perspectives of family carers and GPs. *BMC Palliat Care* 2014; 13: 16.
41. Vernooij-Dassen MJ, Persoon JM, Felling AJ. Predictors of sense of competence in caregivers of demented persons. *Soc Sci Med* 1996; 43: 41–49.
42. Haley WE, LaMonde LA, Han B, *et al.* Family caregiving in hospice: effects on psychological and health functioning among spousal caregivers of hospice patients with lung cancer or dementia. *Hosp J* 2001; 15: 1–18.
43. Gysels M, Higginson IJ. Caring for a person in advanced illness and suffering from breathlessness at home: threats and resources. *Palliat Support Care* 2009; 7: 153–162.
44. Parnell H. Respiratory Disease: Caring for the carers of chronic lung disease sufferers in the community. *J Community Nurs* 2001; 15: 1–4.
45. Goodridge D, Lawson J, Duggleby W, *et al.* Health care utilization of patients with chronic obstructive pulmonary disease and lung cancer in the last 12 months of life. *Respir Med* 2008; 102: 885–891.
46. Williams S. Chronic Respiratory Illness. London, Routledge, 1993.
47. Elkington H, White P, Addington-Hall J, *et al.* The last year of life of COPD: a qualitative study of symptoms and services. *Respir Med* 2004; 98: 439–445.
48. Jones I, Kirby A, Ormiston P, *et al.* The needs of patients dying of chronic obstructive pulmonary disease in the community. *Fam Pract* 2004; 21: 310–313.

49. Seamark DA, Blake SD, Seamark CJ, *et al.* Living with severe chronic obstructive pulmonary disease (COPD): perceptions of patients and their carers. An interpretative phenomenological analysis. *Palliat Med* 2004; 18: 619–625.
50. Kanervisto M, Paavilainen E, Heikkilä J. Family dynamics in families of severe COPD patients. *J Clin Nurs* 2007; 16: 1498–1505.
51. Giacomini M, DeJean D, Simeonov D, *et al.* Experiences of living and dying with COPD: a systematic review and synthesis of the qualitative empirical literature. *Ont Health Technol Assess Ser* 2012; 12: 1–47.
52. Bailey PH. The dyspnea-anxiety-dyspnea cycle – COPD patients' stories of breathlessness: "It's scary/when you can't breathe". *Qual Health Res* 2004; 14: 760–778.
53. Lee E, Lum CM, Xiang YT, *et al.* Psychosocial condition of family caregivers of patients with chronic obstructive pulmonary disease in Hong Kong. *East Asian Arch Psychiatry* 2010; 20: 180–185.
54. Figueiredo D, Gabriel R, Jácome C, *et al.* Caring for relatives with chronic obstructive pulmonary disease: how does the disease severity impact on family carers? *Aging Ment Health* 2014; 18: 385–393.
55. Simpson AC, Young J, Donahue M, *et al.* A day at a time: caregiving on the edge in advanced COPD. *Int J Chron Obstruct Pulmon Dis* 2010; 5: 141–151.
56. Leidy NK, Traver GA. Adjustment and social behaviour in older adults with chronic obstructive pulmonary disease: the family's perspective. *J Adv Nurs* 1996; 23: 252–259.
57. Pinto RA, Holanda MA, Medeiros MM, *et al.* Assessment of the burden of caregiving for patients with chronic obstructive pulmonary disease. *Respir Med* 2007; 101: 2402–2408.
58. Malik FA, Gysels M, Higginson IJ. Living with breathlessness: a survey of caregivers of breathless patients with lung cancer or heart failure. *Palliat Med* 2013; 27: 647–656.
59. Figueiredo D, Gabriel R, Jácome C, *et al.* Caring for people with early and advanced chronic obstructive pulmonary disease: how do family carers cope? *J Clin Nurs* 2014; 23: 211–220.
60. Grande G, Stajduhar K, Aoun S, *et al.* Supporting lay carers in end of life care: current gaps and future priorities. *Palliat Med* 2009; 23: 339–344.
61. Philip J, Gold M, Brand C, *et al.* Facilitating change and adaptation: the experiences of current and bereaved carers of patients with severe chronic obstructive pulmonary disease. *J Palliat Med* 2014; 17: 421–427.
62. Skilbeck J, Mott L, Page H, *et al.* Palliative care in chronic obstructive airways disease: a needs assessment. *Palliat Med* 1998; 12: 245–254.
63. Gore JM, Brophy CJ, Greenstone MA. How well do we care for patients with end stage chronic obstructive pulmonary disease (COPD)? A comparison of palliative care and quality of life in COPD and lung cancer. *Thorax* 2000; 55: 1000–1006.
64. Curtis JR, Engelberg RA, Nielsen EL, *et al.* Patient–physician communication about end-of-life care for patients with severe COPD. *Eur Respir J* 2004; 24: 200–205.
65. Pearlin LI, Mullan JT, Semple SJ, *et al.* Caregiving and the stress process: an overview of concepts and their measures. *Gerontologist* 1990; 30: 583–594.
66. Skaff MM, Pearlin LI. Caregiving: role engulfment and the loss of self. *Gerontologist* 1992; 32: 656–664.
67. Twigg J, Atkin K. Carers Perceived: Policy and Practice in Informal Care. Buckingham, Open University Press, 1994.
68. Payne S, Ellis-Hill C. Chronic and Terminal Illness: New Perspectives on Caring and Carers. Oxford, Oxford University Press, 2001.
69. Cavaye J. Hidden Carers. Edinburgh, Dunedin Academic, 2006.
70. Sampson EL, Lodwick R, Rait G, *et al.* Living with an older person dying from cancer, lung disease, or dementia: health outcomes from a general practice cohort study. *J Pain Symptom Manage* 2016; 51: 839–848.
71. Siegel K. Psychosocial oncology research. *Soc Work Health Care* 1990; 15: 21–43.
72. Heaton J. The gaze and visibility of the carer: a Foucauldian analysis of the discourse of informal care. *Sociol Health Illn* 1999; 21: 759–777.
73. Carduff E, Finucane A, Kendall M, *et al.* Understanding the barriers to identifying carers of people with advanced illness in primary care: triangulating three data sources. *BMC Fam Pract* 2014; 15: 48.
74. Grande GE, Todd CJ, Barclay SI. Support needs in the last year of life: patient and carer dilemmas. *Palliat Med* 1997; 11: 202–208.
75. Currow DC. Caregivers' three-cornered hats: their tricornes. *Palliat Med* 2015; 29: 485–486.
76. Williams LA. Whatever it takes: informal caregiving dynamics in blood and marrow transplantation. *Oncol Nurs Forum* 2007; 34: 379–387.
77. Doherty LC, Fitzsimons D, McIlfatrick SJ. Carers' needs in advanced heart failure: a systematic narrative review. *Eur J Cardiovasc Nurs* 2015; 15: 203–212.
78. Currow DC, Farquhar M, Ward AM, *et al.* Caregivers' perceived adequacy of support in end-stage lung disease: results of a population survey. *BMC Pulm Med* 2011; 11: 55.
79. Moore C, Farquhar M, Gardener C, *et al.* What are the barriers and facilitators to clinicians' ability to meet the needs of patients with advanced COPD and their informal carers? RCN International Nursing Research Conference 2015, abstract 304. www2.rcn.org.uk/__data/assets/pdf_file/0019/620317/RCN-2015-research-Book-of-Abstracts.pdf
80. Bee PE, Barnes P, Luker KA. A systematic review of informal caregivers' needs in providing home-based end-of-life care to people with cancer. *J Clin Nurs* 2009; 18: 1379–1393.

81. Gerrish K. Caring for the carers: the characteristics of district nursing support for family carers. *Prim Health Care Res Dev* 2008; 9: 14–24.
82. Jack B, O'Brien M. Dying at home: community nurses' views on the impact of informal carers on cancer patients' place of death. *Eur J Cancer Care* 2010; 19: 636–642.
83. Greenwood N, Mackenzie A. An exploratory study of anxiety in carers of stroke survivors. *J Clin Nurs* 2010; 19: 2032–2038.
84. Harrop E, Byrne A, Nelson A. "It's alright to ask for help": findings from a qualitative study exploring the information and support needs of family carers at the end of life. *BMC Palliat Care* 2014; 13: 22.
85. Walsh K, Jones L, Tookman A, *et al.* Reducing emotional distress in people caring for patients receiving specialist palliative care. Randomised trial. *Br J Psychiatry* 2007; 190: 142–147.
86. Whitehead B, O'Brien MR, Jack BA, *et al.* Experiences of dying, death and bereavement in motor neurone disease: a qualitative study. *Palliat Med* 2012; 26: 368–378.
87. Grant M, Cavanagh A, Yorke J. The impact of caring for those with chronic obstructive pulmonary disease (COPD) on carers' psychological well-being: a narrative review. *Int J Nurs Stud* 2012; 49: 1459–1471.
88. Hutchinson A, Pickering A, Williams P, *et al.* Emergency department presentations by people with chronic breathlessness. EAPC 2015, 14th World Congress of the European Association of Palliative Care, abstract P2-033. www.eapc-2015.org/tl_files/eapc15/Downloads/EAPC_2015_Abstract_Book.pdf
89. Gray JT, Walker A. Avoiding admissions from the ambulance service: a review of elderly patients with falls and patients with breathing difficulties seen by emergency care practitioners in South Yorkshire. *Emerg Med J* 2008; 25: 168–171.
90. Howard C, Dupont S, Haselden B, *et al.* The effectiveness of a group cognitive–behavioural breathlessness intervention on health status, mood and hospital admissions in elderly patients with chronic obstructive pulmonary disease. *Psychol Health Med* 2010; 15: 371–385.
91. Hsiao PC, Chu CM, Sung PY, *et al.* Differences in COPD patient care by primary family caregivers: an age-based study. *PLoS One* 2014; 9: e107870.
92. Penfold C, Ewing G, Mahadeva R, *et al.* Developing an educational intervention on breathlessness in advanced disease for informal carers. *Palliat Med* 2016; 30: S15.
93. Phillips LR, Reed PG. Into the abyss of someone else's dying: the voice of the end-of-life caregiver. *Clin Nurs Res* 2009; 18: 80–97.
94. Dept of Health. End of Life Care Strategy: Promoting High Quality Care for all Adults at the End of Life. London, Dept of Health, 2008. www.gov.uk/government/uploads/system/uploads/attachment_data/file/136431/End_of_life_strategy.pdf
95. Stoltz P, Andersson EP, Willman A. Support in nursing: an evolutionary concept analysis. *Int J Nurs Stud* 2007; 44: 1478–1489.
96. Peteet JR. A closer look at the concept of support: some application to the care of patients with cancer. *Gen Hosp Psychiatry* 1982; 4: 19–23.
97. Ewing G, Grande G. Development of a Carer Support Needs Assessment Tool (CSNAT) for end-of-life care practice at home: a qualitative study. *Palliat Med* 2013; 27: 244–256.
98. Kamal AH, Dionne-Odom JN. A blue ocean strategy for palliative care: focus on family caregivers. *J Pain Symptom Manage* 2016; 51: e1–e3.
99. University of Nottingham. Supporting carers in end of life care: an introductory programme. Available from: www.nottingham.ac.uk/helm/dev/end_of_life/ Date last accessed: April 1, 2016.
100. Laing M, Sprung S. Working with Health Care Professionals to Increase Carer Awareness, Identification and Referral. Literature Review. London, The Queen's Nursing Institute, 2013. Available from: www.qni.org.uk/supporting_carers/carers_project_resources
101. British Medical Association, NHS England, NHS Employers. 2014/15 General Medical Services (GMS) Contract Quality and Outcomes Framework (QOF). Guidance for GMS Contract 2014/15. NHS England Gateway reference: 01264. Leeds, NHS Employers, 2014. www.hscic.gov.uk/media/14019/QOF-Guidance-GMS-Contract-2014-15/pdf/QOF_guidance_GMS_contract_2014_15.pdf
102. Bradshaw JR. The taxonomy of social need. *In*: McLachlan G, ed. Problems and Progress in Medical Care. Oxford, Oxford University Press, 1971, pp. 69–82.
103. Godfrey M, Callaghan G. Exploring Unmet Need: The Challenge of a User-Centred Response. York, Joseph Rowntree Foundation, 2000. Available from: www.jrf.org.uk/report/exploring-unmet-need-challenge-user-centred-response
104. Knighting K, O'Brien MR, Roe B, *et al.* Development of the Carers' Alert Thermometer (CAT) to identify family carers struggling with caring for someone dying at home: a mixed method consensus study. *BMC Palliat Care* 2015; 14: 22.
105. Knighting K, O'Brien MR, Roe B, *et al.* Gaining consensus on family carer needs when caring for someone dying at home to develop the Carers' Alert Thermometer (CAT): a modified Delphi study. *J Adv Nurs* 2016; 72: 227–239.

106. Ewing G, Brundle C, Payne S, *et al.* The Carer Support Needs Assessment Tool (CSNAT) for use in palliative and end-of-life care at home: a validation study. *J Pain Symptom Manage* 2013; 46: 395–405.
107. Ewing G, Austin L, Diffin J, *et al.* Developing a person-centred approach to carer assessment and support. *Br J Community Nurs* 2015; 20: 580–584.
108. Ewing G, Austin L, Grande G. The role of the Carer Support Needs Assessment Tool in palliative home care: a qualitative study of practitioners' perspectives of its impact and mechanisms of action. *Palliat Med* 2016; 30: 392–400.
109. Edge Hill University. Assessing the Needs of Carers. www.edgehill.ac.uk/carers/ Date last accessed: April 1, 2016.
110. The University of Manchester, University of Cambridge. Carer Support Needs Assessment Tool. http://csnat.org/ Date last accessed: April 1, 2016.
111. Payne S, Hudson P. EAPC task force on family carers: aims and objectives. *Eur J Palliat Care* 2009; 16: 77–81.
112. Candy B, Jones L, Drake R, *et al.* Interventions for supporting informal caregivers of patients in the terminal phase of a disease. *Cochrane Database Syst Rev* 2011; 15: CD007617.
113. Harding R, List S, Epiphaniou E, *et al.* How can informal caregivers in cancer and palliative care be supported? An updated systematic literature review of interventions and their effectiveness. *Palliat Med* 2012; 26: 7–22.
114. Hudson PL, Zordan R, Trauer T. Research priorities associated with family caregivers in palliative care: international perspectives. *J Palliat Med* 2011; 14: 397–401.
115. Hudson PL, Remedios C, Thomas K. A systematic review of psychosocial interventions for family carers of palliative care patients. *BMC Palliat Care* 2010; 9: 17.
116. Corry M, While A, Neenan K, *et al.* A systematic review of systematic reviews on interventions for caregivers of people with chronic conditions. *J Adv Nurs* 2015; 71: 718–734.
117. Caress AL, Luker KA, Chalmers KI, *et al.* A review of the information and support needs of family carers of patients with chronic obstructive pulmonary disease. *J Clin Nurs* 2009; 18: 479–491.
118. Boyle AH. An integrative review of the impact of COPD on families. *South Online J Nurs Res* 2009; 9: 5.
119. Cruz J, Marques A, Figueiredo D. Impacts of COPD on family carers and supportive interventions: a narrative review. *Health Soc Care Community* 2015; in press [DOI: 10.1111/hsc.12292].
120. Farquhar M, Penfold C, Walter FM, *et al.* What are the key elements of educational interventions for lay carers of patients with advanced disease? A systematic literature search and narrative review of structural components, processes and modes of delivery. *J Pain Symptom Manage* 2016; in press [DOI: 10.1016/j.jpainsymman.2015.12.341].
121. Booth S, Chin C, Spathis A. The brain and breathlessness: understanding and disseminating a palliative care approach. *Palliat Med* 2015; 29: 396–398.
122. Zakrisson AB, Theander K, Anderzén-Carlsson A. The experience of a multidisciplinary programme of pulmonary rehabilitation in primary health care from the next of kin's perspective: a qualitative study. *Prim Care Respir J* 2013; 22: 459–465.
123. Cambridge University Hospitals NHS Foundation Trust, Breathlessness Intervention Service. Patient Information Leaflets. Available from: www.cuh.org.uk/breathlessness-intervention-service-bis/resources/patient-information-leaflets Date last accessed: April 1, 2016. Date last updated: 2016.
124. British Lung Foundation. Breathe Easy Support Groups. www.blf.org.uk/support-for-you/breathe-easy Date last accessed: April 1, 2016. Date last updated: 2016.
125. Higginson IJ, Bausewein C, Reilly CC, *et al.* An integrated palliative and respiratory care service for patients with advanced disease and refractory breathlessness: a randomised controlled trial. *Lancet Respir Med* 2014; 2: 979–987.
126. Zimmermann C, Riechelmann R, Krzyzanowska M, *et al.* Effectiveness of specialized palliative care: a systematic review. *JAMA* 2008; 299: 1698–1709.
127. Greer JA, Jackson VA, Meier DE, *et al.* Early integration of palliative care services with standard oncology care for patients with advanced cancer. *CA Cancer J Clin* 2013; 63: 349–363.
128. Zimmermann C, Swami N, Krzyzanowska M, *et al.* Early palliative care for patients with advanced cancer: a cluster-randomised controlled trial. *Lancet* 2014; 383: 1721–1730.
129. Dalgaard KM, Bergenholtz H, Nielsen ME, *et al.* Early integration of palliative care in hospitals: a systematic review on methods, barriers, and outcome. *Palliat Support Care* 2014; 12: 495–513.
130. Gomes B, Calanzani N, Curiale V, *et al.* Effectiveness and cost-effectiveness of home palliative care services for adults with advanced illness and their caregivers. *Cochrane Database Syst Rev* 2013; 6: CD007760.
131. Temel JS, Greer JA, Muzikansky A, *et al.* Early palliative care for patients with metastatic non-small-cell lung cancer. *N Engl J Med* 2010; 363: 733–742.
132. Bakitas M, Lyons KD, Hegel MT, *et al.* Effects of a palliative care intervention on clinical outcomes in patients with advanced cancer: the Project ENABLE II randomized controlled trial. *JAMA* 2009; 302: 741–749.
133. Ewing G, Ngwenya N, Benson J, *et al.* Sharing news of a lung cancer diagnosis with adult family members and friends: a qualitative study to inform a supportive intervention. *Patient Educ Couns* 2016; 99: 378–385.
134. Gaugler JE, Roth DL, Haley WE, *et al.* Modeling trajectories and transitions: results from the New York University caregiver intervention. *Nurs Res* 2011; 60: Suppl. 3, S28–S37.
135. Stroebe M, Schut H, Stroebe W. Health outcomes of bereavement. *Lancet* 2007; 370: 1960–1973.

136. Wendler D, Rid A. Systematic review: the effect on surrogates of making treatment decisions for others. *Ann Intern Med* 2011; 154: 336–346.
137. Cronin P, Hynes G, Breen M, *et al.* Between worlds: the experiences and needs of former family carers. *Health Soc Care Community* 2015; 23: 88–96.
138. Shah SM, Carey IM, Harris T, *et al.* Initiation of psychotropic medication after partner bereavement: a matched cohort study. *PLoS One* 2013; 8: e77734.
139. Carers UK. Bereavement. www.carersuk.org/help-and-advice/practical-support/when-caring-ends/bereavement Date last accessed: April 1, 2016. Date last updated: 2014.
140. Boccaletti L, Efthymiou A, Leonardi B, *et al.* Life After Care: A Handbook to Support Transition to Post-Caring. Dublin, Care Alliance Ireland, 2011. www.carealliance.ie/userfiles/file/LifeAftercareBookletFinalWebVersionOct2011.pdf
141. Age UK. Information for Carers. www.ageuk.org.uk/home-and-care/advice-for-carers/when-your-caring-role-changes/ Date last accessed: July 1, 2016. Date last updated: June 10, 2015.
142. DiGiacomo M, Lewis J, Nolan MT, *et al.* Transitioning from caregiving to widowhood. *J Pain Symptom Manage* 46: 817–825.
143. Sealey M, Breen LJ, O'Connor M, *et al.* A scoping review of bereavement risk assessment measures: implications for palliative care. *Palliat Med* 2015; 29: 577–589.
144. National Institute for Health and Care Excellence (NICE). Guide to the Methods of Technology Appraisal. www.nice.org.uk/article/pmg9/chapter/foreword Date last accessed: June 12, 2016. Date last updated: April, 2013.
145. Goodrich K, Kaambwa B, Al-Janabi H. The inclusion of informal care in applied economic evaluation: a review. *Value Health* 2012; 15: 975–981.

Disclosures: This report is independent research supported by the National Institute for Health Research (Career Development Fellowship, CDF-2012-05-218). The views expressed in this publication are those of the author and not necessarily those of the NHS, the National Institute for Health Research or the Dept of Health.

Chapter 5

Symptom patterns in populations

Magnus Ekström[1], David C. Currow[2] and Katrien Moens[3]

Breathlessness is the cardinal symptom of cardiorespiratory disease. It increases with disease severity and is often associated with other chronic and debilitating symptoms. This chapter reviews the prevalence and consequences of breathlessness in advanced disease and the affected (older) population, associated symptoms, and risk factors for experiencing more severe symptoms, particularly focusing on changes in breathlessness and associated symptoms over time in patients with advanced disease and nearing death.

As we consider the patterns through which symptoms manifest across populations, there are several key considerations. Rarely does any person with an advanced illness have a single symptom. More likely, symptoms occur in clusters that relate to several factors. Many symptoms coexist because: 1) the disease has a predictable burden likely to cause symptoms; 2) symptoms that are expected to simultaneously get worse are not directly related to each other (disease progression) [1], for example, both breathlessness and fatigue are known to worsen as death approaches; 3) the way we experience the pathology to which we are exposed differs from person to person and seemingly similar pathophysiological insults are likely to generate quite different perceptions in patients; thus, the same stimulus may create breathlessness and pain in one person, nausea and breathlessness in another; 4) symptoms are prevalent across the population and symptom burden increases with age, comorbidities and frailty; many people will simply have symptoms that coexist because of multiple morbidities, each with its own symptoms [2].

Despite years of effort using large data sets, it is difficult to develop a full understanding of the patterns or clusters of symptoms that coexist with given underlying pathologies [3]. This is, in part, because most of the symptoms under consideration are entirely subjective. It is also because most people bring to advanced illness a number of comorbidities that also need to be taken into account in the mix of symptoms and symptom progression.

Each symptom will vary in intensity, how this intensity changes over time, and how the person perceives the symptom and the impact it has or will have on their life. Each symptom is also likely to differ somewhat in its response to treatment and the other factors that influence how it is perceived.

Ultimately, the common thread between symptoms is that there is a pathophysiological stimulus, the transmission of that stimulus through the nervous system, an interpretation of

[1]Dept of Clinical Sciences, Division of Respiratory Medicine and Allergology, Lund University, Lund, Sweden. [2]Palliative and Supportive Services, Flinders University, Adelaide, Australia. [3]Belgian Cancer Centre, Scientific Institute of Public Health, Brussels, Belgium.

Correspondence: Magnus Ekström, Dept of Clinical Sciences, Division of Respiratory Medicine and Allergology, Lund University, SE-221 00 Lund, Sweden. E-mail: pmekstrom@gmail.com

 Print ISBN: 978-1-84984-071-2. Online ISBN: 978-1-84984-072-9. Print ISSN: 2312-508X. Online ISSN: 2312-5098.

the sensations the stimulus produces to give them meaning and, finally, a response by that person. Meaning or interpretation is crucial in this. The less in control people feel, the more intensely symptoms are likely to be perceived. For example, when well, each of us can induce severe breathlessness through maximal exertion; however, most of us are perfectly calm about this situation because we know we can stop that exertion at any moment and the breathlessness will settle rapidly. By contrast, people with chronic breathlessness because of a severe underlying pathology are rarely likely to feel in control because there is no end in sight and there is nothing that can help bring this breathlessness under control. This is particularly the case if people experience periodic worsening of their breathlessness with no apparent stimulus.

As such, symptom patterns vary widely; coexisting symptoms will be an amalgam of different underlying pathophysiologies and different interpretations or meanings attributed to those symptoms.

A systematic review by Moens *et al.* [4] stated that there are commonalities in problem prevalence across different cancer and non-cancer diagnostic groups, helping us to conclude that palliative care should be made available based on the problems and needs patients exhibit, and not on the diagnostic group to which a patient belongs or to their prognosis [5, 6].

Most symptoms do not occur in isolation. Interactions between many symptoms and common central nervous system pathways for processing these sensations have been demonstrated. Furthermore, most people with advanced respiratory disease have multiple comorbidities, often bringing long-term symptoms from other illnesses [2]. In this chapter, the focus is not only on "breathlessness" but also on other symptoms that are frequently encountered in people with advanced respiratory diseases: fatigue, anorexia, pain, nausea, insomnia, delirium, constipation, diarrhoea, depression, anxiety, worry, problems related to spirituality, and worsening social isolation as the disease progresses. This highlights the importance of the kind of holistic approach that palliative care embodies and the reality that breathlessness interacts with other symptoms. The impact of palliative care-related problems can be felt at different levels, and in this chapter we will describe both the clinical impact on patients and what the prevalence figures can mean for clinicians.

Breathlessness

Prevalence

Overall

Breathlessness is common in the general population and increases steeply in prevalence with increasing age and in chronic disease [7–11]. Most population-based studies of breathlessness have measured the level of exertion required to induce breathlessness and the functional impact of the symptom using tools such as the modified Medical Research Council (mMRC) dyspnoea scale [12].

In the general population, about 30% of middle-aged and older people report breathlessness that has an impact on daily life [7–11]. In the population-based Burden of Obstructive Lung Disease (BOLD) study of 9484 people aged ⩾40 years from 15 countries, 27% reported breathlessness (mMRC ⩾1; "breathless when hurrying on the level or up a slight hill" or worse) with 13% having marked disability (mMRC ⩾2), and 2% suffering from breathlessness at rest [8]. Breathlessness is persistent in many people. In a South Australian study, 9% of the general population reported chronic breathlessness defined as an mMRC score ⩾2 daily during at least 3 of the previous 6 months [7].

Predictors independently associated with increased disability from breathlessness are: older age, female sex, obesity or underweight, impaired lung function (as measured by FEV_1 or FVC), smoking, lower socioeconomic status, occupational dust exposure, a history of tuberculosis, and childhood hospitalisations [7–9].

Data on the causes of breathlessness in the general population are limited [13]. In a study from South Australia (n=2824, mean age 46 years, 49% males), the main self-reported causes of chronic breathlessness were respiratory disease (64%), heart disease (17%), and being overweight or unfit (6%) [14].

In a large US population-based study, about 50% of people reported breathlessness for ⩾1 month in the last year of life, with a slight increase from 50% in 1998 to 55% in 2010 [15].

Age

The prevalence of breathlessness is highly age-dependent [8, 9]. A meta-analysis of 21 studies in people aged ⩾65 reported a pooled prevalence of 36% for an mMRC score ⩾1, 16% for an mMRC score ⩾2, and 4.1% for an mMRC score ⩾3 [13]. In South Australia, Bowden *et al.* [16] found a striking "50–50" pattern among people aged ⩾50 years; 50% reported breathlessness (mMRC score ⩾1).

Breathlessness is commonly associated with restricted activity in older people. In a study of 548 community-dwelling people aged ⩾70 years with monthly symptom assessments for more than a decade, restricting breathlessness (defined as breathlessness that caused participants to stay in bed at least half a day or cut down on their usual activities) was experienced by 57% of people at some point during the final year of life [17]. Restricting breathlessness was reported alongside anxiety, depression, impaired mobility, previous smoking and cardiorespiratory disease. Prevalence increased markedly in the last 4 months of life across a range of causes of death (figure 1) [17].

The rising number of older people and people with multimorbidities (two or more chronic medical conditions) in many settings has significant implications for the prevalence of breathlessness globally. In a large study of people (n=1 751 841) registered with 314 medical practices in Scotland, multimorbidities were present in 30% of people aged 45–64 years, 65% of people aged 65–84 years, and 82% of people aged ⩾85 years [18]. Morbidity is higher among people with lower socioeconomic status [18]. In the face of increasing age and multimorbidities in many settings, a continuing rise in the prevalence of breathlessness in the coming decades is likely to occur.

Sex

In the general population, there is a striking difference between men and women in the level of disability from breathlessness as measured by the mMRC scale [8, 9]. In population-based studies of COPD in five Latin American cities (the Latin American Project for the Investigation of Obstructive Lung Disease (PLATINO)) and 15 countries (the BOLD study), women reported significantly more breathlessness than men with odds ratios (ORs) of 1.6 and 2.1, respectively [8, 9]. In the BOLD study, 33% of women compared with 20% of men reported an mMRC score ⩾1 [8]. This was also reflected in a

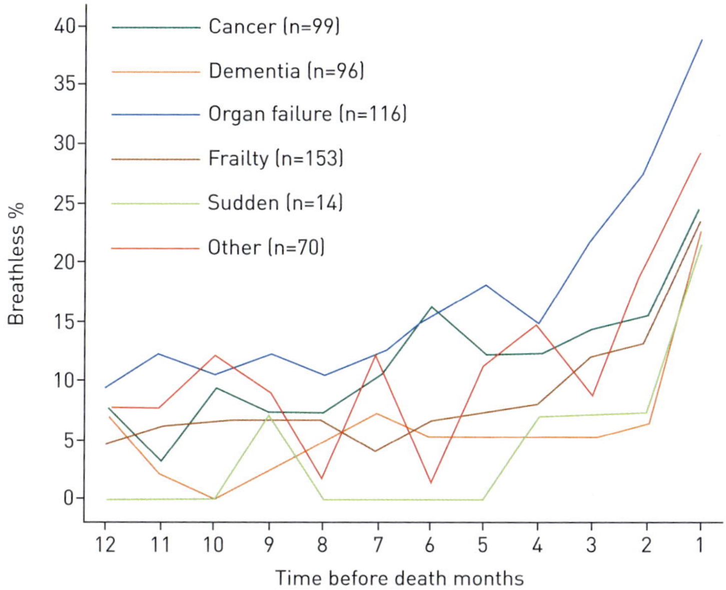

Figure 1. Percentage reporting breathlessness that restricts daily activities in 548 community-dwelling people aged ≥70 years during the last year of life according to the condition leading to death. Reproduced from [17] with permission.

study from South Australia that found women having an adjusted breathlessness OR of 1.9 (95% CI 1.5–2.4) [7].

The causes of higher disability from breathlessness among women in the general population are unknown. The difference between men and women was not explained by discrepancies in age, BMI, smoking, socioeconomic status, heart disease, chronic airflow limitation, or lung function impairment (expressed as FEV_1 or FVC % predicted) [8, 9, 16, 19–22]. One study found that the difference between men and women was attenuated when controlling for mood state, but this was a small study (n=153) and the reported differences were small [23]. A difference between men and women was not found with regard to breathlessness that restricted daily activities during the last year of life in older people [17].

In palliative care, data on any difference in breathlessness between men and women are conflicting. Large studies from Ontario in Canada of the last months of life and an Australian study of the last week of life both found slightly lower breathlessness in women than in men [24, 25]. Differences in breathlessness between men and women warrant further study, including at different points in the disease trajectory.

Different diseases

Breathlessness is common in advanced disease across a range of both malignant and non-malignant diagnoses [4]. A recent systematic review of 73 different studies showed a high prevalence of breathlessness in cancer (16–77%), COPD (56–98%), CHF (18–88%), ESRD (11–82%), dementia (12–52%), advanced AIDS (43–62%), motor neuron disease (MND) (81–88%) and multiple sclerosis (26%) (table 1) [4]. Wide ranges in prevalence are due to when in the disease trajectory breathlessness was sought and which measurement tools were used.

Table 1. Breathlessness# prevalence summary derived from 73 different studies

Characteristics	Cancer	COPD	CHF	ESRD	Dementia	AIDS	Parkinson's	MND	MS
Total patients in all studies	33 175	1835	1230	1031	674	811	No data	52	52
Total studies	40	8	7	11	5	3		1	1
Prevalence range	16–77%	56–98%	18–88%	11–82%	12–52%	43–62%		81–88%	26%
Studies reporting prevalence ⩾50%	16		5	4	1	3			

#: termed "breathlessness", "dyspnoea", "shortness of breath" or "respiratory distress" in different studies. MND: motor neuron disease; MS: multiple sclerosis. Reproduced and modified from [4] with permission.

People with respiratory disease or lung involvement have more common and severe breathlessness. Compared to patients with lung cancer, the odds of experiencing moderate-to-severe breathlessness were markedly lower in patients with gastrointestinal (OR 0.36) or genito-urinary disease (OR 0.41), or breast cancer (OR 0.52; p<0.001 for all comparisons) [24]. In another study, breathlessness during the last week of life in palliative care was highest in patients with respiratory failure followed by patients with lung cancer (figure 2) [25]. Breathlessness is the cardinal symptom of respiratory disease and it is frequently reported as the main symptom in COPD [26]. It worsens as the disease progresses and varies across the course of the day; it is often worst in the morning [27]. Patients with severe COPD have been found to have a similar overall symptom burden and palliative care need when compared with patients with cancer [28, 29].

In recent population-based studies from Sweden, breathlessness in the final week of life was markedly more common in oxygen-dependent patients with COPD compared with patients who were dying from cancer (73% *versus* 22%) [30], and in people with oxygen-dependent ILD compared with patients dying from lung cancer (75% *versus* 42%) [31]. Interestingly, in the majority of symptomatic patients, breathlessness was unrelieved or only partially relieved (spontaneously or with treatment), in contrast to pain which was fully relieved in the majority of patients [30, 31].

Possible contributing causes of breathlessness in patients with cancer have been evaluated in a few studies [32, 33]. A study of 100 patients with advanced cancer (49% lung cancer) reported several potentially reversible contributing factors: impaired lung function (found in 93% of patients: 5% obstructive, 41% restrictive and 47% mixed impairment); hypoxia (40%); anaemia (20%); and bronchospasm (52%) [32]. In a larger study of 923 people with cancer, breathlessness was associated mainly with lung-related factors: a history of smoking; obstructive pulmonary disease; lung irradiation; and a history of exposure to asbestos, coal dust, cotton dust or grain dust [34]. In 125 patients with cancer in their last days of life, anxiety, anaemia,

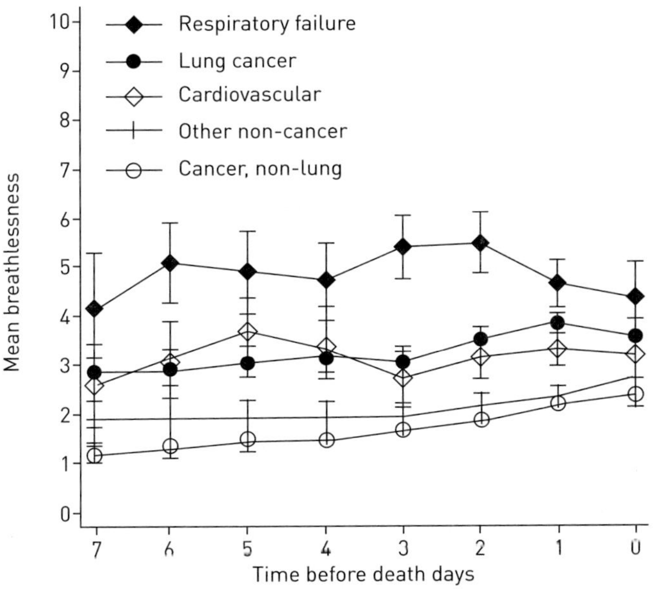

Figure 2. Mean distress from breathlessness (0–10 NRS) in five diagnostic groups during the last week of life (n=12778). Reproduced from [25] with permission.

airway obstruction, cachexia, pleural effusion, infection and lymphangitis were related to more severe breathlessness [33]. Knowledge of the factors contributing to breathlessness in advanced and terminal disease, especially in non-malignant disease, is still limited.

Besides the quantitative intensity or severity, the quality or type of breathlessness may differ according to the underlying cause(s) of the sensation [35, 36]. Breathlessness is thought to consist of at least three different qualities that may be associated with different underlying mechanisms and that can be differentiated by patients: a sensation of increased work or effort of breathing; chest tightness; and air hunger or unsatisfied inspiration [35]. A recent study in a respiratory outpatient clinic (n=109) compared the quality of breathlessness between patients with asthma, COPD, ILD or respiratory muscle weakness [37]. Work/effort was selected as one of the top three qualities in several diseases. Chest tightness was highly specific for asthma (88%) but its sensitivity was only 38%. A similar pattern was observed for the "My breathing is shallow" descriptor in ILD (84% specificity but only 33% sensitivity). More affective qualities were associated with higher anxiety scores [37]. Although the sensory qualities might tell us something about the underlying mechanisms of breathlessness, evidence to date does not suggest that they differ between diseases in a clinically useful way for making a diagnosis, or for guiding the treatments most likely to palliate symptoms.

Trajectories in palliative care

In palliative care, most studies of the severity/intensity and trajectory of breathlessness have used variants of a scale between 0 (none) and 10 (maximum), such as an NRS, or 0–100 mm VAS [38, 39].

Breathlessness is experienced by the majority of palliative care patients and often increases in the last months before death [24, 40]. In a longitudinal study of 5862 patients in a community palliative care programme (Perth, Australia), mean breathlessness intensity increased over time especially in the last 2 weeks of life in patients with cancer (figure 3), whereas breathlessness was at a much higher level that was maintained and failed to lessen over the last 3 months in people with non-malignant disease [40]. Over the same time period, the prevalence of any breathlessness increased from 50% to 65% [40]. The proportion of patients with severe breathlessness (more than seven out of 10) increased from 10% to 26% [40], with the most marked increase in the last days of life.

A similar pattern with mean breathlessness increasing towards death was observed in a large population-based, point-of-care data set of cancer outpatients in Ontario, Canada [24]. Breathlessness increased markedly in the last 4 weeks of life, along with worsening appetite, drowsiness, fatigue, decreased performance status and overall well-being (figure 4) [24].

An interesting analysis using the same database (n=55 883) found that during the last year of life, a patient who reported no breathlessness had a 20–30% probability of developing breathlessness within 1 month, and this probability remained constant throughout the final 12 months [41]. Conversely, breathless patients had a 60–70% probability of reduced breathlessness within 1 month. The change in breathlessness over time differed significantly between individuals, as previously reported [28]. The probability of improvement tended to decrease somewhat as death approached [41].

The trajectory of breathlessness in the last week of life was recently evaluated [25, 42]. A study by Hui *et al.* [42] of patients admitted to an acute palliative care unit (n=203) found that mean breathlessness (measured daily) increased towards death especially in the last

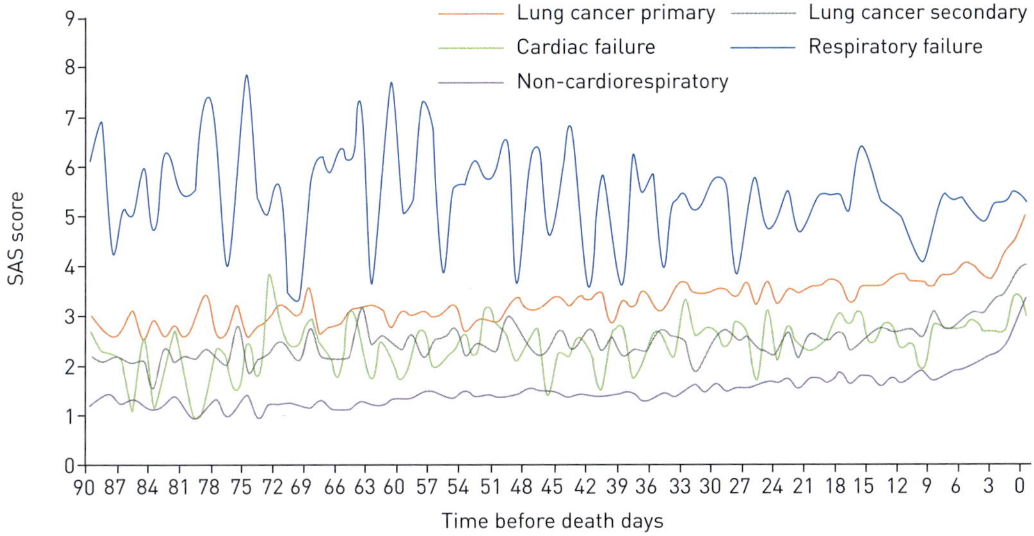

Figure 3. Changes in the mean intensity of breathlessness in five diagnostic groups as death approaches (n=5862). SAS: survival aggregate score. Reproduced from [40] with permission.

2 days. Breathlessness in the last week before death was evaluated in a large study (n=12778) from 87 community and inpatient palliative services, representing >80% of people referred to specialised palliative care in Australia [25]. The results of multivariate analysis showed that breathlessness severity was higher in patients with respiratory failure or lung cancer (figure 2), who were male, had a better performance status (possibly owing to higher activity levels), and concurrent unpleasant sensations (fatigue, nausea and pain) [25]. In contrast to the pattern seen by Hui *et al.* [42], the mean breathlessness level remained relatively

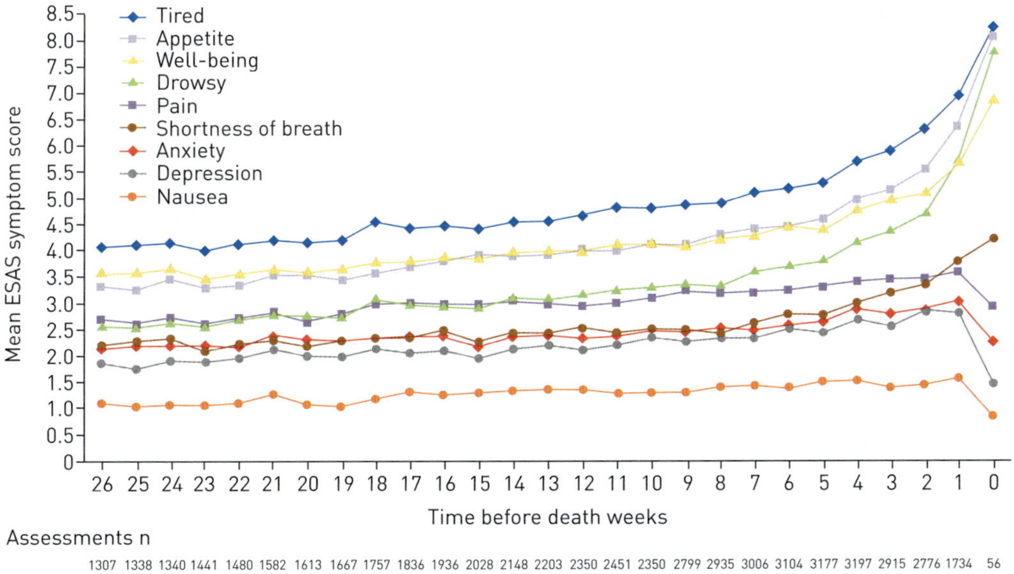

Figure 4. Mean symptom scores towards death in patients with cancer (n=12196). ESAS: Edmonton Symptom Assessment System. Reproduced from [24] with permission.

unchanged during the last week, with only a slight increase towards death (figure 2) [25]. Data from studies on treatments given in the last week of life to palliate breathlessness were unavailable [25, 42].

Of note, the characteristics and temporal patterns of breathlessness were insufficiently captured in the majority of large longitudinal symptom studies [24, 25, 40, 41]. Breathlessness can be categorised as episodic (seconds, minutes or hours) or continuous (days, weeks or months) and as either triggered or not triggered [43]. Common triggers of breathlessness include exertion and emotion [43, 44]. Interestingly, a meta-analysis of 27 studies (7584 patients) across five advanced diseases found that episodic breathlessness was highly prevalent (often daily), commonly lasted <10 min, and was characterised by severe peak intensity [44]. Large-scale studies of the characteristics, duration, and triggers of breathlessness are needed and could have important implications on how to alleviate the distress and negative consequences of different temporal patterns of breathlessness.

Impact on patients

Breathlessness is associated with significant adverse effects for the individual and for society.

Shorter survival

Breathlessness is associated with increased risk of all-cause and cardiorespiratory mortality in the general population [10, 45, 46], including in a twin study [47]. Increased mortality was observed for new-onset and persistent breathlessness, but not in people with transient symptoms [10]. An mMRC score $\geqslant 2$ is a good indicator of decreased survival time in COPD [48]. An mMRC score is a better predictor of mortality in COPD than FEV_1 [48]. Breathlessness is associated with shorter survival in patients admitted to an acute palliative care unit [49].

Impaired health status

Reduced health status and quality of life are strongly related to the patient's symptom burden, including the presence and severity of breathlessness, both in the general population [12, 50] and in people living with an advanced disease such as lung cancer [51].

Impaired activities of daily living

To reduce the distress from breathlessness, patients limit their activities of daily living, such as working, walking, sleeping, sexual intercourse, social relationships, and general activities [52, 53]. Breathlessness is strongly linked to reduced physical activity and capacity, and impaired activities of daily living [52, 54], including physical and physiological domains [53]. Severe breathlessness is associated with loss of the will to live as an individual nears death [55].

Increased health service use and serious events

Breathlessness and especially a breathlessness crisis is a distressing and feared symptom by both patients and caregivers [56, 57] People with worsening breathlessness particularly fear that they may suffocate [58]. In a systematic review of primary care, breathlessness was one of the main reasons for consultation in about 2% of patients [59]. In a recent Norwegian study, this was the third most common symptom presentation (9%) in the ED after abdominal pain (13%) and chest pain (13%) [60].

Moderate-to-severe breathlessness was associated with increased ED visits during the subsequent week in outpatients with cancer in the Ontario Cancer Registry [61]. In the same database, breathlessness was also among the top five reasons for visiting the ED during the last 2 weeks of life in people who died from cancer (n=91 561) [62].

In breathless patients in the ED (n=253), the severity of the worst breathlessness was a good predictor of admission or discharge [63]. The combination of a breathlessness VAS score ⩾6, heart rate ⩾94 beats·min^{-1} at triage, and ambulance arrival predicted admission with 90% sensitivity and 84% specificity in all ED patients [63].

Breathlessness (NRS score ⩾4) has also been associated with an increased risk of serious in-hospital events (need for a special response team, intensive care, or death): 20% compared with 10% in people with no or less severe breathlessness [64].

Interaction with other symptoms

Breathlessness frequently co-occurs with other symptoms. Breathlessness management needs a holistic care approach that takes into account the other symptoms that breathlessness interacts with. The co-occurrence with other symptoms can be termed "symptom clustering" [65, 66]. A definition of symptom clusters that is commonly used is that of two or more interrelated symptoms presenting together with a high level of predictability [65, 66]. The predictive ability of symptom clusters can help to define patient outcomes in much the same way factors like functional status and quality of life can [67]. Two approaches can be used when conducting a symptom cluster analysis: a clinical approach and a statistical approach. Studies that focus on a small number of preselected symptoms use a clinical approach and generally use correlational analysis [68]. Clinically observed associations of symptoms likely to cluster, such as pain, fatigue and depression, are the starting point for this kind of analysis [68]. Studies that use multi-symptom assessment tools or symptom checklists with a large number of symptoms generally use the statistical approach [68]. In this type of analysis, there are no clinical assumptions of symptom associations; factor or cluster analyses are used to discover statistically defined symptom clusters. Analysing multiple symptoms with a statistical approach can identify clusters that may have been overlooked during clinical assessment [69].

Symptom cluster studies are important because they provide clinicians with the information needed to manage symptoms with appropriate treatment plans and thereby help lessen the total symptom burden [69]. Symptoms that belong to a specific cluster may have a common biological mechanism; thus, treating one symptom can help relieve other symptoms in that cluster, although clinical application of this hypothesis is currently limited [68]. When one symptom is detected, knowledge of symptom clusters can instigate the clinical investigation of associated symptoms. A systematic review [70] of symptom clusters in advanced cancer patients identified two studies that reported stable breathlessness-related clusters: a breathlessness–fatigue–anxiety cluster and a fatigue–pain–nausea–drowsiness–breathlessness–loss-of-appetite cluster [71]. The clinical usefulness of these clusters has yet to be established.

Knowledge of symptoms interacting with breathlessness may also facilitate the identification of breathlessness. For these reasons, the following section presents information on the occurrence of a range of other symptoms in patients with advanced cancer and in patients with other life-limiting illnesses.

Other symptoms

Prevalence

The evidence on the prevalence of fatigue, breathlessness, anorexia, pain, nausea, insomnia, delirium, constipation, diarrhoea, depression, anxiety, worry, spirituality problems and social problems in people living with advanced cancer, COPD, CHF, ESRD, dementia, AIDS, Parkinson's disease, MND and multiple sclerosis (MS) was systematically reviewed by Moens *et al.* [4]. This systematic review compared the prevalence of palliative care-related problems in patients with advanced cancer and these eight advanced non-cancer patient groups, and described and compared the characteristics of the prevalence studies.

A total of 143 symptom prevalence studies in advanced disease were included. The greatest number of studies focused on patients with advanced cancer (n=57) and ESRD (n=47), whereas the lowest number of studies focused on patients with MND (n=3) and MS (n=2). Most studies originated from the USA (n=57), the UK (n=20) and Canada (n=13). In the group with advanced cancer, 37 out of 58 studies used a point prevalence to collect data. In the ESRD group, 28 out of 47 studies used a period prevalence with a minimum–maximum time range of "past 2 days" to "the last 2 months". The other diagnostic groups mostly used a period prevalence. With regard to the measurement tools used with the advanced cancer and non-cancer groups, 75 out of 143 studies used validated scales. In the advanced dementia patient group, four out of seven studies used retrospective reviews of patients' charts.

Because of the heterogeneity between studies with regard to the different measurement tools and study designs used, the review could not apply meta-analytic techniques to analyse the prevalence data. For that reason, they reported the prevalence figures using minimum and maximum prevalence ranges and recorded the number of studies that showed the prevalence of a problem in a particular diagnostic group of ⩾50%. Looking at the majority of studies that recorded a prevalence of ⩾50% in comparison to the total number of studies for each problem per diagnostic group, the following problems showed a prevalence ⩾50%: fatigue in advanced cancer, COPD, CHF, ESRD, AIDS and MS; anorexia in advanced cancer, COPD, ESRD and AIDS; pain in advanced cancer, COPD, ESRD, AIDS, Parkinson's disease, MND and MS; dyspnoea in COPD, CHF, ESRD, AIDS and MND; insomnia in COPD, AIDS and Parkinson's disease; constipation in ESRD and MND; diarrhoea in AIDS; depression in COPD and AIDS; anxiety in AIDS and Parkinson's disease; worry in advanced cancer, COPD, ESRD and AIDS; and lack of well-being in advanced cancer. The problems for which they found the widest minimum (<10%) and maximum (⩾50%) prevalence ranges were: nausea/vomiting in advanced cancer and ESRD; insomnia in advanced cancer and ESRD; delirium in advanced cancer; constipation in advanced cancer and ESRD; depression in advanced cancer, CHF and ESRD; anxiety in advanced cancer, dementia and Parkinson's disease; and worry in advanced cancer. Within the group of 143 articles, only five studies directly compared the prevalence of palliative care-related problems to another diagnostic group while using the same measurement tool. In these studies, the range of the minimum and maximum prevalence was not wide. They identified only four studies on problems related to spirituality, and one study on palliative care-related problems of a social nature.

Differences in data collection time-points (point *versus* period prevalence, or a mix of both), period prevalence time ranges, definitions for a problem, sample size, and the measurement methods used across studies probably caused wide variations in the minimum and maximum prevalence ranges. In light of these variations and because of the methodological heterogeneity across studies, there is as much variation in prevalence between diagnostic groups as there is similarity. Understanding the prevalence of palliative care-related symptoms in patients with non-malignant disease compared to patients with cancer is complex because of the often different trajectories of functional decline and dependency in patients with non-malignant disease [72], their comorbidities, and the changing stages of disease progression.

Clinical impact

There is an urgent need to intensify the measurement and reporting of palliative care-related problems of a spiritual and social nature. Pain, fatigue, anorexia, dyspnoea and anxiety are highly prevalent in advanced cancer and non-cancer diagnostic groups [20]. Therefore, healthcare providers should be more aware and more sensitive when assessing and treating these problems.

Palliative care practitioners should be encouraged to use existing patient reported outcome measures (PROMs) to assess, measure, evaluate or monitor different aspects of their provided care. Specific PROMs are recommended because they are developed to measure outcomes in palliative care, are more responsive to clinically meaningful changes, and can be used in specific domains or for specific conditions, *e.g.* symptoms, function, or palliative care needs [73]. Examples of such outcome measures are the Palliative care Outcome Scale and the Edmonton Symptom Assessment System.

Conclusion

Chronic breathlessness is prevalent across the community and is more prevalent in people with advancing, life-limiting illnesses, especially in the last weeks and days of life. Treating the reversible underlying cause(s) is the first essential step in establishing the diagnosis of chronic breathlessness, but despite treatment efforts, breathlessness persists for many people. People with respiratory disease or lung involvement and heart failure are particularly prone to experience worsening breathlessness. Importantly, most advancing illnesses at the EOL are associated with breathlessness in a large percentage of the population, even in the absence of demonstrated cardiorespiratory disease, suggesting that avenues for future research should include understanding whether there is a central nervous system common pathway for the perception of breathlessness and whether the changes associated with cachexia in advanced disease contribute to difficulty in the physical process of breathing.

When multiple symptoms are considered, breathlessness and anxiety are often associated and can create a cycle of worsening for both symptoms as each intensifies. The opportunity to address each of these symptoms simultaneously is likely to provide specific benefits for patients and their caregivers.

References

1. Aktas A, Walsh D, Hauser K, *et al.* Should we cluster patients or symptoms? The myth of symptom clusters based on 'depression, insomnia, pain' and 'depression, fatigue, pain'. *BMJ Support Palliat Care* 2016; 6: 210–218.
2. Currow DC, Clark K, Kamal A, *et al.* The population burden of chronic symptoms that substantially predate the diagnosis of a life-limiting illness. *J Palliat Med* 2015; 18: 480–485.
3. Walsh D, Rybicki L. Symptom clustering in advanced cancer. *Support Care Cancer* 2006; 14: 831–836.

4. Moens K, Higginson IJ, Harding R. Are there differences in the prevalence of palliative care-related problems in people living with advanced cancer and eight non-cancer conditions? A systematic review. *J Pain Symptom Manage* 2014; 48: 660–677.
5. Waller A, Girgis A, Currow D, *et al.* Development of the palliative care needs assessment tool (PC-NAT) for use by multi-disciplinary health professionals. *Palliat Med* 2008; 22: 956–964.
6. Waller A, Girgis A, Lecathelinais C, *et al.* Validity, reliability and clinical feasibility of a Needs Assessment Tool for people with progressive cancer. *Psychooncology* 2010; 19: 726–733.
7. Currow DC, Plummer JL, Crockett A, *et al.* A community population survey of prevalence and severity of dyspnea in adults. *J Pain Symptom Manage* 2009; 38: 533–545.
8. Grønseth R, Vollmer WM, Hardie JA, *et al.* Predictors of dyspnoea prevalence: results from the BOLD study. *Eur Respir J* 2014; 43: 1610–1620.
9. Lopez Varela MV, Montes de Oca M, Halbert RJ, *et al.* Sex-related differences in COPD in five Latin American cities: the PLATINO study. *Eur Respir J* 2010; 36: 1034–1041.
10. Figarska SM, Boezen HM, Vonk JM. Dyspnea severity, changes in dyspnea status and mortality in the general population: the Vlagtwedde/Vlaardingen study. *Eur J Epidemiol* 2012; 27: 867–876.
11. Voll-Aanerud M, Eagan TM, Wentzel-Larsen T, *et al.* Changes in respiratory symptoms and health-related quality of life. *Chest* 2007; 131: 1890–1897.
12. Bestall JC, Paul EA, Garrod R, *et al.* Usefulness of the Medical Research Council (MRC) dyspnoea scale as a measure of disability in patients with chronic obstructive pulmonary disease. *Thorax* 1999; 54: 581–586.
13. van Mourik Y, Rutten FH, Moons KG, *et al.* Prevalence and underlying causes of dyspnoea in older people: a systematic review. *Age Ageing* 2014; 43: 319–326.
14. Johnson MJ, Bowden JA, Abernethy AP, *et al.* To what causes do people attribute their chronic breathlessness? A population survey. *J Palliat Med* 2012; 15: 744–750.
15. Singer AE, Meeker D, Teno JM, *et al.* Symptom trends in the last year of life from 1998 to 2010: a cohort study. *Ann Intern Med* 2015; 162: 175–183.
16. Bowden JA, To TH, Abernethy AP, *et al.* Predictors of chronic breathlessness: a large population study. *BMC Public Health* 2011; 11: 33.
17. Johnson MJ, Bland JM, Gahbauer EA, *et al.* Breathlessness in elderly adults during the last year of life sufficient to restrict activity: prevalence, pattern, and associated factors. *J Am Geriatr Soc* 2016; 64: 73–80.
18. Barnett K, Mercer SW, Norbury M, *et al.* Epidemiology of multimorbidity and implications for health care, research, and medical education: a cross-sectional study. *Lancet* 2012; 380: 37–43.
19. Lindström M, Kotaniemi J, Jönsson E, *et al.* Smoking, respiratory symptoms, and diseases: a comparative study between northern Sweden and northern Finland: report from the FinEsS study. *Chest* 2001; 119: 852–861.
20. de Torres JP, Casanova C, Montejo de Garcini A, *et al.* Gender and respiratory factors associated with dyspnea in chronic obstructive pulmonary disease. *Respir Res* 2007; 8: 18.
21. Neuman A, Gunnbjörnsdottir M, Tunsäter A, *et al.* Dyspnea in relation to symptoms of anxiety and depression: a prospective population study. *Respir Med* 2006; 100: 1843–1849.
22. Lamprecht B, Vanfleteren LE, Studnicka M, *et al.* Sex-related differences in respiratory symptoms: results from the BOLD Study. *Eur Respir J* 2013; 42: 858–860.
23. Gijsbers van Wijk CM, Huisman H, Kolk AM. Gender differences in physical symptoms and illness behavior. A health diary study. *Soc Sci Med* 1999; 49: 1061–1074.
24. Seow H, Barbera L, Sutradhar R, *et al.* Trajectory of performance status and symptom scores for patients with cancer during the last six months of life. *J Clin Oncol* 2011; 29: 1151–1158.
25. Ekström M, Allingham SF, Eagar K, *et al.* Breathlessness during the last week of life in palliative care: an Australian prospective, longitudinal study. *J Pain Symptom Manage* 2016; 51: 816–823.
26. Miravitlles M, Ferrer J, Baró E, *et al.* Differences between physician and patient in the perception of symptoms and their severity in COPD. *Respir Med* 2013; 107: 1977–1985.
27. Kessler R, Partridge MR, Miravitlles M, *et al.* Symptom variability in patients with severe COPD: a pan-European cross-sectional study. *Eur Respir J* 2011; 37: 264–272.
28. Bausewein C, Booth S, Gysels M, *et al.* Individual breathlessness trajectories do not match summary trajectories in advanced cancer and chronic obstructive pulmonary disease: results from a longitudinal study. *Palliat Med* 2010; 24: 777–786.
29. Weingaertner V, Scheve C, Gerdes V, *et al.* Breathlessness, functional status, distress, and palliative care needs over time in patients with advanced chronic obstructive pulmonary disease or lung cancer: a cohort study. *J Pain Symptom Manage* 2014; 48: 569–581.e1.
30. Ahmadi Z, Lundström S, Janson C, *et al.* End-of-life care in oxygen-dependent COPD and cancer: a national population-based study. *Eur Respir J* 2015; 46: 1190–1193.
31. Ahmadi Z, Wysham NG, Lundström S, *et al.* End-of-life care in oxygen-dependent ILD compared with lung cancer: a national population-based study. *Thorax* 2016; 71: 510–516.
32. Dudgeon DJ, Lertzman M. Dyspnea in the advanced cancer patient. *J Pain Symptom Manage* 1998; 16: 212–219.

33. Chiu TY, Hu WY, Lue BH, *et al.* Dyspnea and its correlates in Taiwanese patients with terminal cancer. *J Pain Symptom Manage* 2004; 28: 123–132.
34. Dudgeon DJ, Kristjanson L, Sloan JA, *et al.* Dyspnea in cancer patients: prevalence and associated factors. *J Pain Symptom Manage* 2001; 21: 95–102.
35. Laviolette L, Laveneziana P. Dyspnoea: a multidimensional and multidisciplinary approach. *Eur Respir J* 2014; 43: 1750–1762.
36. Parshall MB, Schwartzstein RM, Adams L, *et al.* An official American Thoracic Society statement: update on the mechanisms, assessment, and management of dyspnea. *Am J Respir Crit Care Med* 2012; 185: 435–452.
37. Chang AS, Munson J, Gifford AH, *et al.* Prospective use of descriptors of dyspnea to diagnose common respiratory diseases. *Chest* 2015; 148: 895–902.
38. Bausewein C, Farquhar M, Booth S, *et al.* Measurement of breathlessness in advanced disease: a systematic review. *Respir Med* 2007; 101: 399–410.
39. Dorman S, Jolley C, Abernethy A, *et al.* Researching breathlessness in palliative care: consensus statement of the National Cancer Research Institute Palliative Care Breathlessness Subgroup. *Palliat Med* 2009; 23: 213–227.
40. Currow DC, Smith J, Davidson PM, *et al.* Do the trajectories of dyspnea differ in prevalence and intensity by diagnosis at the end of life? A consecutive cohort study. *J Pain Symptom Manage* 2010; 39: 680–690.
41. Jia J, Barbera L, Sutradhar R. Using Markov multistate models to examine the progression of symptom severity among an ambulatory population of cancer patients: are certain symptoms better managed than others? *J Pain Symptom Manage* 2016; 51: 232–239.
42. Hui D, dos Santos R, Chisholm GB, *et al.* Symptom expression in the last seven days of life among cancer patients admitted to acute palliative care units. *J Pain Symptom Manage* 2015; 50: 488–494.
43. Simon ST, Higginson IJ, Benalia H, *et al.* Episodic and continuous breathlessness: a new categorization of breathlessness. *J Pain Symptom Manage* 2013; 45: 1019–1029.
44. Simon ST, Bausewein C, Schildmann E, *et al.* Episodic breathlessness in patients with advanced disease: a systematic review. *J Pain Symptom Manage* 2013; 45: 561–578.
45. Knuiman MW, James AL, Divitini ML, *et al.* Lung function, respiratory symptoms, and mortality: results from the Busselton Health Study. *Ann Epidemiol* 1999; 9: 297–306.
46. Pesola GR, Ahsan H. Dyspnea as an independent predictor of mortality. *Clin Respir J* 2016; 10: 142–152.
47. Waller K, Kaprio J, Kujala UM. Dyspnea and all-cause mortality: 28-yr follow-up study among adult twins. *Med Sci Sports Exerc* 2014; 46: 1538–1545.
48. Nishimura K, Izumi T, Tsukino M, *et al.* Dyspnea is a better predictor of 5-year survival than airway obstruction in patients with COPD. *Chest* 2002; 121: 1434–1440.
49. Mori M, Parsons HA, De la Cruz M, *et al.* Changes in symptoms and inpatient mortality: a study in advanced cancer patients admitted to an acute palliative care unit in a comprehensive cancer center. *J Palliat Med* 2011; 14: 1034–1041.
50. Hsu KY, Lin JR, Lin MS, *et al.* The modified Medical Research Council dyspnoea scale is a good indicator of health-related quality of life in patients with chronic obstructive pulmonary disease. *Singapore Med J* 2013; 54: 321–327.
51. Iyer S, Roughley A, Rider A, *et al.* The symptom burden of non-small cell lung cancer in the USA: a real-world cross-sectional study. *Support Care Cancer* 2014; 22: 181–187.
52. Ho SF, O'Mahony MS, Steward JA, *et al.* Dyspnoea and quality of life in older people at home. *Age Ageing* 2001; 30: 155–159.
53. Tanaka K, Akechi T, Okuyama T, *et al.* Prevalence and screening of dyspnea interfering with daily life activities in ambulatory patients with advanced lung cancer. *J Pain Symptom Manage* 2002; 23: 484–489.
54. Troosters T, Sciurba F, Battaglia S, *et al.* Physical inactivity in patients with COPD, a controlled multi-center pilot-study. *Respir Med* 2010; 104: 1005–1011.
55. Chochinov HM, Tataryn D, Clinch JJ, *et al.* Will to live in the terminally ill. *Lancet* 1999; 354: 816–819.
56. Janssens T, De Peuter S, Stans L, *et al.* Dyspnea perception in COPD: association between anxiety, dyspnea-related fear, and dyspnea in a pulmonary rehabilitation program. *Chest* 2011; 140: 618–625.
57. Gysels MH, Higginson IJ. The lived experience of breathlessness and its implications for care: a qualitative comparison in cancer, COPD, heart failure and MND. *BMC Palliat Care* 2011; 10: 15.
58. Nauck F, Alt-Epping B. Crises in palliative care: a comprehensive approach. *Lancet Oncol* 2008; 9: 1086–1091.
59. Viniol A, Beidatsch D, Frese T, *et al.* Studies of the symptom dyspnoea: a systematic review. *BMC Fam Pract* 2015; 16: 152.
60. Langlo NM, Orvik AB, Dale J, *et al.* The acute sick and injured patients: an overview of the emergency department patient population at a Norwegian University Hospital Emergency Department. *Eur J Emerg Med* 2014; 21: 175–180.
61. Barbera L, Atzema C, Sutradhar R, *et al.* Do patient-reported symptoms predict emergency department visits in cancer patients? A population-based analysis. *Ann Emerg Med* 2013; 61: 427–437.e5.
62. Barbera L, Taylor C, Dudgeon D. Why do patients with cancer visit the emergency department near the end of life? *CMAJ* 2010; 182: 563–568.

63. Saracino A, Weiland TJ, Jolly B, *et al.* Verbal dyspnoea score predicts emergency department departure status in patients with shortness of breath. *Emerg Med Australas* 2010; 22: 21–29.
64. Banzett RB, Howell MD, O'Donnell CR, *et al.* Dyspnea prevalence and risk of adverse event in a general hospital population. *Am J Respir Crit Care Med* 2013; 187: A2508.
65. Aktas A. Cancer symptom clusters: current concepts and controversies. *Curr Opin Support Palliat Care* 2013; 7: 38–44.
66. Miaskowski C, Dodd M, Lee K. Symptom clusters: the new frontier in symptom management research. *J Natl Cancer Inst Monogr* 2004; 17–21.
67. Dong ST, Costa DS, Butow PN, *et al.* Symptom clusters in advanced cancer patients: an empirical comparison of statistical methods and the impact on quality of life. *J Pain Symptom Manage* 2016; 51: 88–98.
68. Kirkova J, Aktas A, Walsh D, *et al.* Cancer symptom clusters: clinical and research methodology. *J Palliat Med* 2011; 14: 1149–1166.
69. Aktas A, Walsh D, Rybicki L. Symptom clusters: myth or reality? *Palliat Med* 2010; 24: 373–385.
70. Dong ST, Butow PN, Costa DS, *et al.* Symptom clusters in patients with advanced cancer: a systematic review of observational studies. *J Pain Symptom Manage* 2014; 48: 411–450.
71. Chan CW, Richardson A, Richardson J. A study to assess the existence of the symptom cluster of breathlessness, fatigue and anxiety in patients with advanced lung cancer. *Eur J Oncol Nurs* 2005; 9: 325–333.
72. Addington-Hall J, Fakhoury W, McCarthy M. Specialist palliative care in nonmalignant disease. *Palliat Med* 1998; 12: 417–427.
73. Bausewein C, Daveson B, Benalia H, *et al.* Outcome Measurement in Palliative Care. The Essentials. Milan, European Association for Palliative Care, 2011. www.eapcnet.eu/LinkClick.aspx?fileticket=-T62WTgTHtU%3D&tabid=1577

Disclosures: D.C. Currow is an unpaid advisory board member for Helsinn Pharmaceuticals. He is also a paid consultant and received payment for intellectual property with Mayne Pharma, and is a consultant with Specialised Therapeutics Australia Pty Ltd.

Chapter 6

The construct of breathlessness

Sara Booth[1] and Robert Lansing[2]

We will discuss the "construct for breathlessness" in its broadest sense to reflect the fact that breathlessness is a symptom indirectly measured and highly dependent upon a complex combination of physical sensations, thoughts, perceptions, cultural conditioning and emotional states. We will consider our progress in obtaining a common scientific understanding as well as developing a working "construct" in its clinical management. Definitions and descriptions of breathlessness have focused mostly on how clinicians and scientists understand this symptom to the neglect of formulations directly related to the implementation of clinical management and relief. We consider the need to relate the language and findings of clinical and laboratory research to the patient's need to understand and respond to their own experience of breathlessness. To this end, we will consider the diversity and evolving concepts of the nature of the symptom in the scientific community and the practicalities of applying these to patients, particularly those faced with a lifetime of suffering.

Julius Comroe, the eminent cardiologist, showed great prescience when he stated that breathlessness "involves both the perception of the sensation by the patient and his reaction to it…" [1]. This insight remains the foundation of the current clinical management of chronic, refractory breathlessness in advanced disease. It may even be called a "construct of breathlessness".

It is now more usual to express this original construct as the importance of managing both the perceptual and affective dimensions of the symptom. Paying attention to these aspects of care is recognised as crucial in reducing the impact of breathlessness, thus improving the quality of life not only of those who suffer from breathlessness but also of those closest to them. The lives of those close to someone affected by breathlessness are also profoundly constrained, both emotionally and physically, by the symptom. Breathlessness is now recognised as a complex experience of the mind and body [2], with wide-ranging, damaging effects on everyone connected to the person living with it.

When Comroe defined breathlessness, he was speaking at the first symposium on the symptom in 1965 [1]. This was convened with the purpose of bringing together general medical clinicians and scientists to improve understanding of this disabling, often invisible, symptom [3]. Although it quickly focused on pathophysiology, this landmark meeting laid

---

[1]Cambridge University Hospitals NHS Foundation Trust, Cambridge, UK. [2]Beth Israel Deaconess Medical Center, Boston, MA, USA.

Correspondence: Sara Booth, Box 63, Elsworth House, Cambridge University Hospitals NHS Foundation Trust, Hills Road, Cambridge CB2 2OO, UK. E-mail: sb628@cam.ac.uk

 Print ISBN: 978-1-84984-071-2. Online ISBN: 978-1-84984-072-9. Print ISSN: 2312-508X. Online ISSN: 2312-5098.

a foundation for the progress that has been made in the last 50 years in understanding not only the causes but also the consequences of this devastating symptom. It also represented recognition that the effective investigation and management of breathlessness required clinicians and scientists from a range of disciplines and backgrounds to work together.

Palliative care was not a specialty at this time. Healthcare systems did not recognise the need to care actively for people who were dying or had symptomatic advanced disease. Cicely Saunders was the pioneer in this field and had been working to develop her ideas into a coherent philosophy that could be translated into clinical care. Effective symptom control was at its heart, and the first modern hospice, St Christopher's in south London, UK, opened in 1967, 2 years after the breathlessness symposium [4, 5]. It became a place where research into symptom control was supported: one of the first clinical trials in the management of breathlessness was carried out there, led by Abe Guz, who had been at that first meeting [6].

Much of the work recognising the immensely distressing impact of breathlessness has been carried out in palliative care. Increasingly, however, "advanced disease clinics", encompassing symptom relief, are being set up in departments of respiratory medicine and cardiology (N. Smallwood, Royal Melbourne Hospital, Parkville, Australia; personal communication). Recently, statements from the heart of academic respiratory medicine have called for palliative care to be provided for patients with respiratory disease [7], and for breathlessness to be named the "first vital symptom" that should be measured in every patient [8, 9]. It seems to us that this is a propitious time to review the breadth and depth of the applications of Comroe's construct, and to understand any need for its further development to make it useful to those with an interest in shortness of breath, particularly patients and families.

It is clear to us that any useful construct of breathlessness must resonate with clinicians and scientists in the ward, clinic and laboratory, and with those engaged in psychosocial research; in other words, it must have "face validity". We have interpreted this brief quite widely using historical as well as contemporary ideas of breathlessness, highlighting areas that we consider need further examination, without reviewing them fully. The complex effects of breathlessness, its assessment, general management, the personal experience of living with it and other related areas, are well described and are reviewed in detail elsewhere in this issue of the *Monograph*.

A useful construct should synthesise the latest research and best historical thinking on this subject. We name under-researched aspects of breathlessness that offer opportunities to make significant contributions to our understanding and management of the symptom. We will discuss the diversity and range of the construct's many possible applications and the special difficulties in relating ideas and findings from different fields, particularly between scientific research and clinical care.

Comroe's early insight remains critically important: that the way an individual patient reacts to his or her experience of breathlessness is central to its severity. We would now understand that this reaction can be modified. Help is often necessary, using approaches that stem from a growing understanding of the genesis of breathlessness and the evidence accumulating in the arts and sciences of central nervous system functioning, psychology, the humanities and physical activity.

Diversity of application

The most widely accepted current definition of pathological breathlessness defines it as "A subjective experience of breathing discomfort that consists of qualitatively distinct sensations that vary in intensity. The experience derives from interactions among multiple physiologic, psychological, social and environmental factors and may induce secondary physiological and behavioural responses" [10]. This has served the science of breathlessness well but cannot, and was not intended to, form a construct of breathlessness that meets patients' and families' needs for greater understanding of the symptom. It may also be of limited application in the fields of philosophy and the other humanities [11]; it does not consider life before breathlessness.

Patients often seek help outside mainstream medicine, as they may receive little support with managing this all-encompassing symptom. Any construct would ideally be comprehensible in all spheres of society so that everyone can understand the difficulties of living with chronic breathlessness, a symptom without the social notoriety of pain. Greater general understanding of breathlessness could reduce the social isolation and guilt that many with the symptom experience. It is not uncommon for patients, particularly smokers, to demonstrate a feeling of being unworthy or undeserving of help, feeling that they have brought the symptom on themselves.

Health service managers have a profound impact on the likelihood of effective management of the breathless patient, so the construct needs to speak to this constituency too. We therefore hope that any general construct can be of use to people from any background who live with the symptom, or who wish to investigate it or help others manage it.

A general construct of breathlessness used by investigators and clinicians in their many separate fields can provide both a shared language and methodologies of assessing breathlessness. It will facilitate the integration of information and promote the cross-fertilisation of ideas developed in various specialties, both of which are aspirations of the American Thoracic Society statement [10] and the original symposium [1]. A continuing challenge is to relate the findings and ideas developed in special fields, for example those obtained with healthy subjects in the special conditions of the laboratory with those obtained from patients in clinical settings. In what ways are these similar or different? Is breathlessness from chest strapping in the laboratory a good model of breathlessness in restrictive lung disease [12, 13]?

It is important to recognise the limitations of our current construct and to view it as still evolving. It must be able to accommodate corrections and incorporate new findings and ideas. Variations and modifications will emerge from the special requirements of these separate fields: different populations, experimental manipulations, ways of measuring breathlessness and new theoretical approaches. New or apparently novel ideas and findings, given time to develop, could be of value and later incorporated into a general construct.

Assessing breathlessness by the patient's report: the *sine qua non* of the construct of breathlessness

Descriptions

For too long, patients' reports of breathlessness were unheard or overlooked [14], possibly because clinicians' uncertainties about how to treat the symptom discouraged them from eliciting it or "noticing" it in patients' stories. Unlike pain, breathlessness has not been frequently and consistently assessed, in spite of evidence that it is a better predictor of clinical outcomes than other parameters [15]. It seems to us that the patients' reports of the private experience of breathing discomfort are the core of any breathlessness construct. As their reports are available to us primarily through language (conversations, interviews and questionnaires), our present construct has developed largely through a better understanding of the words and expressions used to describe it. Inferring breathlessness from observation of breathing behaviour is now being studied [16, 17] but still requires verbal reports for validation.

The transition from simple terms, such as "breathlessness" and "shortness of breath", to our present understanding of the several dimensions of the experience has largely been through the systematic study of patients' own words in relation to physiological and clinical states, using sophisticated statistical methods to analyse their frequency and grouping [18–21]. These studies have shown a remarkable similarity in their use among diverse groups and populations, in spite of cultural and individual differences, and form the basis of our conversation with subjects, as well as our professional interactions. Chest tightness, air hunger and increased work of breathing (or their synonyms) have emerged as the most common descriptors used. Their relationship to physiological stimuli and respiratory pathology provides a working framework for current research and clinical management. Combining these descriptions of breathlessness with quantitative measures such as questionnaires and rating scales has permitted the systematic study of the quality and intensity of these perceptions.

Assessment tools

For many years, there was no assessment tool for breathlessness of any aetiology, only disease-specific quality-of-life tools. This meant that palliative care clinicians, who see patients with any illness, had no accurate way of gauging the impact of their interventions or understanding the course of an individual's symptom. Single-dimension rating scales, such as the Borg scale, VASs and NRSs, have been the quantitative tools responsible for forming the present construct of breathlessness (covered in another chapter of this *Monograph* [22]).

Recently, two additional instruments for the measurement of breathlessness in clinical practice (Dyspnoea-12) and in clinical research and laboratory settings (the MDP) have been validated, as described elsewhere [23, 24]. These developments represent a major advance in both enhancing communication between patients and clinicians and enabling the completion of good clinical and laboratory research. Both tools encapsulate Comroe's construct of understanding the sensory and affective dimensions of the symptom.

Assessment and prognosis

The prognostic importance of breathlessness for longer-term survival has been known for some time [15]: now the availability of the MDP has enabled researchers to demonstrate that it is also related to short-term prognosis [25]. This increasing recognition that the severity of an individual's breathlessness gives a better indication of their prognosis than other measurable variables, such as lung function [26–28], gives additional weight to Comroe's interpretation of breathlessness as linked to outcome. Predictive tools are available for accurately establishing the short and longer term prognostic implications of the state of being breathless (covered in another chapter of this *Monograph* [29]). This will help clinicians to understand the importance of assessing breathlessness and patients to understand the importance of personally actively managing their disease [30]. It is clear that patients do not always understand that breathlessness is a serious long-term symptom until they are severely disabled. People with poorly managed breathlessness make extensive and often futile use of medical services; this may bring the symptom higher up the list of managerial priorities in a way that descriptions of individual suffering have not. All health systems are keen to reduce unscheduled use of services, particularly admissions to hospitals and attendances at EDs. The communication with a patient about breathlessness will be distinct from that with a colleague in another medical specialty, or with a scientist or a manager; the language needs to be chosen to give the message the best chance of being heard.

Some work in progress

Many different aspects of our understanding of breathlessness are still developing and are in need of further investigation. A few of these are discussed below.

Qualities of the experience

The present general agreement that there are three distinct qualities of breathlessness, "air hunger", "work and effort" and "tightness", is based on population studies of diverse groups using statistical clustering and factor analysis [31, 32]. These terms and their synonyms are selected by both healthy people and patients, with air hunger being the most prominent. Yet people in these groups also described their experience with a variety of other words and expressions, some of which may be unique to a culture or individual [33]. As many different sensory inputs are activated together in normal and pathological breathing, and their separate contributions are not well understood, the present classification is subject to extension and refinement. Individual patients, through experience, have become sensitive to many changes in their breathing that are not revealed in population studies, yet their verbal descriptions may be useful in their clinical management. We still cannot currently link descriptors of chronic breathlessness reliably to discrete pathologies [34, 35], although "chest tightness" is always linked to asthma. Future studies may find apparently idiosyncratic descriptions to be common to certain clinical conditions. The construct of breathlessness will be enriched by continued studies of the variety of verbal descriptions available to patients and carers.

Intensity of the experience

At one time, doctors did not recognise the range of possible individual responses and some talked (some still do) about "disproportionate breathlessness" [36], because it was not understood that a defined level of disease severity (commonly measured by pulmonary function tests) did not equate to a consistent level of breathlessness in different individuals. Breathlessness severity has been shown to correlate better with prognosis than lung function in those with COPD [15], the general population [26] and other disease groups [27]. In carefully selected individuals given lung volume reduction surgery, only 50% are significantly improved symptomatically, in spite of increases of lung function of 25% of more [37]. This suggests the need to study the contribution of many factors other than lung function to the intensity of the symptom, such as a patient's general health (both psychological and physical) and their social support, health beliefs and cultural influences. Breathlessness may well correlate better with mortality because it represents the cumulative impact of a number of individual characteristics. The relative contribution of different qualities of breathlessness to its overall intensity, as measured on a single-dimension scale, is also in need of further study [31, 38].

Accessing the experience

Our evolving construct depends on the way an individual's private experience is accessed and interpreted in their interaction with the investigator or clinician. What we tell them and what they tell us in our continuing dialogue is at the heart of all our efforts to understand and relieve their discomfort. The nature of this interaction in relation to patient compliance and treatment outcomes needs more study. Bridging the gap between the patient's and clinician's separate understanding of the symptom is especially important where communication is difficult, as in palliative care. There are a number of barriers to communication because of problems such as fatigue, cognitive deficits, somnolence, being on a ventilator or language difficulties. This may require the development of new ways for patients to rate and express their breathlessness, perhaps including picture scales [39], or hand or facial gestures, as well as a better understanding of the relationship of observed signs (*e.g.* respiratory, postural, facial) to breathlessness.

As important as the present validated measures are in providing uniformity and comparisons across studies, there may still be a need to extend them to groups or situations quite different from those used in the validation [31, 40]. The history of the most widely used measures of breathlessness and pain (*e.g.* Borg scale, McGill pain questionnaire) shows that they have been modified and supplemented to meet such needs.

Individual differences

The personal differences that can influence a person's ratings or verbal reports of breathlessness are still poorly understood, such as differences in stoicism, sensitivity and somatisation (*i.e.* the expression of distress through bodily sensations and symptoms, common in those who have had traumatic early life experiences). There is evidence that individuals can vary widely in their interpretation and use of validated rating scales [41]. These variations might be revealed with the use of systematic debriefings and studies of the effect of instructions on the use of rating scales.

Situational differences

There is a need to continue to understand the relationship between laboratory studies of breathlessness and the "real life" experiences: in what ways are they similar or different [42]? The former allows the control necessary to separate and understand the various contributions to the experience but cannot duplicate the results of a patient's altering their behaviour to reduce their discomfort. A good example of these difficulties is comparing the results of imaging studies with their necessary constraints to life situations [43–45]. Those in a laboratory know that the experience of breathlessness will end and that it has no relationship to an underlying disease, which may be life threatening. They do not experience the interaction of their family's response to their breathlessness. In the laboratory situation, breathlessness is expected and the atmosphere is calm. Nonetheless, those who have experienced extreme "air hunger" under laboratory conditions have reported that they found the experience unbearable.

Opportunities for exploration

There are a number of areas in which we need a better understanding of breathlessness in its biological and psychophysiological context. Some of these are discussed below.

Role of systemic inflammation and ageing

Chronic, systemic inflammation is now linked to many disease and symptom states where it was not recognised previously, such as schizophrenia, depression, cardiovascular disease, COPD and cancer. The degree of inflammation measured as the level of a simple acute-phase protein (C-reactive protein) may be a reliable guide to prognosis in these illnesses [46], as well as in more obviously inflammatory illness such as the vasculitides.

It is sometimes uncertain whether chronic inflammation is a cause of ill-health or an effect [47]. It is well established that an individual's emotional status can affect and be affected by chronic inflammation, and it is clear that inflammation worsens symptom severity in, for example, pain. This work has not yet been carried out in breathlessness or extensively in respiratory medicine, although its importance has been suggested [48, 49]. It is interesting to note that "accelerated ageing" from an imbalance of the inflammatory response ("imflammaging" [50]) or abnormal activation of the inflammatory response is now considered important in many apparently diverse areas of medicine, such as depression [46], schizophrenia [51] and cardiovascular disease [52], as well the ageing process itself [50], and in many symptoms, such as cachexia [53] and pain [54]. Age-related changes in a patient's response to breathlessness are especially important in palliative care. Promoting healthy ageing as well as active disease management is now recognised to require a multidimensional approach, encompassing attention to diet, psychological approaches that enhance a sense of agency and resilience [55], and the promotion of physical and mental exercise.

Understanding the placebo effect

Benedetti and co-workers [56, 57] considered the study of the placebo effect to be contiguous with "studying the psychosocial context around the patient" at the time of the treatment, and that "it is a psychobiological phenomenon that can be attributable to different mechanisms, including expectation of clinical improvement and Pavlovian conditioning".

As we understand that shortness of breath is generated in the central nervous system and influenced and conditioned by psychological, social and environmental factors, it becomes obvious that it is essential to understand and utilise the placebo effect when trying to maximise the impact of the few treatments that there are for breathlessness. It also makes it easier to understand why the "way treatments are delivered" is central to their effectiveness [58]. The ability of any of the current treatments to reduce breathlessness can probably be enhanced by understanding the principles that produce and enhance the placebo effect: these include the importance of social reinforcement, information about demonstrated effectiveness and positive feedback for any success [59].

This effect may be particularly important for non-pharmacological treatments. An example is use of a hand-held fan to relieve breathlessness. This is one of the central management strategies used by the Cambridge Breathlessness Intervention Service (BIS). This cheap, portable, safe, everyday piece of equipment has the potential to increase self-efficacy, encourage exercise and reduce anxiety by increasing the internal locus of control of breathless patients. Its very strengths may also be its weaknesses, as it is not a drug and does not look like a sophisticated piece of medical equipment. It can only be transformed into this if explanations of the most effective ways for it to be used are given by a convinced clinician. The evidence of its efficacy needs to be cited [60, 61] and a demonstration given: the art of medicine needs to be employed [62]. In a longitudinal study of patients with COPD who were not advised about the use of the fan, it added nothing to standard care [63].

The many likely mechanisms and the impact and effective use of the placebo effect need urgent investigation. It is clear from pain research that placebos may exert their analgesic effects through the same spinal pathways involved in pain relief by opioid therapy [64, 65]. These effects are likely to be at least as useful as the few drugs available for breathlessness palliation and much safer in those with chronic conditions, who may live for many years.

Evolutionary role of the perception of breathlessness

Most of our life-sustaining physiological systems continue automatically, without any indication of change reaching consciousness. Breathlessness is controlled both voluntarily and automatically. The needed behavioural responses require perceptual and cognitive processes that are dependent on cortical structures. Changes in breathlessness are also often linked to a feeling, such as fear, joy or anxiety. Damasio and Carvalho [66] postulated that "the addition of a felt experiential component to sensory mapped body afferent signals emerged and prevailed in evolution because of the benefits it conferred on life regulation" and that "felt experiences permit more flexible and effective corrective measures than somatic mapping alone, especially in the realm of complex behaviour". The authors suggested that an accompanying feeling could be of evolutionary advantage in that it gives a necessary motivational edge to experiences that require adaptive changes in behaviour to correct homeostatic imbalances. They postulated that it may be helpful to regard chronic breathlessness (and pain) as "pathologies of feeling" in trying to develop more effective treatment strategies. This interpretation of breathlessness lends support to the use of complex interventions in treatment [58, 67]. It is noticeable that patients in the Cambridge BIS evaluation stated that "the way the intervention was delivered", and thus the feelings evoked by the treatment strategies, was important in its success [58].

Neuroscience research is delineating in more detail the contributions of different areas of the brain to the sensation of breathlessness. Recent work has demonstrated that separate parts of the periaqueductal grey matter may be responsible for different aspects of the complex feeling, with one area subserving the intensity of the sensation and one anticipating it [68]. Progress in our understanding of the biological-evolutionary role of breathlessness will require research strategies relating human brain studies of the possible substrates of breathlessness with animal studies of similar neural systems. Of great advantage would be the development of animal models similar to those used successfully in studying pain. This is discussed further in another chapter in this *Monograph* [69]. Behavioural techniques using operant or conditioned learning techniques still need to be developed, perhaps in collaboration with workers in veterinary science for whom animal breathlessness is a major concern [70, 71]. Such behavioural techniques may also be applicable in assessing and control of breathlessness in noncommunicative patients.

Breathing practice as a way to better general physical and psychological health

There has been a recent rediscovery in the west of ancient Eastern traditions of breathing training, martial arts and yoga movement, and interest in their possible relationship to improved health [72, 73]. Research into mindfulness-based stress reduction and cognitive therapy is growing rapidly, and some evidence strongly suggests that it can have an equal impact to standard drug therapy regimens in preventing relapse in severe depression [74] and that it may be beneficial in other conditions in helping to improve the quality of life. There is also evidence to suggest that "yoga breathing" can have beneficial effects on oxygen saturation and general health in those with severe heart failure [75, 76]. There is very little discussion, and much less research, on any potential for these ideas to help severe breathlessness in advanced disease, and any construct of breathlessness needs to encompass future evidence and understanding in these areas.

Our construct in action: patient-centred symptom management

A scientific analysis of the construct of breathlessness is a sterile academic exercise if divorced from the human need from which it arose. The two essential questions of "What do we know about it?" and "What do we do about it?" cannot be separated. Our understanding of the many aspects of breathlessness should guide our management of the symptom, but our success in this depends largely on the active participation of the patient.

As in all good medical practice, an interactive rather than a didactic clinician-to-patient approach will help us make patients collaborators in their care, rather than passive recipients. To some extent, this ideal "standard of practice" is followed in many facilities and institutions. There may still be a need for formal training and investigation of this collaborative process because it is so important in long-term care of chronic breathlessness. The following are just three examples of directions this might take.

Understanding and changing a patient's "personal construct" of breathlessness

According to the psychotherapeutic theory of "personal construct", developed by George Kelly [77, 78], a person's mental construct is the lens through which they see the world: understanding it, explaining events and making predictions about it. These can be changed or corrected by further experiences and by getting new information. The individual is seen as continually testing, modifying and enlarging this view. Although clinicians may use our current conception of breathlessness to help the patient cope with the symptom, the patient comes with his or her own "personal construct" of breathlessness. This is based on what they have learned during their life and from many other sources during the course of their treatment (which may have lasted years), as well as being derived from their experiences with their disease. This forms the basis for their way of living and coping with breathlessness, but may also consist of misinformation and making intuitive but counterproductive responses, or responding to conflicting advice from different clinicians. The ability of people to revise and enlarge their personal construct makes it likely that clinicians and caretakers can reshape the patient's understanding of their symptom, thereby helping them participate more effectively in its management. Clinicians' personal constructs of breathlessness need to be similarly informed.

The translation of the formal elements of our scientific construct into a form that is helpful to a patient is an important part of this process. Thought must be given to creating scripts that can be used, tested and revised, such as the following:

> Chronic breathlessness, the shortness of breath you feel when you have an illness that cannot be cured, is very different from the sensation you feel when you are healthy and run up a hill, or swim, or do something athletic or joyful. This shortness of breath has no happy associations; it is often frightening, upsetting and very disabling. It is also stressful for those closest to us: they want to help but don't know how to. It is usual to feel anxious, even panicky, when you feel breathless. Often those closest to you will feel helpless, and sometimes frightened, when you are having a bad attack of breathlessness.
>
> We feel frightened because our bodies are programmed, like a machine, to need to breathe. This drive to breathe is very strong for all of us, and not being able to breathe properly is associated with very serious anxiety, caused by our brains trying to put things right. Being short of breath is so horrible that often we try to avoid it by resting; this makes our muscles weak and we become unfit. We will get more and more breathless if we simply rest all the time, trying to avoid being short of breath.
>
> We know now, from medical research, that we need to use both our muscles and our minds to improve our own shortness of breath when we are ill. We need to change our behaviour and react differently to being breathless. We can alter the way we feel about breathlessness, making it less frightening and restricting. Changes in the way we feel can be as powerful as a drug in helping our illness improve. We often need help from other people to change our reactions to being breathless and to start to feel less frightened by it.

This may be the beginnings of a construct for patients, families and lay people affected by breathlessness or trying to help someone who is. These are therapeutic tools that, to the best of our knowledge, have not been studied or exploited in the management of breathlessness.

Understanding and interrupting the spiral of disability

The benefits for health of exercise and a nonsedentary lifestyle are becoming irrefutable, with evidence from all areas of medicine, even in those with advanced disease [79]. Breathlessness research is rich in studies that demonstrate that "deconditioned muscles" have a different structure to those that are exercised regularly, leading to the earlier onset of lactic acidosis and leg fatigue on walking. This "breathlessness→rest→deconditioning→more breathless at lower levels of exertion" has been called the "spiral of disability" (figure 1).

By the time many patients have advanced disease, this downward spiral is well established and difficult to reverse. Those close to a breathless person may instinctively feel that it is better for them to rest, particularly when breathlessness is so unpleasant. It was also customary, until relatively recently, for doctors to advise bed-rest for many conditions (*e.g.* myocardial infarction, back pain, following surgery, during and after cancer treatment) where early mobilisation and increased activity is now favoured. Cultural changes within medicine, and the rationale for them, need to be communicated more effectively to the general population and specifically to the breathless patient.

Medical advice to exercise, including exercise prescriptions and exhortations for the continuance of activity after pulmonary rehabilitation, is generally ineffective. We believe that the science of behaviour change, for example the use of motivational interviewing [80] and the use of psychological interventions [81], needs more investigation in the context of advanced disease. Clinicians need to know how to discern which methods to use for each individual to help them to mobilise and continue to be active in a way that enhances their quality of life, harnessing the support of family members who may otherwise remain sceptical. An example of this is the system used in the Cambridge BIS [82] called

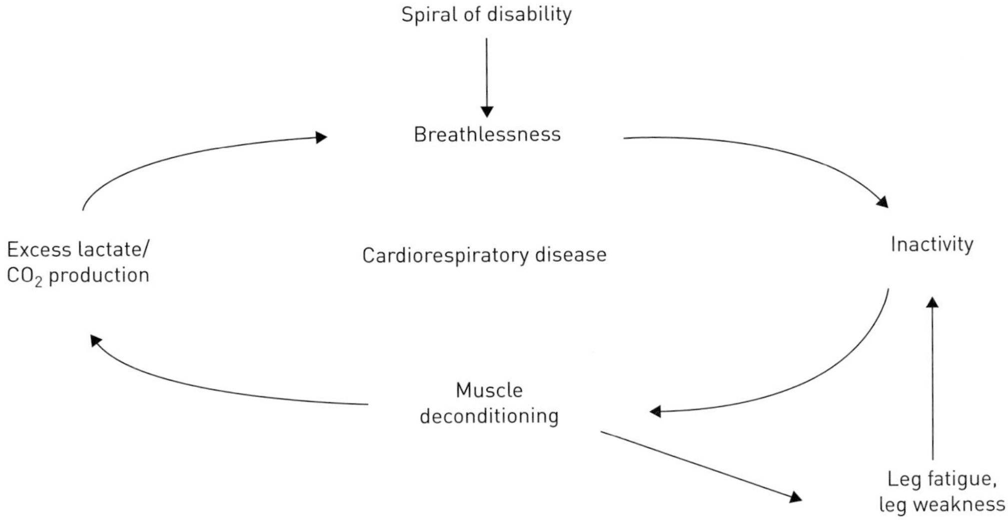

Figure 1. The "spiral of disability".

"Breathing, Thinking, Functioning" for linking non-pharmacological treatments to specific aspects of pathophysiology that may be causing or worsening breathlessness (figure 2). At the initial assessment, the clinician seeing the patient (and carer) will assess which "vicious circle" is the strongest driver of breathlessness (in most people, all the spirals operate to some degree) and target their initial treatment strategy towards overcoming this.

Breathing cycle

Patients for whom this cycle predominates have dysfunctional breathing patterns, and breathing retraining and other interventions that target breathing control may be most useful.

Thinking cycle

People for whom this cycle predominates have unhelpful beliefs or previously unpleasant experiences, or sometimes even a single "trigger event" that has coloured their thoughts and feelings about breathlessness. Giving them correct information about what generates, or will help, shortness of breath, such as correcting the impression that because breathlessness feels so awful it is important to avoid it, will help avoid deconditioning.

Functioning cycle

When patients have become very inactive, their muscles need to be reconditioned, so helping them to become active again, perhaps with the use of mobility aids, is the priority.

The "Breathing, Thinking, Functioning" diagram (figure 2) has been used with great success with patients by providing a rationale for the institution of certain treatment approaches and increasing concordance (A. Spathis, Cambridge BIS, Cambridge, UK; personal communication). We would urge that the preliminary work done in the area of personalised medicine in people with advanced disease is built upon, so that patients and carers are offered treatment with a high likelihood of success [83].

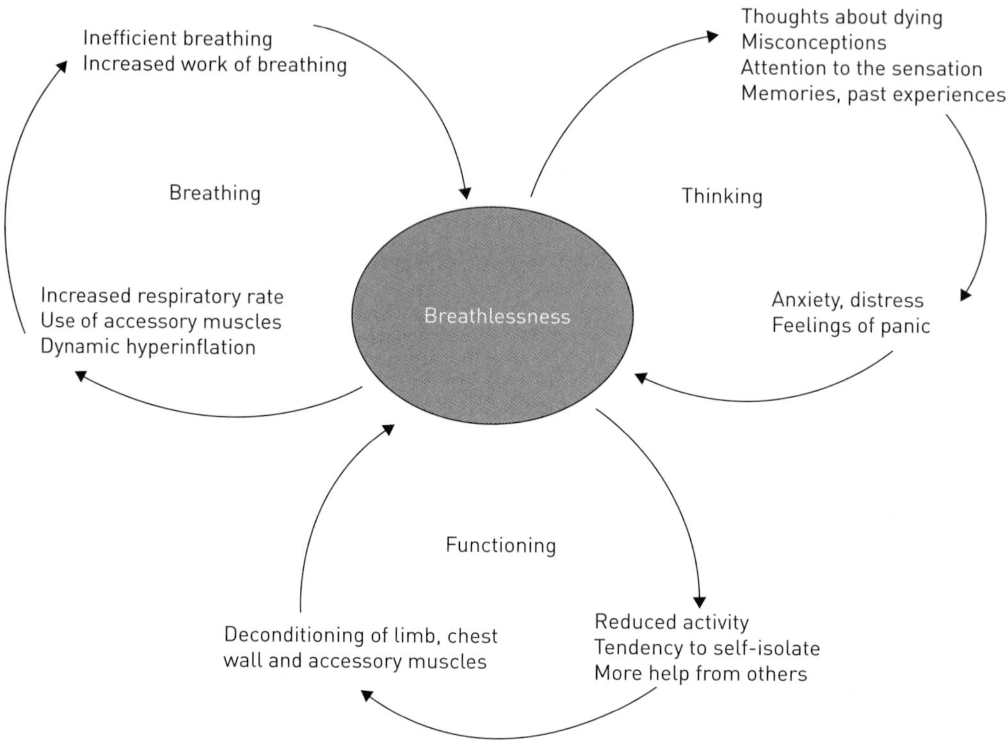

Figure 2. The "Breathing, Thinking, Functioning" diagram used by the Cambridge Breathlessness Intervention Service. ©2014 Cambridge Breathlessness Intervention Service.

Providing evidence of non-pharmacological and lifestyle interventions

Patients may be told, on enquiring about any one of a range of non-pharmacological interventions, that "There is no evidence for it." In breathlessness work, this is often due to a lack of research on that particular question. This may be because it is difficult to look for reliable evidence in non-pharmacological treatments due to the complexities and uncertainties of investigating diet, psychological strategies, and social and societal interventions. There are, however, at least three interpretations of this statement, applicable in a number of situations, and these interpretations of the same phrase have quite different meanings.

There may be no evidence because no evidence has been sought and there are no trials in this area. There may be no evidence because good trials have been done and they have shown that the intervention (using current investigative techniques) is not supported by evidence. "There is no evidence" can also mean that the available evidence is equivocal or incomplete.

In these circumstances, doctors and other clinicians must make a distinction between these three states of evidence and be prepared to guide patients, taking into account evidence from across the whole medical, psychological and basic science fields, taking advice where necessary, and giving a rationale for their recommendation, particularly bearing in mind the patient's goals. The patient may accept or reject the advice given.

Simply saying that "there is no evidence", or failing to make a recommendation in a difficult area, leaves the patient isolated in trying to make sense of conflicting or absent evidence.

For example, the authors in one textbook of respiratory medicine were not prepared to support the use of a fan in breathlessness in 2012 "because there is no evidence" [84]. In fact, this safe, cheap, self-efficacy-promoting intervention had a rationale based on work in normal volunteers, some possible physiological mechanisms, a clinical trial [6] and the likelihood of it being helpful psychologically. It also has no adverse effects. Given these facts, it would seem a reasonable approach to support the use of a fan while further investigation is completed. The balance towards using or not using an intervention would be the other way if the approach was hazardous.

Although there is no definitive evidence in diet, nutritional supplementation, psychosocial care, and some psychological or complementary interventions, we can suggest what is likely to be most helpful without being dogmatic, and emphasising the need to keep an open mind, using evidence from other specialties, where appropriate. We should be in a better position to help people make decisions in areas of uncertainty than people trying to find their way around the internet. Instead of saying "don't google this", help people to find the two or three good papers or sites with evidence on breathlessness if they want to look at the evidence themselves. It may be possibly in the future to "personalise medicine" using a more systematic approach including genomic data [83].

Conclusion

The time for nihilism in the management of breathlessness is past, although this distressing and disabling symptom remains an enigma in many ways [85]. The increased numbers of people involved in breathlessness research and the variety of backgrounds from which they come give hope that very significant progress may soon be made in reducing the impact of shortness of breath on the lives of those affected. It is astonishing that a symptom that affects millions, possibly billions, of people across the world, and that is going to become more common as COPD, lung cancer, ischaemic heart disease and asbestosis continue to rise in incidence, has been relatively invisible until recently.

The most effective treatments currently available depend on the individual affected by the symptom changing their reaction to this instinctively terrifying sensation. Sufferers primarily have to train themselves to use their minds [86] and their muscles [87] to overcome the many limitations that shortness of breath imposes on them and those closest to them. Like many with chronic illness, they need to develop more inner resources than those fortunate enough to be healthy. They are often given no help to do this complex task. They are required to understand, modify and then harness their thoughts, feelings, learned responses and cultural beliefs to overcome the unpleasantness of breathlessness. This is no small task.

Many clinicians who look after patients with diseases associated with shortness of breath underrate its importance and severity, or remain uncertain about how to manage it, and therefore avoid it. They do not actively elicit the sensation [8], leaving patients to manage as best they can alone. This may soon be seen as completely unacceptable practice.

One of the barriers to effective management is that our current construct of symptom management is still focused on finding a single effective drug therapy that will reverse the sensation in everyone, without the necessity for behavioural change. In pain, a sensation that is in many ways similar neurophysiologically and about which there is much more research, this has not been possible This focus on finding a single therapy distracts clinicians and scientists from exploiting the effective therapies that do exist, including exercise, the placebo effect [88, 89], psychological interventions, the hand-held fan and other non-pharmacological approaches [91–92], and from trying to advance methodologies for studying complex and non-pharmacological interventions [93]. They have forgotten Comroe.

We believe that Comroe's original construct of breathlessness has not yet been surpassed for its pithy summary of what patients need to know from their clinicians and what they can be helped to achieve by an interested, informed clinical team who are abreast of the research in a very complex area, albeit summed up by Comroe's few words: "...dyspnoea is difficult, laboured, uncomfortable breathing; it is an unpleasant type of breathing, though it is not painful in the usual sense of the word. It is subjective and, like pain, it involves both perception of the sensation by the patient and his reaction to the sensation." [1]

If clinicians are going to be effective in helping patients manage their "reaction to the sensation" and scientists are to increase our understanding of it, both must look beyond simple, single-pronged approaches. Shortness of breath and an individual's reaction to it involve many different physical sensations, affected by cognitions, beliefs, motivation, and social and cultural influences. Clinicians must embrace a construct that harnesses patients' creativity and imagination to use every resource (both internal and external) available to them, many of which have no financial but significant personal cost, to defer the onset of breathlessness and, when it becomes inevitable, live the best life possible in company with this complex and remorseless symptom.

References

1. Comroe JH Jr. Some theories of the mechanisms of dyspnoea. *In*: Howell JBL, Campbell EJM, eds. Breathlessness. Oxford, Blackwell Scientific, 1966; pp. 1–5.
2. Booth S, Moosavi S, Higginson IJ. The etiology and management of intractable breathlessness in patients with advanced cancer: a systematic review of pharmacological therapy. *Nat Clin Pract Oncol* 2008; 5: 90–100.
3. Gysels M, Higginson IJ. Access to services for patients with chronic obstructive pulmonary disease: the invisibility of breathlessness. *J Pain Symptom Manage* 2008; 36: 451–460.
4. Clark D. Cicely Saunders. Founder of the Modern Hospice Movement. Selected Letters 1949–1999. Oxford, Oxford University Press, 2005.
5. Clark D. 2014. Early Origins of St Christopher's Hospice. http://endoflifestudies.academicblogs.co.uk/early-origins-of-st-christophers-hospice/ Date last updated: June 19, 2014. Date last accessed: April 2016.
6. Booth S, Kelly M, Cox NPG. Does oxygen help dyspnea in cancer patients? *Am J Respir Crit Care Med* 1996; 153: 1515–1518.
7. Brown CE, Jecker NS, Randall Curtis J. Inadequate palliative care in chronic lung disease. An issue of health care inequality. *Ann Am Thorac Soc* 2016; 13: 311–316.
8. Banzett RB, O'Donnell D. Should we measure dyspnea in everyone? *Eur Respir J* 2014; 43: 1547–1550.
9. Currow DC, Johnson MJ. Distilling the essence of breathlessness – the first vital symptom. *Eur Respir J* 2015; 45: 1526–1528.
10. Parshall MA, Schwartzstein R, Adams L, *et al.* An official American Thoracic Society Statement: update on the mechanisms, assessment, and management of dyspnea. *Am J Respir Crit Care Med* 2012; 185: 435–452.
11. Carel H. Illness (The Art of Living). London, Routledge, 2008.
12. Scano G, Innocenti-Bruni G, Stendardi L. Do obstructive and restrictive lung diseases share common underlying mechanisms of breathlessness? *Respir Med* 2010; 104: 925–933.
13. Faisal A, Alghamdi BJ, Ciavaglia CE, *et al.* Common mechanisms of dyspnea in chronic interstitial and obstructive lung disorders. *Am J Respir Crit Care Med* 2016; 193: 299–309.
14. Roberts DK, Thorne SE, Pearson C. The experience of dyspnea in late stage cancer: patients' and nurses' perspectives. *Cancer Nurs* 1993; 16: 310–320.

15. Nishimura K, Izumi T, Tsukino M, *et al.* Dyspnea is a better predictor of 5-year survival than airway obstruction in patients with COPD. *Chest* 2002; 121: 1434–1440.
16. Campbell ML. Caring for dying patients in the intensive care unit: managing pain, dyspnea, anxiety, delirium, and death rattle. *AACN Adv Crit Care* 2015; 26: 110–120.
17. Persichini R, Gay F, Schnidt M, *et al.* Diagnostic accuracy of respiratory distress observation scales as surrogates of dyspnea self-report in intensive care unit patients. *Anesthesiology* 2015; 123: 830–837.
18. Simon PM, Schwartzstein RM, Weiss JW, *et al.* Distinguishable types of dyspnea in patients with shortness of breath. *Am Rev Respir Dis* 1990; 142: 1009–1014.
19. Elliott MW, Adams L, Cockcroft A, *et al.* The language of breathlessness. Use of verbal descriptors by patients with cardiopulmonary disease. *Am Rev Respir Dis* 1991; 144: 826–832.
20. Harver A, Mahler DA, Schwartzstein RM, *et al.* Descriptors of breathlessness in healthy individuals: distinct and separable constructs. *Chest* 2000; 118: 679–690.
21. Smith J, Albert P, Bertella E, *et al.* Qualitative aspects of breathlessness in health and disease. *Thorax* 2009; 64: 713–718.
22. Parshall MB, Yorke J. Measurement of breathlessness. *In*: Bausewein C, Currow DC, Johnson MJ, eds. Palliative Care in Respiratory Disease (ERS Monograph). Sheffield, European Respiratory Society, 2016; pp. 134–152.
23. Yorke J, Moosavi SH, Shuldham C, *et al.* Quantification of dyspnoea using descriptors: development and initial testing of the Dyspnoea-12. *Thorax* 2010; 65: 21–26.
24. Banzett RB, O'Donnell CR, Guilfoyle TE, *et al.* Multidimensional Dyspnea Profile: an instrument for clinical and laboratory research. *Eur Respir J* 2015; 45: 1681–1691.
25. Banzett RB, Howell MD, O'Donnell CR, *et al.* Dyspnea prevalence and risk of adverse event in a general hospital population. *Am J Respir Crit Care Med* 2013; 187: A2508.
26. Figarska SM, Marike Boezen H, Vonk JM. Dyspnoea severity, changes in dyspnea status and mortality in the general population: the Vlagtwedde/Vlaardingen study. *Eur J Epidemiol* 2012; 27: 867–876.
27. Argulian E, Agarwal V, Bangalore S, *et al.* Meta-analysis of prognostic implications of dyspnea versus chest pain in patients referred for stress testing. *Am J Cardiol* 2014; 113: 559–564.
28. Zoumot Z, Jordan S, Hopkinson N. Emphysema; time to say farewell to therapeutic nihilism. *Thorax* 2014; 69: 973–975.
29. Ekström M, Currow DC, Moens K. Symptom patterns in populations. *In*: Bausewein C, Currow DC, Johnson MJ, eds. Palliative Care in Respiratory Disease (ERS Monograph). Sheffield, European Respiratory Society, 2016; pp. 70–84.
30. Gysels M, Higginson IJ. The experience of breathlessness: the social course of chronic obstructive pulmonary disease. *J Pain Symptom Manage* 2010; 39: 555–563.
31. Lansing RW, Gracely RH, Banzett RB. The multiple dimensions of dyspnea: review and hypotheses. *Respir Physiol Neurobiol* 2009; 167: 53–60.
32. Lansing RW, Im BS, Thwing JI, *et al.* The perception of respiratory work and effort can be independent of the perception of air hunger. *Am J Respir Crit Care Med* 2000; 162: 1690–1696.
33. Petersen S, Orth B, Ritz T. Awareness of breathing: the structure of language descriptors of respiratory sensations. *Health Psychol* 2008; 27: 1234–1127.
34. Chowienczyk S, Javadzadeh S, Booth S, *et al.* Association of descriptors of breathlessness with diagnosis, self-reported severity of breathlessness and self-reported distress due to breathlessness in patients with advanced cancer or advanced COPD. *J Pain Symptom Manage* 2016; in press [DOI: 10.1016/j.jpainsymman.2016.01.014].
35. Chang A, Munson J, Gifford AH, *et al.* Prospective use of descriptors of dyspnea to diagnose common respiratory diseases. *Chest* 2015; 148: 895–902.
36. Burns BH, Howell JB. Disproportionately severe breathlessness in chronic bronchitis. *Q J Med* 1969; 38: 277–294.
37. Zoumot Z, Davey C, Jordan S, *et al.* A randomised controlled study of bronchoscopic lung volume reduction with endobronchial valves for patients with heterogeneous emphysema and intact interlobar fissures: the BeLieVeR-HIFi study. *Efficacy Mech Eval* 2015; 2, 2.5.
38. Von Leupoldt A, Balewski S, Petersen S, *et al.* Verbal descriptors of dyspnea in patients with COPD at different intensity levels of dyspnea. *Chest* 2007; 132: 141–147.
39. McGrath PJ, Pianosi PT, Unru AM, *et al.* Dalhousie dyspnea scales: construct and content validity of pictorial scales for measuring dyspnea. *BMC Pediatr* 2005; 5: 33.
40. Javadzadeh S, Chowienczyk S, Booth S, *et al.* Comparison of respiratory health-related quality of life in patients with intractable breathlessness due to advanced cancer or advanced COPD. *BMJ Support Palliat Care* 2016; 6: 105–108.
41. de Williams AC, Davies HTO, Chadury Y. Simple pain rating scales hide complex idiosyncratic meanings. *Pain* 2000; 85: 457–463.
42. O'Donnell CR, Schwartzstein RM, Lansing RW, *et al.* Dyspnea affective response: comparing COPD patients with healthy volunteers and laboratory model with activities of daily living. *BMC Pulm Med* 2013; 13: 27.

43. Higashimoto, Honda N, Yamagata T, *et al.* Exertional dyspnoea and cortical oxygenation in patients with COPD. *Eur Respir J* 2015; 46: 1615–1624.
44. Binks A. Measuring the breathless brain: is real life too noisy? *Eur Respir J* 2015; 46: 1554–1556.
45. Mularski R, Campbell ML, Asch M. A review of quality of care evaluation for the palliation of dyspnea. *Am J Respir Crit Care Med* 2010; 181: 534–538.
46. Lamb GW, McArdle PA, Ramsey S, *et al.* The relationship between the local and systemic inflammatory responses and survival in patients undergoing resection for localized renal cancer. *BJU Int* 2008; 102: 756–761.
47. Berk M, Williams LJ, Jacka F, *et al.* So depression is an inflammatory disease, but where does the inflammation come from? *BMC Med* 2013; 11: 200.
48. Mahler DA, Huang S, Tabrizi M, *et al.* Efficacy and safety of a monoclonal antibody recognizing interleukin in COPD: a pilot study. *Chest* 2001; 26: 926–934.
49. Veen JC, Smits HH, Ravensberg AJ, *et al.* Impaired perception of dyspnea in patients with severe asthma: relation to sputum eosinophils. *Am J Respir Crit Care Med* 1998; 158: 1134–1141.
50. Franceschi C, Capri M, Monti D, *et al.* Inflammaging and anti-inflammaging. A systemic perspective on aging and longevity emerged from studies in humans. *Mech Age Dev* 2007; 128: 92–105.
51. Bloomfield PS, Selveraj S, Veronese M, *et al.* Microglial activity in people at ultra high risk of psychosis and in schizophrenia: an [^{11}C]PBR28 PET brain imaging study. *Am J Psych* 2016; 173: 44–52.
52. Hansson GK. Inflammation, atherosclerosis and coronary artery disease. *N Engl J Med* 2005; 352: 1685–1695.
53. Tsoli M, Robertson G. Cancer cachexia: malignant inflammation, tumorkines, and metabolic mayhem. *Trends Endocrinol Metab* 2013; 24: 174–183.
54. DeLeo JA, Yezierski RJ. The role of neuroinflammation and neuroimmune activation in persistent pain. *Pain* 2001; 90: 1–6.
55. Hoffman AJ. Enhancing self-efficacy for optimized patient outcomes through the theory of symptom self-management. *Cancer Nurs* 2013; 36: E16–E26.
56. Benedetti F, Mayburg HS, Wager TD, *et al.* Neurobiological mechanisms of the placebo effect. *J Neurosci* 2005; 25: 10390–10402.
57. Benedetti F, Carlino E, Pollo A. How placebos change the patient's brain. *Neuropsychopharmacology* 2011; 36: 339–354.
58. Farquhar MC, Prevost AT, McCrone P, *et al.* Is a specialist breathlessness service more effective and cost-effective for patients with advanced cancer and their carers than standard care? Findings of a mixed-method randomised controlled trial. *BMC Med* 2014; 12: 194.
59. Hoffman G, Harrington A, Fields HA. Pain and the placebo: what we have learned. *Perspect Biol Med* 2005; 48: 248–265.
60. Galbraith S, Fagan P, Perkins P, *et al.* Does the use of a handheld fan improve chronic dyspnea? A randomized, controlled, crossover trial. *J Pain Symptom Manage* 2010; 39: 831–838.
61. Swan F, Booth S. The role of airflow for the relief of chronic breathlessness. *Curr Opinion Support Pall Care* 2015; 9: 206–211.
62. Booth S. Science supporting the art of medicine, improving the management of breathlessness. *Palliat Med* 2013; 27: 483–485.
63. Bausewein C, Booth S, Gysels M, *et al.* The effectiveness of a hand-held fan for breathlessness: a randomised phase II trial. *BMC Palliative Care* 2010; 9: 22.
64. Eippert F, Bingel U, Schoell ED. Activation of the opioidergic descending pain control system underlies placebo. *Analgesia Neuron* 2009; 63: 533–543.
65. Eippert F, Finterbusch J, Bingel U. Direct evidence for spinal cord involvement in placebo analgesia. *Science* 2009; 326: 404.
66. Damasio A, Carvalho GB. The nature of feelings: evolutionary and neurobiological origins. *Nat Rev Neurosci* 2013; 14: 143–152.
67. Higginson IJ, Bausewein C, Reilly C, *et al.* An integrated palliative and respiratory care service for patients with advanced disease and refractory breathlessness: a randomised controlled trial. *Lancet Respir Med* 2014; 2: 979–987.
68. Faull AK, Jenkinson M, Ezra M, *et al.* Conditioned respiratory threat in the subdivisions of the human periaqueductal gray matter. *Elife* 2016; 5, e12047.
69. Jensen D, Pattinson K, Jolley C. Mechanisms of breathlessness. *In*: Bausewein C, Currow DC, Johnson MJ, eds. Palliative Care in Respiratory Disease (ERS Monograph). Sheffield, European Respiratory Society, 2016; pp. 111–133.
70. Beausoliel NJ, Mellor DJ. Introducing breathlessness as a significant animal welfare issue. *New Zealand Vet J* 2015; 63: 44–51.
71. Johnson MS, Martin M. Investigation of dyspnoea in dogs. *In Practice* 2008; 30: 558–566.
72. Kabat-Zinn J. Full Catastrophe Living. New York, Dell Publishing, 1991.
73. Brown RP, Gerber PL. The Healing Power of the Breath. Boston, Shambhala Publications, 2012.
74. Kuyken W, Byford S, Taylor R, *et al.* Mindfulness-based cognitive therapy to prevent relapse in recurrent depression. *J Consult Clin Psychol* 2008; 76: 966–978.

75. Spicuzza L, Gabutti A, Porta C, *et al.* Yoga and chemoreflex response to hypoxia and hypercapnia. *Lancet* 2000; 356: 1495–1496.
76. Coats ASJ. Teaching heart failure patients how to breathe. *Lancet* 1998; 358: 1299–1300.
77. Kelly GA. A Theory of Personality: the Psychology of Personal Constructs. New York, W.W. Norton & Company, 1963.
78. Carver CS, Scheier MF. Perspectives on Personality. Needham Heights, Allyn & Bacon, 2000.
79. Goodlin SJ. Palliative care in congestive heart failure. *J Am Coll Cardiol* 2009; 54: 386–396.
80. Rollnick S, Heather N, Bell A. Negotiating behaviour change in medical settings: the development of brief motivational interviewing. *Mental Health* 2009; 1: 25–37.
81. Deter HC. Psychosocial interventions for patients with chronic disease. *Biopsychosoc Med* 2012; 6: 2.
82. Spathis A. Genesis of breathlessness. *In*: Booth S, Burkin J, Moffat C, *et al.*, eds. Managing Breathlessness in Clinical Practice. London, Springer, 2014.
83. Radder JE, Shapiro S, Berndt A. Medicine for chronic, complex diseases: chronic obstructive pulmonary disease as an example. *Personal Med* 2014; 11: 669–679.
84. Ahmedzai S, Baldwin D, Currow D, eds. Supportive Care in Respiratory Disease. 2nd Edn. Oxford, Oxford University Press, 2012.
85. Anon. The enigma of breathlessness. *Lancet* 1986; 1: 891–892.
86. Benzo P, Kirsch Dulohery P, *et al.* Emotional intelligence: a novel outcome associated with wellbeing and self-management in chronic obstructive airways disease. *Ann Am Thorac Soc* 2015; 13: 10–16.
87. Jolley CJ, Moxham J. A physiological model of patient-reported breathlessness during daily activities in COPD. *Eur Respir Rev* 2009; 18: 66–79.
88. Lucas V, Booth S. The importance of placebo effects in enhancing palliative care interventions. *BMJ Support Palliat Care* 2014; 4: 212–216.
89. Tracey I. Getting the pain you expect: mechanisms of placebo, nocebo and reappraisal effects in humans. *Nature* 2010; 16: 1277–1283.
90. Bausewein C, Booth S, Gysels M, *et al.* Non-pharmacological interventions for breathlessness in advanced stages of malignant and non-malignant diseases. *Cochrane Database Syst Rev* 2008; 2: CD005623.
91. Booth S, Fallon M, Chin C, *et al.* Listening to patients: ensuring that younger people living with chronic symptomatic illness have access to responsive palliative care services. *Palliat Med* 2016; 30: 3–5.
92. Booth S, Chin C, Spathis A. Breathlessness and the brain. *Palliat Med* 2015; 29: 396–398.
93. Booth S, Galbraith S, Ryan R, *et al.* The importance of the feasibility study: lessons from a study of the hand-held fan used to relieve dyspnoea in people who are breathless at rest. *Palliat Med* 2016; 30: 504–509.

Disclosures: None declared.

Chapter 7

Patient and carer experience of breathlessness

Ann Hutchinson

Chronic breathlessness has wide-ranging, interrelated, physical, psychological, social and existential consequences for those living with it, and for family and friends who care for them. Despite this, the symptom often remains invisible to others. Recognition that breathlessness is a multifaceted symptom with extensive effects is necessary for the symptom to be managed effectively. A full assessment of the effects of breathlessness by a health professional is needed so that the patient and carer are aware that these are legitimate concerns to present to their clinician, thus countering the invisibility of the symptom.

Chronic breathlessness is a common symptom of cardiorespiratory conditions and cancer (covered in another chapter of this issue of the *Monograph* [1]) and has wide-ranging effects on the lives of people who live with it and of those who care for them (also covered elsewhere in this *Monograph* [2]). The considerable qualitative literature of patient and carer experiences of breathlessness due to COPD and heart failure demonstrates that this symptom not only imposes considerable physical limitations but also results in psychological distress, changes to social relationships and existential concerns [3, 4]. There is a clear need to raise the profile of breathlessness as a therapeutic target in its own right to ensure that it is assessed and managed effectively, recognising the wide-reaching effects that breathlessness has. The experience of breathlessness described in this chapter is contextualised with reference to the model of quality of life (QoL) from Raphael *et al.* [5] and the concept of "total dyspnoea" [6].

Disability, dependency, QoL and breathlessness

Breathlessness greatly affects the QoL of both patients and carers. QoL has been defined as "the degree to which a person enjoys the important possibilities of his or her life" [5]. One model of QoL encompasses the three domains of Being, Belonging and Becoming, each domain having physical, psychological, social and spiritual dimensions [5]. Thus, health is not merely the absence of illness but encompasses existential possibilities valued by people: being able to manage daily activities and cope mentally, belonging to family and community groups, and becoming what is important to them by being able to pursue their

Hull York Medical School, University of Hull, Hull, UK.

Correspondence: Ann Hutchinson, Hull York Medical School, Hertford Building, University of Hull, Cottingham Road, Hull, HU6 7RX, UK. E-mail: hyah6@hyms.ac.uk

 Print ISBN: 978-1-84984-071-2. Online ISBN: 978-1-84984-072-9. Print ISSN: 2312-508X. Online ISSN: 2312-5098.

own goals. The model is derived from the work of philosophers in the phenomenological tradition such as Heidegger [7] and Merleau-Ponty [8] who argue that, as our body is the basis of our interaction with the world, "being able to" carry out our activities and projects in the world is central to our view of ourselves, without which we can feel lost and useless. Thus, living with breathlessness can affect whether we see ourselves as "being able to" or "not being able to" and can affect the quality of our existence as a whole.

The QoL of both patients and their carer can be severely affected by breathlessness [9]. Disability caused by breathlessness and restriction of activities that make life meaningful can result in feelings of worthlessness and loss of self-respect:

> "Well basically it's all gone [referring to QoL] . . . I was a dancer, I can't dance, I was a singer, I can't sing and I used to play sport. In fact I can't have a bath by myself now. The quality of life that you see is gone, so now I'm in my bed, I've got a laptop and things around the bed, but that's it, just watching everything go." [10]

This model of QoL is particularly applicable to the experience of chronic breathlessness, as its structure has much in common with the concept of "total dyspnoea", both of which take into account physical, psychological, social and existential aspects and can be used to describe fully the experience of breathlessness.

Total dyspnoea

Chronic breathlessness not only affects people's physical abilities but also can cause psychological and existential distress, and thereby dramatically alter the QoL of both patients and their carers. Rather than focusing on the physical signs of breathlessness, breathlessness can be better understood when considered as "total dyspnoea" [6]: a subjective experience with physical, psychological, social and existential dimensions. This approach to breathlessness is modelled on the concept of "total pain" pioneered by Saunders [11], and is an example of the biopsychosocial approach pioneered by Engel [12]. The concept of "total dyspnoea" allows us to see the wide-ranging effects that breathlessness can have on a person and their family, from limitations in physical activity, disability and dependency to changes in their social relationships and the consequent psychological and existential distress caused by these losses and restrictions. This framework of "total dyspnoea" will be used to describe in detail the wide-ranging effects breathlessness has on the lives of patients and carers.

Physical effects of breathlessness

> "The worst thing I think is the stairs, going up and down the stairs. Ordinary household chores I find difficult. Very restrictive, because of your breathing. And now of late . . . even simple things like having a shower and getting dressed." [13]

Chronic breathlessness, irrespective of underlying cause, makes engagement in physical activities such as walking, lifting and climbing difficult. Physical activity is involved in many activities of daily living, such as walking to the shops, preparing meals, bathing, cleaning, gardening, working, performing hobbies and socialising. Therefore, a reduced ability to be physically active has major implications for the breathless patient and their carer.

Patients describe the increasing restriction of their daily activities as a result of breathlessness, becoming increasingly disabled and dependent on others for help and support. This curtailment of the ability to carry out activities of daily living results in dependency on others, which can be difficult to come to terms with.

An ethnographic study of Canadian COPD patients [14] found many examples of disability due to breathlessness. These included not being able to mow the lawn, carry heavy bags, do the shopping, vacuum the house or walk across a car park, all of which caused considerable limitations and reduced independent living.

Breathlessness imposes physical limitations on patients but also on their family or carer, to the extent that the carer's health may also suffer as a result of taking on many of the patient's former roles, but this is superseded by concern for the patient.

The effect of breathlessness on physical activity has been explored from a phenomenological perspective by Carel [15]. She describes how breathlessness makes many things impossible and causes a shrinking "lifeworld", and argues that the physical world becomes altered for breathless people, as the effort required to manage physical activities means that they are forced to attend to the environment around them in a different way from those who are not impeded by illness. As Carel [15] describes: "The trail that seemed so inviting and beautiful is now harsh and endless."

The physical limitations imposed by breathlessness have extensive effects on people's daily lives. These, in turn, may have psychological, social and existential effects on both patients and those caring for them. It is important to note that these effects may be interrelated; for example, psychological impacts of breathlessness are likely to influence physical limitations (*e.g.* as a result of confidence), as well as *vice versa*.

The ups and downs of breathlessness

> "In other words if it's too hot or too cold, if it's humid or it's damp, you're in trouble. . . . Then of course there's windy weather, I just can't make it in windy weather at all. I have great difficulty breathing if I happen to go against it. . . . Also, if there's any kind of smoke, fumes or smog when you're out, especially exhaust fumes from the cars and buses and what have you, then it's murder to breathe." [16]

Variability in breathlessness severity, even within the same day, is a major challenge. Unless very severe, most patients have stable, manageable or no breathlessness at rest but experience breathlessness induced by exertion and/or other triggers, such as emotion or a change in the environment. Breathlessness usually returns to baseline levels on rest or removal/cessation of the triggers. Consequently, a common coping strategy is to avoid exertion [17]. If the symptom intensity does not return to baseline levels or patients experience increased breathlessness of unknown cause that occurs "out of the blue", they can find this very distressing.

A wide variety of environmental factors may trigger breathlessness, including physical exertion, anxiety, hot or cold air, weather, humidity, smoke, air pollution and time of day. Although many patients describe breathlessness triggered by one or another environmental trigger, there are also occasions when there is no obvious trigger, and patients report five different types of episodic breathlessness [18].

The variability of breathlessness leads to uncertainty for both the patient and their carer, leading to difficulties in planning, as the patient may not be well enough on the day to carry out the planned activity. As breathlessness can change even within a day, they become vigilant at monitoring their levels of breathlessness.

Alongside this variability in the daily experience of breathlessness, patients may have exacerbations of their underlying condition, often accompanied by worse breathlessness, which may then trigger an emergency presentation to their GP or the ED [19]. A meta-synthesis of the qualitative literature of the experience of exacerbations of COPD identified significant acute and long-term effects [20]. Acutely, there is often intense fear, heightened vigilance of bodily sensations and an urgent need for "rescue". In the long term, exacerbations interrupt the daily pattern of the patient's life and are a serious cause of uncertainty. Thus, the trajectory of functional decline for people with COPD is one of many ups and downs, with accompanying uncertainty [19].

Psychological effects of breathlessness

Anxiety, fear and panic

> "It's like a vicious circle. Your breathing gets bad so you get anxious, then you get afraid, and your breathing gets worse, which makes you more afraid. The COPD feeds the anxiety and the anxiety feeds the fear." [21]

For both the patient and carer, breathlessness is a distressing and frightening symptom. The distressing nature of breathlessness is illustrated by the highly emotive language of breathlessness commonly used by patients to describe the sensation, such as "choking", "smothering", "couldn't get air", "deathly sick" and "fighting for breath" [22].

Anxiety, breathlessness and panic are commonly described in terms of a vicious circle, and the link between breathlessness and anxiety is clearly described by patients. This vicious cycle has been described as the "dyspnoea–anxiety–dyspnoea cycle" by Bailey [23], who reported how patients find it "scary when you can't breathe", a very natural feeling when fighting for air.

The close relationship of breathlessness, anxiety and panic often leaves patients feeling vulnerable and open to attack by their breathlessness. Not only do patients feel anxiety due to breathlessness but so do those who care for them, as they may be frightened by seeing their loved one very breathless.

Patients find their breathlessness terrifying and unpredictable. Distress during episodes of breathlessness may be so severe that the patient fears they will suffocate. The manner of dying is clearly a concern, with patients fearing suffocating to death alone in their home [16]. Equally, carers may experience fear about their loved one's death, constantly fearing that they may stop breathing, and so feeling the need to sleep near the patient in case something happens. This may lead to exhaustion on the part of the carer, as they "sleep with one eye open" and so suffer regular interruption to their sleep [24].

Depression

> "Depression is the biggest problem. It is the worst, because if you were an active person all your life and now you're inactive, it's hard to accept." [25]

Depression is also commonly experienced by breathless patients and may result from the long-term disability and loss resulting from the physical limitations imposed by breathlessness. The depression associated with chronic breathlessness may lead to feelings of hopelessness where patients feel that they no longer have anything to live for.

Carers may also suffer from depression, helplessness and exhaustion when faced with the relentless task of caring for someone who is chronically breathless, due to the unremitting nature of the care needed [26]. The strain of looking after someone who is depressed can exact a toll on those who care for them. Understanding the psychological difficulties that are faced by breathless patients and their carers is key to helping them manage breathlessness. However, this is an area that is often overlooked.

Social effects of the experience of breathlessness

Social isolation and changes to relationships, identity and roles often accompany the physical and psychological effects of the experience of breathlessness.

Social isolation

> "We often feel lonely and on the edge of things." [27]

The physical limitations imposed by breathlessness (*e.g.* problems with walking, speaking and lifting) result in great difficulty in taking part in activities, which in turn leads to limitations of social life and social isolation. The inability to go shopping has more far-reaching effects than being unable to buy things; in addition, patients miss the everyday social interactions that go along with shopping, such as walking along the street and having a chat with people they know.

Leisure activities, such as walking, dancing and fishing, which all involve considerable physical activity, become impossible for breathless patients and often, by association, for their partner/carer. No longer being able to take part in these activities limits the social lives of both the patient and carer, and results in a sense of loss and isolation [28]. Lifestyle inevitably changes, with consequent loss and marginalisation.

Changes to relationships

> "Gradually we have had less and less to talk about . . . gives the impression that he has no interest anymore, neither in myself nor in his surroundings. I think this is some kind of envy of me, in my heart I can feel it. . . . After he started to go in and out of hospitals we stopped being good friends like we used to be. . . . The disease has isolated him from the family and myself, and now we have restricted issues to talk about . . . it makes me sad when I think about it." [29]

As a result of these changes, it is unsurprising that breathlessness can alter the relationship of the patient and carer. The social changes that can happen to breathless patients affect the way they relate to others, and this can strain patient/carer relationships. Life may become "just being with each other, putting up with each other… I would give anything to just get out of the house" [9].

Often, the carer of a breathless patient is a spouse/partner, and breathlessness takes its toll on intimate relationships, for example with difficulties over maintaining a sexual relationship, an issue that may not be addressed routinely [29].

As well as intimate relationships, relationships with the wider family may also be affected by living with breathlessness, for example limitations in playing with children and grandchildren [30].

Changes to social identity and roles

> "It's the silly thing . . . not being able to carry the shopping . . . I was brought up in the Victorian school . . . the man always carries the bags. . . ." [26]

A person's identity is made up partly by their own individual traits and partly by the social groups with which they identify. Social groupings may be formed on the basis of categories, such as gender, ethnicity, socioeconomic status, religious affiliation and occupational group.

The many limitations on the physical activities caused by chronic breathlessness can lead to a person no longer being able to fulfil certain roles and may lead to a change in their identity. The roles that are commonly affected by living with breathlessness include gender, partner, carer and worker. Roles related to social activities and hobbies such as dancing, gardening and walking also become restricted for both patient and carer.

When breathless people feel unable to do the activities they associate with their gender role, such as carrying the shopping or cooking meals, they feel less of a man/woman, which can be very distressing [26].

Carers also undergo changes in their roles, often moving away from being a partner with an intimate relationship (*e.g.* spouse) to becoming a carer and having to take on many other new roles, such as nurse, cook and gardener [31].

The role of worker is frequently challenged by breathlessness, as it can lead to patients and their carers having to stop work due to their own breathlessness or to the pressures of caring for a breathless person [16].

These changes in role may adversely affect the relationship between the patient and carer, and may lead the carer to put their life on hold and re-evaluate aspects of their life together [26].

Existential aspects of the experience of breathlessness

> "I've always said I'm not afraid of dying 'cause I know where I'm going. But when I get short of breath I get scared – I don't know why – I shouldn't. I think smothering to death is a hard way to go." [32]

Existential or spiritual concerns are an intrinsic part of being human and may be expressed through an organised religion or in other ways that are meaningful to the individual [33]. Existential concerns, such as being at peace, having a sense of purpose and connection to others, and holding beliefs about the meaning of life, lead to a sense of well-being. However, existential distress can arise due to a sense of suffering and loss, with distress about relationships, loss of control, being a burden on others and impending death [34].

Existential distress may therefore arise from living and dying with chronic breathlessness, and may include challenges to faith, difficulty finding meaning and purpose, relationship difficulties, uncertainty, problems in maintaining a sense of identity, and isolation and hopelessness.

Some patients find solace in their religious convictions and practices, which enable them to live with their breathlessness and cope with their suffering [16, 35]. However, physical limitations may make it difficult for them to continue with any form of religious observance. This may affect them adversely, isolating them from the support of their religious community at the time when they need it [36].

Uncertainty is due not only to the variability of breathlessness and the unpredictability of exacerbations but also to uncertainty about progression, decline and death. This uncertainty can lead to feelings of hopelessness, and some patients begin to wonder if it is worth continuing to live at all, even if such thoughts would normally be out of character [16]. Some may desire to end their lives in order "to end the struggle to breathe" [37].

The manner of their death may also be a concern, with many patients unaware of how their underlying condition may bring about their death or that there may be effective palliative care. A lack of knowledge may mean that patients (and also carers) believe and fear that they may die with the feeling of suffocating that they regularly experience with increased breathlessness [32].

The invisibility of breathlessness

Interviews of COPD patients about their access to healthcare services found that access was poor [38]. The insidious onset of breathlessness, the perceived stigma and the lack of responsiveness to breathlessness from healthcare professionals if accessed led to both an intentional hiding of the symptom and a perception that the symptom and its effects were not legitimate concerns to bring to the doctor [39]. Thus, chronic breathlessness could be "invisible" to healthcare professionals.

Challenges and recommendations for clinical practice

The experience of chronic breathlessness affects all aspects of life and interaction with other people, including healthcare professionals, and thus influences how well the patient makes use of health services in primary, secondary and tertiary care.

A full assessment of the physical, psychological, social and existential effects of breathlessness, covering aspects including the variability of breathlessness and the impact on mood, QoL and isolation of patients and carers by the health professional, is needed so that the patient and carer are aware that such concerns are legitimate to present to their clinician, thus helping to counter the invisibility of the symptom.

Healthcare professionals need to be up to date on the current management of breathlessness and to be aware that there are evidence-based interventions targeting breathlessness in its own right (covered in another chapter of this issue of the *Monograph* [40]), and should liaise with other colleagues as necessary.

Healthcare professionals need the communication skills to discuss the future, including fears about the mode of dying, so that the patient can make well-informed decisions about their treatment options at the EOL.

Conclusion

Daily breathlessness has wide-ranging effects for both the patient and their family carers. Much of this experience remains invisible to others both in the general public and in the healthcare profession. Recognition that breathlessness is a multifaceted symptom with extensive psychological, social and existential effects is necessary for the symptom to be assessed properly and then managed effectively.

References

1. Ekström M, Currow DC, Moens K. Symptom patterns in populations. *In*: Bausewein C, Currow DC, Johnson MJ, eds. Palliative Care in Respiratory Disease (ERS Monograph). Sheffield, European Respiratory Society, 2016; pp. 70–84.
2. Farquhar M. Supporting informal carers. *In*: Bausewein C, Currow DC, Johnson MJ, eds. Palliative Care in Respiratory Disease (ERS Monograph). Sheffield, European Respiratory Society, 2016; pp. 51–69.
3. Disler RT, Green A, Luckett T, *et al.* Experience of advanced chronic obstructive pulmonary disease: metasynthesis of qualitative research. *J Pain Symptom Manage* 2014; 48: 1182–1199.
4. Yu DS, Lee DT, Kwong AN, *et al.* Living with chronic heart failure: a review of qualitative studies of older people. *J Adv Nurs* 2008; 61: 474–483.
5. Raphael D, Brown I, Renwick R, *et al.* Measuring the quality of life of older persons: a model with implications for community and public health nursing. *Int J Nurs Stud* 1997; 34: 231–239.
6. Abernethy AP, Wheeler JL. Total dyspnoea. *Curr Opin Support Palliat Care* 2008; 2: 110–113.
7. Heidegger M. Being and Time. New York, Harper, 1962.
8. Merleau-Ponty M. Phenomenology of Perception. London, Routledge, and Henley, Kegan Paul, 1962.
9. Boyle AH. Living with a spouse with chronic obstructive pulmonary disease: the meaning of wives' experiences. *J Nurs Healthcare Chron Illn* 2009; 1: 273–282.
10. Hallas CN, Howard C, Theadom A, *et al.* Negative beliefs about breathlessness increases panic for patients with chronic respiratory disease. *Psychol Health Med* 2012; 17: 467–477.
11. Saunders C. The treatment of intractable pain in terminal cancer. *Proc R Soc Med* 1963; 56: 195–197.
12. Engel GL. The clinical application of the biopsychosocial model. *Am J Psychiatry* 1980; 137: 535–544.
13. Caress A, Luker K, Chalmers K. Promoting the health of people with chronic obstructive pulmonary disease: patients' and carers' views. *J Clin Nurs* 2010; 19: 564–573.
14. Boyles CM, Bailey PH, Mossey S. Chronic obstructive pulmonary disease as disability: dilemma stories. *Qual Health Res* 2010; 21: 187–198.
15. Carel H. Illness: the Cry of the Flesh. Stocksfield, Acumen, 2008.
16. Williams SJ. Chronic Respiratory Illness. London, Routledge, 1993.
17. Gysels M, Higginson IJ. The experience of breathlessness: the social course of chronic obstructive pulmonary disease. *J Pain Symptom Manage* 2010; 39: 555–563.
18. Simon ST, Higginson IJ, Benalia H, *et al.* Episodes of breathlessness: types and patterns – a qualitative study exploring experiences of patients with advanced diseases. *Palliat Med* 2013; 27: 524–532.
19. Giacomini M, DeJean D, Simeonov D, *et al.* Experiences of living and dying with COPD: a systematic review and synthesis of the qualitative empirical literature. *Ont Health Technol Assess Ser* 2012; 12: 1–47.
20. Harrison SL, Apps L, Singh S, *et al.* 'Consumed by breathing' – a critical interpretive meta-synthesis of the qualitative literature. *Chronic Illn* 2014; 10: 31–49.
21. Willgoss TG, Yohannes AM, Goldbart J, *et al.* "Everything was spiraling out of control": experiences of anxiety in people with chronic obstructive pulmonary disease. *Heart Lung* 2012; 41: 562–571.
22. Parshall MB, Welsh JD, Brockopp DY, *et al.* Dyspnea duration, distress, and intensity in emergency department visits for heart failure. *Heart Lung* 2001; 30: 47–56.
23. Bailey PH. The dyspnea-anxiety-dyspnea cycle – COPD patients' stories of breathlessness: "It's scary/when you can't breathe". *Qual Health Res* 2004; 14: 760–778.
24. Hearson B, McClement S, McMillan DE, *et al.* Sleeping with one eye open: the sleep experience of family members providing palliative care at home. *J Palliat Care* 2011; 27: 69.
25. Wilson JS, O'Neill B, Reilly J, *et al.* Education in pulmonary rehabilitation: the patient's perspective. *Arch Phys Med Rehabil* 2007; 88: 1704–1709.
26. Booth S, Silvester S, Todd C. Breathlessness in cancer and chronic obstructive pulmonary disease: using a qualitative approach to describe the experience of patients and carers. *Palliat Support Care* 2003; 1: 337–344.
27. Guthrie S, Hill K, Muers M. Living with severe COPD. A qualitative exploration of the experience of patients in Leeds. *Respir Med* 2001; 95: 196–204.
28. Gysels MH, Higginson IJ. Caring for a person in advanced illness and suffering from breathlessness at home: threats and resources. *Palliat Support Care* 2009; 7: 153–162.
29. Bergs D. "The Hidden Client" – women caring for husbands with COPD: their experience of quality of life. *J Clin Nurs* 2002; 11: 613–621.

30. Nicolson P, Anderson P. Quality of life, distress and self-esteem: a focus group study of people with chronic bronchitis. *Br J Health Psychol* 2003; 8: 251–270.
31. Seamark DA, Blake SD, Seamark CJ, *et al.* Living with severe chronic obstructive pulmonary disease (COPD): perceptions of patients and their carers. An interpretative phenomenological analysis. *Palliat Med* 2004; 18: 619–625.
32. Wortz K, Cade A, Menard JR, *et al.* A qualitative study of patients' goals and expectations for self-management of COPD. *Prim Care Respir J* 2012; 21: 384–391.
33. Henoch I, Bergman B, Danielson E. Dyspnea experience and management strategies in patients with lung cancer. *Psycho Oncology* 2008; 17: 709–715.
34. Morita T, Kawa M, Honke Y, *et al.* Existential concerns of terminally ill cancer patients receiving specialized palliative care in Japan. *Support Care Cancer* 2004; 12: 137–140.
35. Nicholls DA. The experience of chronic breathlessness. *Physiother Theory Pract* 2003; 19: 123–136.
36. Ryan M, Farrelly M. Living with an unfixable heart: a qualitative study exploring the experience of living with advanced heart failure. *Eur J Cardiovasc Nurs* 2009; 8: 223–231.
37. Barnett M. Chronic obstructive pulmonary disease: a phenomenological study of patients' experiences. *J Clin Nurs* 2005; 14: 805–812.
38. Gysels MH, Higginson IJ. Access to services for patients with chronic obstructive pulmonary disease: the invisibility of breathlessness. *J Pain Symptom Manage* 2008; 36: 451–460.
39. Gysels MH, Higginson IJ. Self-management for breathlessness in COPD: the role of pulmonary rehabilitation. *Chron Respir Dis* 2009; 6: 133–140.
40. Johnson MJ, Barbetta C, Currow DC, *et al.* Management of chronic breathlessness. *In*: Bausewein C, Currow DC, Johnson MJ, eds. Palliative Care in Respiratory Disease (ERS Monograph). Sheffield, European Respiratory Society, 2016; pp. 153–171.

Disclosures: None declared.

Chapter 8

Mechanisms of breathlessness

Dennis Jensen[1,2], Kyle Pattinson[3,4] and Caroline Jolley[5]

The perception of breathlessness in the sensory (intensity) and affective (unpleasantness) domains involves the integration of respiratory efferent and afferent sensory information within cortical and subcortical neural networks. Recent advances in the visualisation of the neurobiology of breathing and physiological measurement of the neural respiratory drive (NRD) have furthered our understanding of breathlessness through the investigation of: 1) altered pulmonary physiology in symptomatic patients; and 2) the mechanisms of action of established and novel interventions. Irrespective of the underlying pathophysiology, the findings of such studies support the hypothesis that breathlessness intensity in obstructive and restrictive lung disorders reflects the awareness of increased NRD required to support ventilation, consequent to intrinsic respiratory mechanical loading and/or increased ventilatory demand. Qualitatively distinct descriptors of breathlessness (*e.g.* work/effort, air hunger, unsatisfied inspiration) probably involve the integration of discrete afferent inputs relative to the prevailing level of NRD. Conditioned responses are likely to underlie learned behaviours driving physical activity avoidance and breathlessness-related anticipatory fear and anxiety, contributing to the vicious cycle of functional decline in CRD.

Breathlessness is a prevalent and distressing symptom of pulmonary, cardiovascular, malignant and neuromuscular diseases [1]. Breathlessness has been defined as "a subjective experience of breathing discomfort that consists of qualitatively distinct sensations that vary in intensity. The experience derives from interactions among multiple physiological, psychological, social, and environmental factors, and may induce secondary physiological and behavioural responses." [1] From this definition, it is clear that the mechanisms of breathlessness are highly complex and multifactorial. Using evidence from both experimental and clinical studies, this chapter focuses specifically on the central and peripheral physiological mechanisms of breathlessness and its key domains: the perceived intensity of breathlessness (sensory domain), unpleasantness (affective domain) and subsequent cognitive and emotional responses [2]. In particular, the chapter provides a review and discussion of: 1) the critical role of the neural respiratory drive (NRD) in causing and relieving breathlessness; 2) the role of central feedback from respiratory sensory afferent receptors in the neuromodulation of breathlessness and its clinical management; and 3) the central neuroanatomical structures underlying the perception of breathlessness in humans.

[1]Clinical Exercise and Respiratory Physiology Laboratory, Dept of Kinesiology and Physical Education, McGill University, Montreal, QC, Canada. [2]Research Institute of the McGill University Health Centre, Translational Research in Respiratory Diseases Program, Montreal, QC, Canada. [3]Nuffield Dept of Clinical Neurosciences, University of Oxford, John Radcliffe Hospital, Oxford, UK. [4]Nuffield Dept of Anaesthetics, Oxford University Hospitals NHS Foundation Trust, John Radcliffe Hospital, Oxford, UK. [5]Centre of Human and Aerospace Physiological Sciences, Faculty of Life Sciences and Medicine, King's College London, London, UK.

Correspondence: Dennis Jensen, Dept of Kinesiology and Physical Education, McGill University, Montreal, QC, H2W 1S4, Canada. E-mail: dennis.jensen@mcgill.ca

 Print ISBN: 978-1-84984-071-2. Online ISBN: 978-1-84984-072-9. Print ISSN: 2312-508X. Online ISSN: 2312-5098.

Neurophysiological mechanisms of breathlessness

NRD: the proximate cause of breathlessness

The output from the respiratory centres of the brainstem, the NRD, is tightly controlled to achieve the levels of minute ventilation (V'_E) required to maintain blood gas homeostasis. Increases in the load imposed on the respiratory muscles and/or a reduction in their force-generating capacity, such as occurs in chronic obstructive and restrictive pulmonary disease, results in higher levels of NRD needed to support any given level of V'_E at rest and during exercise (figure 1) [3–9]. Breathing is also under volitional cortical control, *e.g.* during talking and eating.

An increase in breathing implies not only an increase in NRD, but also generation of distinct patterns of sensory feedback from vagal afferents (innervating the lung and respiratory tract), and cervical and thoracic dorsal root afferents (innervating the proprioceptors of the chest wall and respiratory muscles) in response to thoracic volume expansion, respiratory muscle tension development and changes in respired flow and pressure (figure 2). Central feedback from respiratory sensory nerves contributes to the neuromodulation of breathlessness. For example,

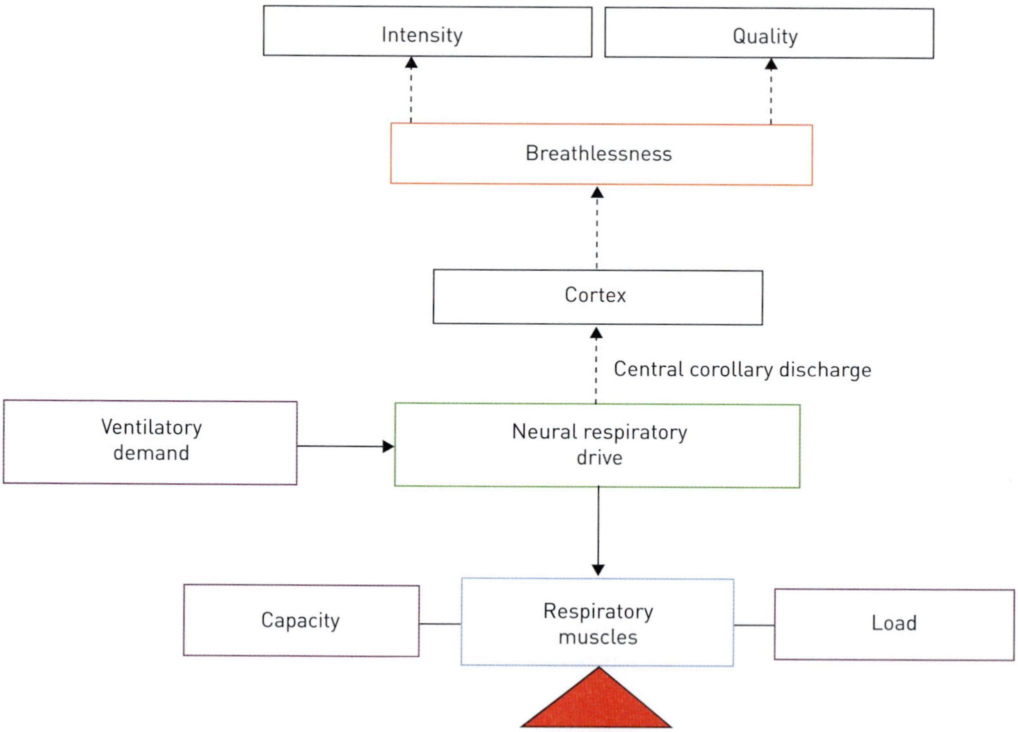

Figure 1. A physiological model of breathlessness in health and disease. Breathlessness, in both health and disease, can be rated quantitatively, in terms of intensity, and qualitatively in distinct sensory and affective domains (*e.g.* respiratory work/effort, air hunger, unsatisfied inspiration). Increased intrinsic mechanical loading, reduced capacity of the respiratory muscles and/or increased ventilatory demand leads to increased levels of neural respiratory drive to support ventilation. Increased neural respiratory drive results in increased breathlessness intensity. Thus, breathlessness intensity in cardiorespiratory disorders can be understood in the context of an appropriate integrated response to the combined effects of increased ventilatory demand and impaired ventilatory mechanics, which increase the mechanical load on the respiratory muscle pump and/or reduce respiratory muscle force-generating capacity. Adapted and modified from [9] with permission.

resumption of spontaneous breathing at the "break point" of a maximal voluntary breath-hold manoeuvre causes rapid relief of breathlessness (presumably *via* increased activity of vagal, cervical and/or thoracic dorsal root afferents), despite persistent or even increased chemostimulation (*i.e.* NRD) by hypoxia and hypercapnia [10, 11]. Moreover, an inverse relationship exists between tidal volume (V_T) expansion and intensity ratings of air hunger at fixed elevated levels of end-tidal carbon dioxide tension (P_{ETCO_2}) in mechanically ventilated, quadriplegic patients with high-level cervical injuries, an effect attributed to changes in pulmonary stretch receptor activity [12]. Afferent receptors of the pulmonary system most widely implicated in the neuromodulation of breathlessness include: central and peripheral chemoreceptors; slowly and rapidly adapting stretch receptors; bronchopulmonary C-fibres, including juxtacapillary or J-receptors; and chest wall and respiratory muscle spindles and Golgi tendon organs [13–16]. A detailed description of the morphological and functional features of these afferent receptors and their effective stimuli have been reviewed in detail elsewhere [16, 17].

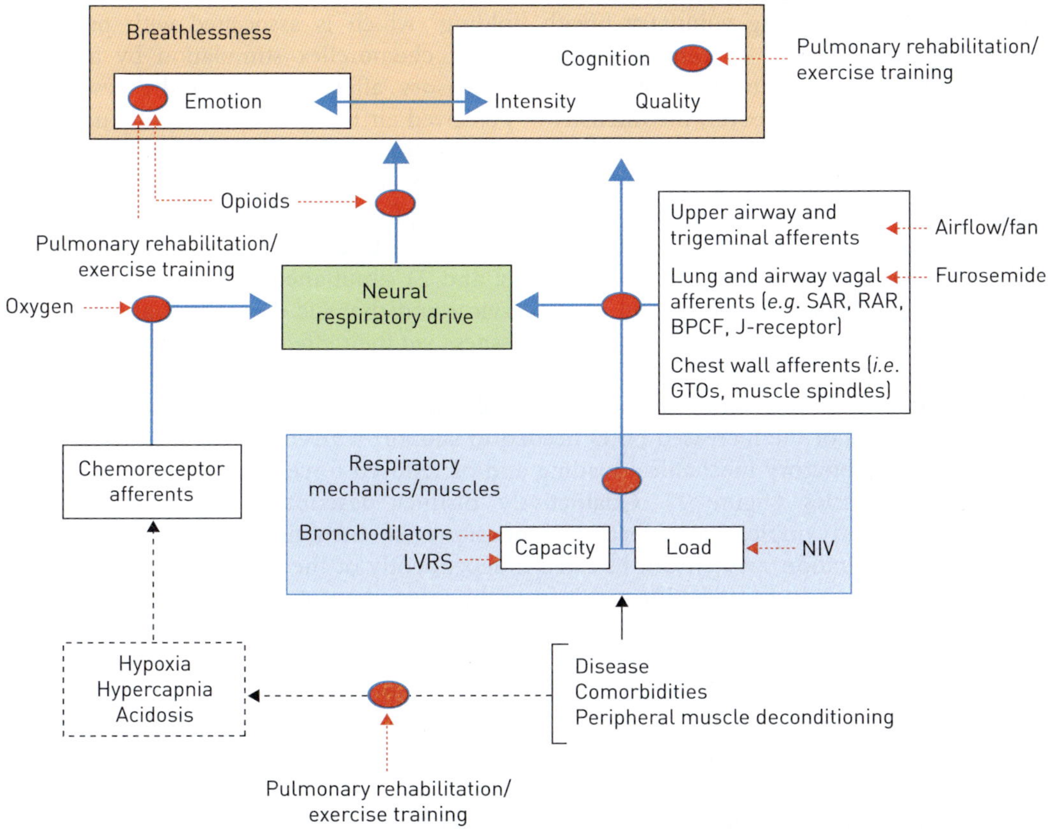

Figure 2. A simplified conceptual neurophysiological model of breathlessness in the sensory (intensity), affective (unpleasantness) and emotional domains, with selected pharmacological and non-pharmacological targets and their proposed mechanism(s) of action. As illustrated in figure 1, increased intrinsic respiratory mechanical loading, reduced respiratory muscle force-generating capacity and/or increased ventilatory demand result in increased neural respiratory drive, which is perceived as increased breathlessness intensity. The corollary of this is that any intervention capable of reducing neural respiratory drive by improving the load–capacity balance of the respiratory muscle pump (*e.g.* bronchodilators, LVRS, NIV) and/or decreasing ventilatory demand (*e.g.* oxygen, rehabilitative exercise training) has the potential to alleviate breathlessness intensity in patients with respiratory disease. Refer to the text for further details. LVRS: lung volume reduction surgery; SAR: slowly adapting stretch receptor; RAR: rapidly adapting stretch receptor; BPCF: bronchopulmonary C-fibre; J-receptor: juxtacapillary receptor; GTO: Golgi tendon organ.

Transmission of sensory afferent information to higher cortical centres provides a potential mechanism by which afferent feedback can modulate breathlessness perception directly [18, 19]. However, the homeostatic function of sensory feedback from afferent receptors, in concert with central and peripheral chemoreceptor inputs, is to modulate efferent motor output to the respiratory muscles, *i.e.* NRD [19]. "Central corollary discharge" refers to the simultaneous projection of resultant neural signals from the motor cortex and/or respiratory centres of the brainstem to the respiratory pump muscles and sensory areas of the brain. Studies by Chen *et al.* [20, 21] in unanaesthetised, decerebrated, vagus- and carotid sinus-denervated, paralysed and ventilated cats reported that thalamic and mesencephalic neurons demonstrate phasic respiratory activity, which increased as a function of increasing phrenic nerve discharge and thus NRD. These findings were interpreted as evidence of respiratory-related central corollary discharge and led to the hypothesis that the perception of breathlessness in humans is mechanistically linked to the awareness of increased NRD as sensed by increased central corollary discharge. Support for this hypothesis comes from studies in healthy adults wherein breathlessness intensity ratings increased swiftly to intolerable levels during voluntary breath holding (which is associated with progressive increases in NRD due to central and peripheral chemoreflex stimulation by asphyxia), despite little or no activation of respiratory sensory afferents due to the cessation of breathing [10, 22]. Moreover, the intensity of perceived air hunger, an inherently unpleasant form of breathlessness [23], increases in direct proportion to elevations in $P_{\mathrm{ETCO_2}}$ (reflecting increased chemostimulation and thus NRD) at fixed levels of V'_{E} in mechanically ventilated quadriplegic patients with complete paralysis resulting from high-level cervical injuries [24] or neuromuscular blockade [23, 25]. Collectively, these findings suggest that: 1) increased NRD is the proximate cause of breathlessness; and 2) simultaneous feedback from central and peripheral chemoreceptors, and vagal, cervical and thoracic dorsal root afferent nerves contribute to the neuromodulation of breathlessness *via* their effects on NRD.

In this context, the intensity of perceived breathlessness in disease states can be understood as the awareness of the increased NRD needed to support a given level of V'_{E} in the setting of increased respiratory mechanical loading and/or reduced force-generating capacity of the respiratory muscles (figure 1). Qualitatively distinct descriptors (*e.g.* chest tightness, work/effort) and unpleasant affective dimensions of breathlessness (*e.g.* air hunger, unsatisfied inspiration), which can be rated independently of the sensory intensity domains of breathlessness, are considered to result from the integration of distinct afferent sources [1, 2, 23, 26–28]. For example, Demediuk *et al.* [27] found that increasing NRD by increasing $P_{\mathrm{ETCO_2}}$ at a constant V'_{E} decreased the intensity ratings of respiratory work/effort and simultaneously increased the intensity ratings of air hunger. Lansing *et al.* [28] similarly reported that the intensity ratings of air hunger (not respiratory work/effort) increased when NRD was increased *via* increased $P_{\mathrm{ETCO_2}}$ at a constant V'_{E}, whereas the intensity ratings of respiratory work/effort (not air hunger) increased when V'_{E} was increased at a constant $P_{\mathrm{ETCO_2}}$. In keeping with these observations, Banzett *et al.* [23] showed that air hunger is far more unpleasant than respiratory work/effort at matched levels of intensity.

Central neuroanatomical substrates of breathlessness

As outlined earlier, the conscious perception of breathlessness reflects a complex integration of efferent and afferent sensory information shaped by conscious and unconscious processes in the brain (figure 2). Visualisation of the neurobiology of breathlessness through functional neuroimaging is a relatively new field of research [29, 30]. The brain area most commonly identified during laboratory-induced breathlessness is the insular cortex (often extending into the operculum) [31–42]. The insular cortex is associated with emotion processing, self-awareness and consciousness [43, 44], and is part of a network that integrates sensory information with conscious and unconscious processes such as decision-making, emotions, suffering, memory, motivation and arousal. The prefrontal cortex, anterior and posterior cingulate cortices, cerebellum, amygdala, striatum and periaqueductal grey matter (PAG) have all been inconsistently identified in the various neuroimaging studies of breathlessness [18, 34, 37–42, 45–52].

The interpretation and generalisability of findings of functional neuroimaging studies of breathlessness is limited because of the varying methodologies used and the relatively small number (*i.e.* <20) of original research articles. Furthermore, the extent to which the findings of studies investigating the mechanisms of acute laboratory-induced breathlessness in healthy adults [18, 49] are applicable to understanding the neurobiology of chronic breathlessness in advanced disease is unclear; however, studies in symptomatic patients with COPD are starting to emerge (figure 3) [48]. The discussion that follows proposes how the aforementioned areas of the brain may contribute to breathlessness, although in most cases definitive neuroimaging studies are required.

By driving breathlessness-related fear and anxiety, maladaptive learning may be a key mechanism underlying the severity of chronic breathlessness, regardless of disease status [53]. Learned associations between otherwise innocuous cues (*e.g.* the ring of a doorbell) and breathlessness during the behavioural response (*e.g.* walking to answer the door) exemplify the psychological process known as conditioning. Conditioned responses are likely to underlie learned behaviours driving physical activity avoidance and breathlessness-related anticipatory fear and anxiety, contributing to the well-described vicious cycle of functional decline in CRD. Drawing on observations in the pain literature [54, 55], the insular, prefrontal and anterior cingulate cortices may possibly work together to prepare the brain for an impending breathlessness stimulus. To this end, a recent report by Faull *et al.* [56] provided new evidence for a role of the PAG, which gates neural traffic to and from the periphery (*e.g.* vagal afferent receptors), in conditioned breathlessness anticipation in healthy adults.

Depression is known to worsen pain *via* actions in the prefrontal cortex [57] as part of a "suffering" network that interacts with the insular cortex [58]. Depression is also associated with heightened symptoms of breathlessness [59]. In a recent study of brain responses to breathlessness-related word cues in patients with COPD [48], activity in the prefrontal and paracingulate cortices was correlated with ratings of breathlessness (figure 3) and partly explained by depression levels. Another study by von Leupoldt *et al.* [39] used a focused region of interest approach to investigate the impact of mood on activity in the amygdala and insular cortex of healthy volunteers. In that study, mood was manipulated by presenting happy and sad faces during resistive load breathing, with stronger breathlessness-related activation of the amygdala and insular cortex occurring during sad *versus* happy face presentation [39]. It is worth considering, however, that happy or sad faces might activate the amygdala and insular cortex, in a manner independent of the breathlessness stimulus.

One new technology that might help advance our understanding of breathlessness processing is magnetoencephalography (MEG), which measures brain activity by detecting magnetic fields generated by neuronal currents [60, 61]. The particular advantages of MEG for the study of breathlessness are that it has a high temporal resolution and experiments

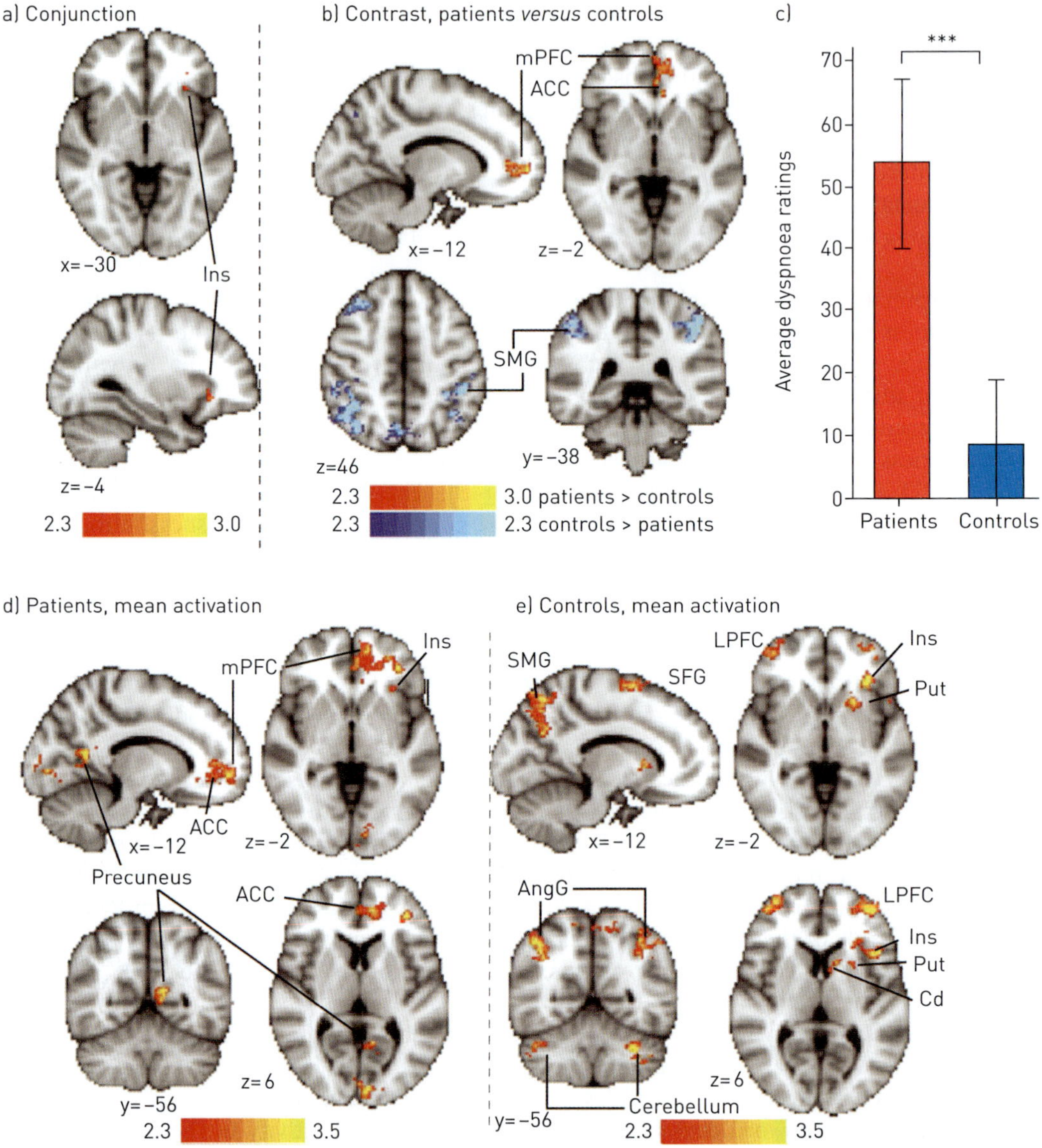

Figure 3. Activation (contrasts and conjunction) correlating with VAS ratings to breathlessness-related word cues in people with COPD and age-sex matched healthy controls. This demonstrates activation of many emotion-regulating areas. Maps are cluster-level corrected for multiple comparisons at $p<0.05$ across the whole brain. Maps represent conjunction analysis (activations common to both groups), comparisons between groups (patients *versus* controls in red-yellow, controls *versus* patients in blue-light blue), and mean activations in patients and controls. Bar graph is mean±SD breathlessness ratings for each group. ***: $p<0.001$. Cerebellum is crus I and VI. ACC: anterior cingulate cortex; AngG: angular gyrus; Cd: caudate; Ins: insular cortex; LPFC: lateral prefrontal cortex; MFG: middle frontal gyrus; mPFC: medial prefrontal cortex; Put: putamen; SMG: supramarginal gyrus; SFG: superior frontal gyrus. Reproduced from [48] with permission.

are conducted in the sitting position. Johnson *et al.* [61] recently confirmed that MEG is a feasible method to investigate exercise-induced breathlessness in adults with chronic lung disease. Future work using MEG would be particularly suited to investigating the dynamics of brain networks that process breathlessness and its response to therapy.

Understanding breathlessness through pulmonary disease pathophysiology

Obstructive lung disease

In diseases characterised by expiratory airflow limitation (*e.g.* COPD, asthma, cystic fibrosis (CF)), NRD is elevated at rest and during exercise compared to healthy individuals to compensate for the increased respiratory mechanical load relative to reduced respiratory muscle force-generating capacity, these being consequences of impaired respiratory mechanics (figures 4 and 5a) [3–9, 62]. Ventilatory demand is also increased to overcome ventilation–perfusion mismatch [63], hypoxaemia, hypercapnia and early-onset metabolic (lactic) acidosis during exercise as a consequence of the reduced aerobic capacity of the locomotor muscle [64, 65].

The capacity of the respiratory system to respond to the increased ventilatory demands of exercise is grossly impaired in adults with COPD, particularly those with advanced disease [65]. This impairment is due to static and dynamic lung hyperinflation (figure 6) [66], which positions V_T on the upper alinear (noncompliant) extreme of the respiratory system's sigmoid pressure–volume relationship. Under these circumstances, V_T expansion becomes mechanically constrained early in exercise as inspiratory capacity (IC) and inspiratory reserve volume (IRV) decrease from their relatively reduced resting values (figure 7c–e) [66]; breathing frequency increases (tachypnoea) (figure 7d) [66]; the inspiratory muscles (*e.g.* diaphragm) shorten, functionally weaken and become less contractile [67–70]; respiratory muscle effort requirements and the work of breathing increase [62, 71]; and breathlessness intensity ratings rapidly escalate to intolerable levels (figure 8) [66].

The progressive shortening, weakening and mechanical loading of the inspiratory muscles that accompany exercise-induced decreases in IC and IRV necessitate, in the face of increased ventilatory demand, a compensatory increase in NRD to generate the intrathoracic pressures and respiratory flow rates needed to achieve or maintain any given V_T and V'_E during exercise in patients with COPD *versus* healthy individuals (figures 4, 7a and 7b) [5, 6, 62, 67, 72]. The resultant disparity between increasing NRD and increasing mechanical/muscular output of the respiratory system (figures 5b and 7b) has been termed neuromechanical/neuroventilatory uncoupling or dissociation.

A growing body of evidence suggests that higher breathlessness intensity ratings at equivalent power outputs and levels of V'_E during exercise in patients with CF and COPD (figure 8a and 8b) *versus* healthy controls are mechanistically linked to higher NRD, quantified as diaphragm electromyogram (EMG_{di}) activity expressed as a percentage of volitional maximum ($EMG_{di\%max}$) (figure 8c) [4, 5, 62, 72]. MURPHY *et al.* [73] similarly reported that changes in NRD, quantified as parasternal intercostal EMG activity expressed as a percentage of volitional maximum, following an acute exacerbation of COPD correlated positively with concurrent changes in breathlessness intensity ratings, further substantiating the role of increased NRD as the proximate cause of breathlessness in patients with obstructive lung disease.

ILD

Pulmonary reserve in ILD is limited by mechanical and gas exchange abnormalities. This results in increased NRD as a consequence of increased ventilatory demand and increased

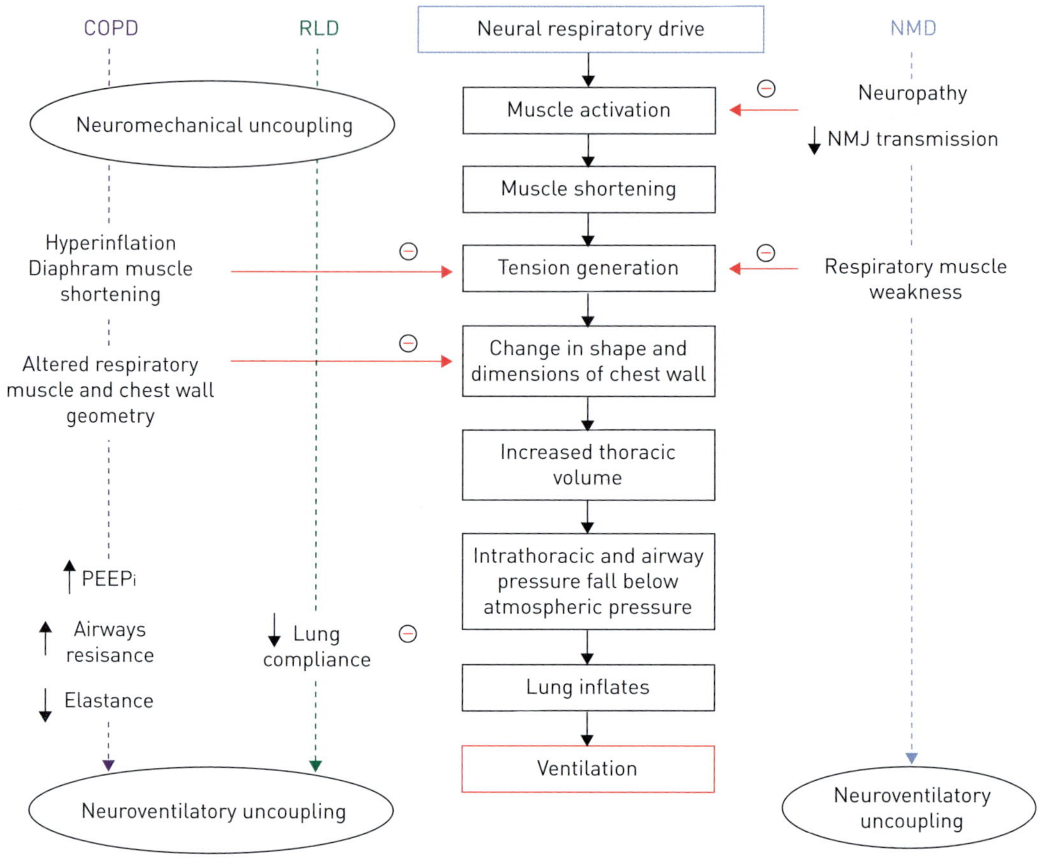

Figure 4. Impact of COPD, restrictive lung disease (RLD, *e.g.* ILD) and neuromuscular disease complicated by respiratory muscle weakness (*e.g.* amyotrophic lateral sclerosis (ALS)) on the translation of neural respiratory drive to ventilation. Disordered ventilatory mechanics in patients with COPD and RLD progressively uncouple the neural respiratory drive from generation of respiratory muscle tension, intrathoracic pressure and ventilation, *i.e.* neuromechanical and neuroventilatory uncoupling. In neuromuscular diseases, respiratory muscle weakness causes neuroventilatory uncoupling as a result of neuropathy (*e.g.* ALS), impaired neuromuscular junction (NMJ) transmission (*e.g.* myasthenia gravis), a primary muscle disorder (*e.g.* Duchenne's muscular dystrophy) or a mixed neuropathic/myopathic disorder (*e.g.* critical illness neuromyopathy). PEEPi: intrinsic positive end-expiratory pressure; NMD: neuromuscular disease. Adapted and modified from [9] with permission.

mechanical load on the respiratory muscles, increasing the work of breathing [5, 74–76]. Respiratory muscle weakness should also be considered as a cause of reduced ventilatory capacity in ILD [74, 77–79], particularly in the context of inflammatory myopathies [80].

In persons with ILD, the sigmoid pressure–volume curve of the respiratory system typically shifts downwards and to the right (*i.e.* contracts along its volume axis), which is consistent with a stiff, noncompliant lung (figure 4) [81]. As a result, pulmonary function tests in ILD are consistent with a restrictive ventilatory defect (*i.e.* reduced total lung capacity, vital capacity, IC and IRV) without reductions in isovolume flow rates [5, 77, 81, 82]. Lung gas transfer is frequently reduced and its decline may precede abnormalities in lung volume [83]. The main cause for exercise-induced hypoxaemia is ventilation–perfusion mismatch [84].

Compared with healthy controls, patients with ILD report higher levels of breathlessness intensity at any given V'_E, power output and rate of oxygen uptake (V'_{O_2}) during exercise

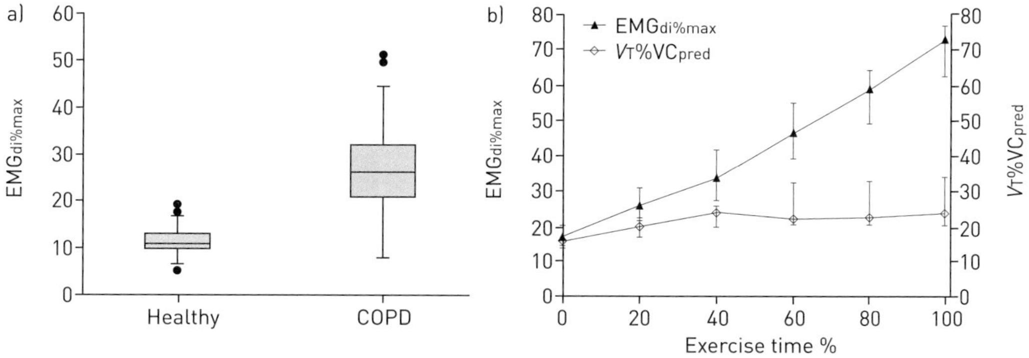

Figure 5. a) Box-and-whisker plots comparing resting measures of neural respiratory drive (*i.e.* diaphragm electromyogram activity expressed as a percentage of volitional maximum (EMGdi%max)) in 30 patients with COPD, with 26 healthy individuals matched for age, height and BMI ($p<0.001$ by independent samples t-test). The box length is the interquartile range (IQR). Closed circles are outliers, *i.e.* cases with values between 1.5 and 3 IQRs from the upper and lower edge of the box. Reproduced from [3] with permission. b) Relationship between increasing neural respiratory drive (EMGdi%max) and increasing thoracic volume displacement (tidal volume (V_T) expressed as a percentage of predicted vital capacity (VCpred) (V_T%VCpred)) during symptom-limited incremental cycle or treadmill exercise testing in 12 patients with COPD. Data points represent median and IQR. Reproduced from [72] with permission.

(figure 8a and 8b) [5, 82]. In addition to increasing the intrinsic mechanical loading of the respiratory muscles, these impairments in static and dynamic ventilatory mechanics (*e.g.* reduced IC and IRV) also serve to limit V_T expansion early in exercise despite increasing NRD (figure 7c–e) [5, 82]. The inability to further expand V_T means that increases in V'_E can only be achieved through increases in breathing frequency (tachypnoea) (figure 7f). Using EMGdi%max to quantify NRD, FAISAL *et al.* [5] recently elucidated the extent of the resultant neuromechanical uncoupling during exercise in patients with mild-to-moderate ILD. In that study, higher breathlessness intensity ratings at any given V'_E and power output during exercise in patients with ILD compared with healthy controls were closely related to greater EMGdi%max as a result of greater restrictive constraints on V_T expansion, *i.e.* reduced IRV or increased V_T/IC (figure 8) [5]. Interestingly, relationships between breathlessness intensity and EMGdi%max were almost identical during exercise in patients with ILD compared with patients with COPD and healthy controls (figure 8c) [5]. The key interpretation of these findings is that disease-specific differences in static and dynamic ventilatory mechanics (and presumably also respiratory afferent feedback) did not influence the fundamental association between increasing breathlessness intensity ratings and increasing NRD, lending support to the hypothesis that increased NRD is the final common pathway in the genesis of increased breathlessness intensity in health and respiratory disease (figures 1 and 2).

Descriptor phrases alluding to unsatisfied inspiration (*e.g.* "I cannot get enough air in") are selected more frequently at end-exercise by COPD and ILD patients than healthy controls [5, 71, 82, 85]. Accumulating evidence suggests that these differences in the quality of perceived breathlessness may have their origins in neuromechanical uncoupling [85, 86], thus implicating a role for the central processing of mismatch between NRD and sensory feedback from vagal, cervical and thoracic afferent receptors in shaping the quality of breathlessness.

Neuromuscular respiratory weakness

In neuromuscular respiratory muscle weakness, the mechanical properties of the respiratory system are frequently normal, but a higher level of NRD is needed to achieve levels of

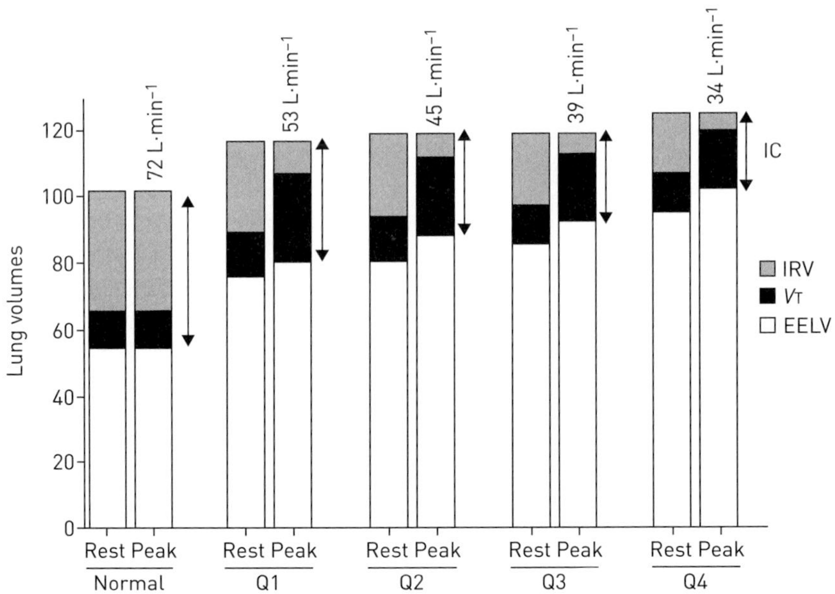

Figure 6. Progressive hyperinflation, shown by increasing end-expiratory lung volume (EELV), expressed as % predicted total lung capacity, is illustrated at rest and peak exercise as FEV_1 quartile worsens in patients with COPD. Peak values of dynamic inspiratory capacity (IC), tidal volume (V_T) and ventilation (values shown above peak exercise bars) decreased with worsening disease severity, although similar peak ratings of breathlessness intensity were reached (data not shown). Normative data are shown for comparison (n=21). Data across groups of patients with COPD (n=427) were divided into quartiles based on FEV_1 expressed as a percentage of predicted normal values, where Q1=54.5–85.1%; Q2=43.8–54.1%; Q3=34.9–43.6%; and Q4=16.5–34.9%. IRV: inspiratory reserve volume. Reproduced from [66] with permission.

respiratory muscle activation and V'_E required to meet homeostatic demands (figure 4) [87]. A rapid and shallow breathing pattern characterised by a reduced V_T (associated with lung atelectasis), decreased inspiratory time and increased breathing frequency (*i.e.* increased velocity of shortening) [88], further increases demand on the weakened respiratory muscles. Patients with more severe respiratory muscle weakness, commonly seen in advanced amyotrophic lateral sclerosis (ALS), recruit accessory muscles of respiration even at rest [89, 90]. GEORGES *et al.* [89] recently reported that relief of breathlessness in the A1 (immediate affective) component of the MDP correlated with reductions in neck inspiratory muscle EMG activity on application of NIV support in ventilator-dependent ALS patients with severe diaphragm weakness/paralysis (figure 2).

Understanding breathlessness through its management

Bronchodilator therapy

Although inhaled bronchodilators are the mainstay of the pharmacotherapy for obstructive lung diseases (*e.g.* COPD, asthma), consequent reductions in exertional breathlessness are poorly related to improvements in FEV_1, but correlate well with indices of improved V_T expansion (*e.g.* increased IC and IRV) and enhanced neuromechanical coupling [91–93]. In patients with COPD, single-dose inhalation of terbutaline, albuterol, fenoterol, salbutamol, ipratropium bromide and fluticasone/salmeterol propionate have all been shown to reduce indices of NRD (*e.g.* EMG_{di}, mouth-occlusion pressure at 0.1-s of inspiration ($P_{0.1}$), and

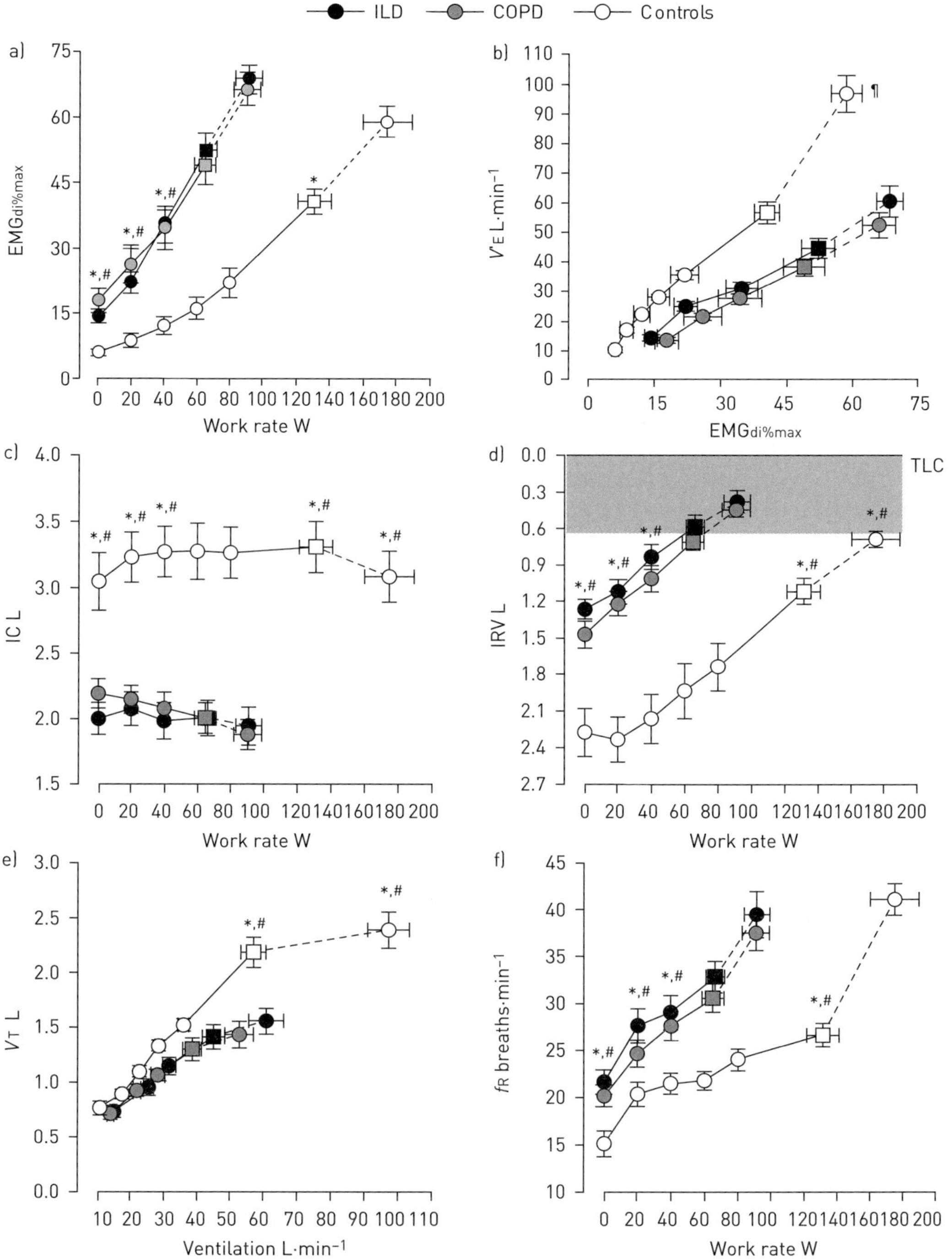

Figure 7. a) Neural respiratory drive, b) neuroventilatory coupling, c) and d) operating lung volumes, and e) and f) breathing pattern during symptom-limited incremental cycle exercise testing in patients with ILD (n=16), patients with COPD (n=16), and age-matched healthy controls (n=16). The shaded area in d) represents the minimal inspiratory reserve volume (IRV) reached by all groups at the end of exercise. Square symbols represent tidal volume (V_T)-minute ventilation (V'_E) inflection points. Values are mean±SEM. *: $p<0.05$ for ILD *versus* controls; #: $p<0.05$ for COPD *versus* controls; ¶: $p<0.05$ for differences in V'_E-neural respiratory drive slopes between patient groups and healthy controls. $EMG_{di\%max}$: root mean square of the crural diaphragm electromyogram activity expressed as a percentage of volitional maximum; IC: inspiratory capacity; f_R: breathing frequency; TLC: total lung capacity. Adapted from [5] with permission.

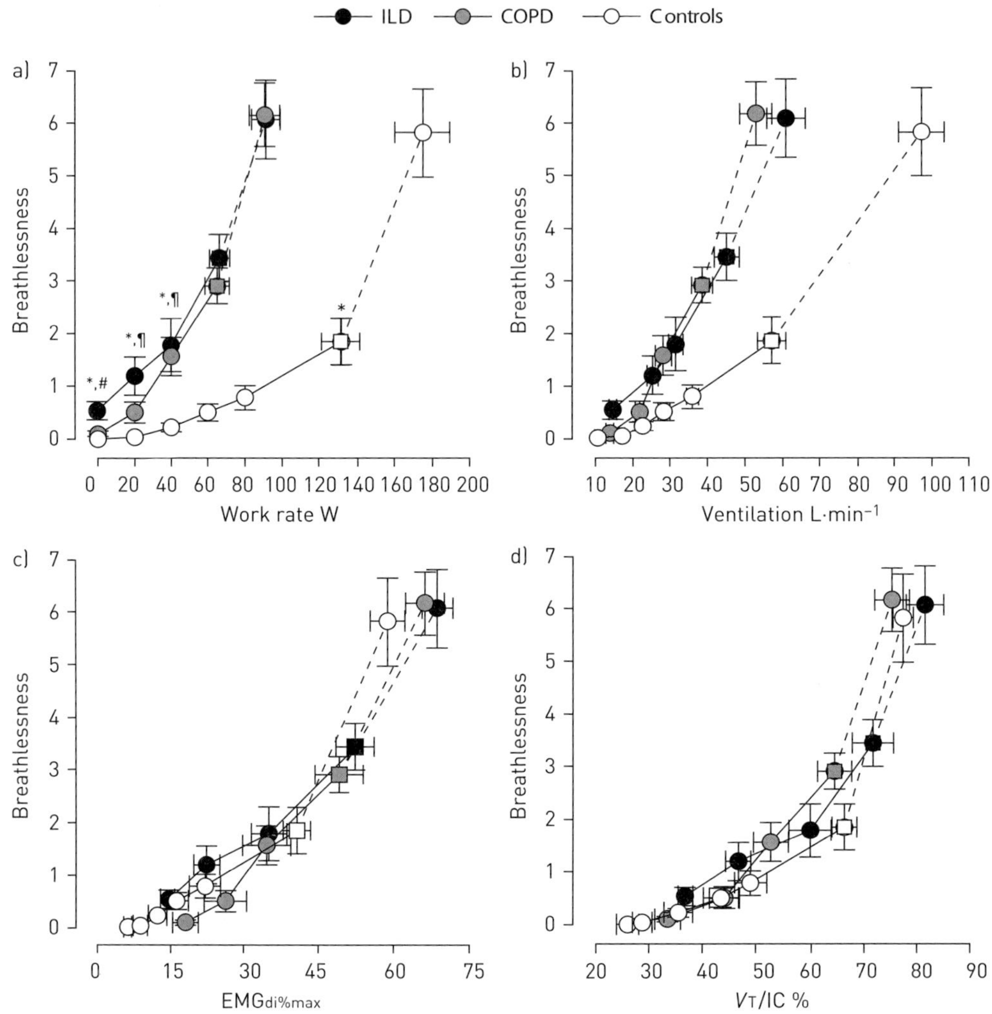

Figure 8. Exertional breathlessness (breathlessness) intensity ratings during symptom-limited incremental cycle exercise testing in patients with ILD (n=16), patients with COPD (n=16), and age-matched healthy controls (n=16). Breathlessness intensity ratings (Borg scale) are presented relative to: a) work rate; b) ventilation; c) neural respiratory drive; and d) tidal volume (V_T) to inspiratory capacity (IC) ratio. Square symbols represent the V_T-ventilation inflection points. Values are mean±SEM. *: p<0.05 for ILD *versus* controls; #: p<0.05 for ILD *versus* COPD; ¶: p<0.05 for COPD *versus* controls. $EMG_{di\%max}$: root mean square of the crural diaphragm electromyogram activity expressed as a percentage of volitional maximum. Reproduced from [5] with permission.

surface EMG activity of the diaphragm and parasternal intercostal muscles) and to improve neuroventilatory coupling (defined as the ratio of V'_E to EMG_{di} (V'_E/EMG_{di})) at rest and during increased chemostimulation by hypercapnia [94–98], particularly in patients with marked improvements in static lung hyperinflation (*i.e.* resting IC) [96]. Qin *et al.* [99] recently reported that addition of tiotropium bromide to usual therapy for 1 month in patients with severe COPD significantly reduced $EMG_{di\%max}$ at rest and enhanced neuroventilatory coupling during exercise. Moreover, Pino-García *et al.* [97] and Li *et al.* [98] reported that acute, bronchodilator-induced relief of breathlessness intensity at rest correlated with concurrent changes in $P_{0.1}$, EMG_{di} and V'_E/EMG_{di} ratio in patients with moderate-to-severe COPD. The collective results of these studies suggest that inhaled bronchodilators, by decreasing static and dynamic lung hyperinflation and improving the load–capacity balance of the respiratory muscle pump, contribute to the relief of breathlessness at rest and during exercise through a reduction in NRD (figure 2). Similar mechanisms underlying breathlessness relief are observed after surgical lung volume reduction techniques in selected patients with heterogeneous emphysema (figure 2) [100–106].

NIV

As discussed in another chapter in this *Monograph* [107], NIV is a method of breathing support delivered *via* a mouthpiece, nasal pillow or mask worn over the nose and/or mouth. In patients with COPD, the use of NIV during a single bout of exercise has been shown to alleviate breathlessness and improve breathing pattern, gas exchange and exercise tolerance compared to exercise without NIV or exercise with sham NIV [108–113]. Research also suggests that acute and long-term use of NIV decreases breathlessness at rest and during exercise in patients with CF [114, 115], restrictive lung disease [116, 117], end-stage cancer [118] and motor neuron disease [119, 120]. In COPD patients, NIV unloads the inspiratory pump muscles and decreases the work (effort) of breathing during exercise [110, 121, 122], with reductions in breathlessness correlating positively with reductions in both inspiratory muscle effort [121] and NRD assessed by transcutaneous recordings of intercostal, scalene and diaphragmatic EMG activity (figure 2) [113]. Through this mechanism of respiratory muscle unloading and reduced inspiratory neural drive, the use of NIV during pulmonary rehabilitation may allow people with COPD (and perhaps also other chronic pulmonary disorders) to exercise at higher intensities than otherwise possible and to achieve greater relief of breathlessness and improvements in exercise tolerance [123].

Supplemental oxygen

Supplemental oxygen is an effective therapy for relief of breathlessness at rest and during exercise in many hypoxaemic patients and in selected non-hypoxaemic patients, with chronic obstructive and restrictive pulmonary disease [107, 124–127]. Ambulatory oxygen therapy is defined as supplemental oxygen during exercise or during activities of daily living. Despite demonstration of acute benefit during laboratory-based exercise tests, improvements in breathlessness- and fatigue-related quality of life domains are small, and long-term use of ambulatory oxygen therapy has not been shown to consistently confer sustained benefits to exercise capacity or prognosis for those not meeting the criteria for prescription of long-term oxygen therapy (LTOT) [128]. Thus, in patients who desaturate during exercise, but do not meet the criteria for LTOT, ambulatory oxygen therapy is considered only after specialist review if clinically significant improvements in breathlessness and/or functional exercise capacity during a field exercise test (*e.g.* 6-min walk test) are achieved using supplemental oxygen. Typical criteria are: ⩾10% increase in walking distance from baseline; and/or ⩾1 unit decrease in breathlessness on the Borg 0–10 scale, where arterial oxygen saturation measured by pulse oximetry is maintained >90% throughout exercise by supplemental oxygen [129].

The use of palliative oxygen therapy (POT) to reduce distressing refractory breathlessness in end-stage disease is frequently controversial given the lack of evidence of benefit over alternative interventions [129]. There is a poor correlation between breathlessness ratings and blood oxygen levels in patients with end-stage cardiorespiratory disease or cancer, with no evidence of symptomatic benefit over entrained air or opiates in hypoxaemic or non-hypoxaemic patients [130, 131]. However, POT is considered in hypoxaemic patients after individual specialist assessment, when significant breathlessness persists despite trials of alternative pharmacological and non-pharmacological treatment options [129].

In normoxic and hypoxaemic COPD patients who respond, relief from breathlessness during exercise while breathing supplemental oxygen *versus* room air is most likely the result of reduced NRD in association with improved arterial blood and peripheral locomotor muscle oxygen levels, decreased circulating levels of lactate, and reduced chemostimulation of the aortic and carotid bodies (figure 2) [113, 127, 132–139]. To this end, slopes of breathlessness, V'_E, $P_{0.1}$, surface inspiratory muscle (scalene, intercostal and diaphragm) EMG activity and lactate over time are reduced during constant-load cycle exercise testing in COPD while breathing supplemental oxygen *versus* room air, whereas breathlessness/V'_E, breathlessness/lactate and V'_E/lactate slopes are unaffected by supplemental oxygen [113, 134–136]. However, stimulation of facial and upper airway sensory afferents by supplemental airflow is likely to contribute significantly to breathlessness relief even in the absence of improved of blood oxygen levels [131, 140].

Pulmonary rehabilitation/exercise training

Rehabilitative exercise training is arguably the most effective therapeutic intervention to relieve breathlessness in patients with chronic obstructive and restrictive pulmonary disease [141, 142]. Although the mechanisms of breathlessness relief following exercise training in these patients involve numerous physiological, psychological and behavioural adaptations, reductions in peripheral locomotor muscle metabolic requirements and NRD play a central role (figure 2). In patients with COPD, rehabilitative exercise training improves the oxidative capacity of peripheral locomotor muscles [143]. The resultant effect is a delay in the onset of metabolic (lactic) acidosis with attendant reductions in V'_E (presumably *via* reduced peripheral chemoreceptor stimulation) (figure 2), respiratory muscle pressure development and consequently breathlessness at any standardised submaximal time, power output and V'_{O_2} during exercise [64, 144–146]. GAGNON *et al.* [147] recently reported that pharmacological inhibition of central feedback from type III (mechanoreceptors) and type IV (metaboreceptors) sensory nerves in the lower limb muscles of 13 men with moderate-to-severe COPD significantly reduced both V'_E and breathlessness intensity responses to high-intensity, constant-load cycle exercise testing. It follows that exercise training-induced improvements in peripheral locomotor muscle metabolic and contractile function may contribute to reductions in NRD, and consequently breathlessness, during exercise in patients with chronic pulmonary disease *via* reduced afferent signalling from type III and IV sensory nerves in the lower limbs. This possibility requires scientific validation.

Interestingly, pulmonary rehabilitation has more profound benefits on breathlessness anxiety than breathlessness intensity, even in the absence of consistent physiological training adaptations [47, 148, 149]. As such, an important outcome of pulmonary rehabilitation is empowerment to exercise harder by decreasing breathlessness-related fear and anxiety (figure 2). This might reflect the benefits of education and other cognitive-behavioural interventions that form the complex intervention of pulmonary rehabilitation on catastrophic misinterpretations of ambiguous physical sensations (*e.g.* increased V'_E and/or heart rate) and perceived control over the disease and breathlessness (*i.e.* increased self-efficacy) [150–153]. It is reasonable to speculate from studies in chronic pain [154, 155] and one study in breathlessness [47] that the prefrontal cortex may play a role in the relief of breathlessness intensity and breathlessness-related anxiety following pulmonary rehabilitation.

Nebulised furosemide

As reviewed in detail elsewhere [156, 157], including in another chapter in this *Monograph* [107], inhalation of nebulised furosemide (20–40 mg), a loop diuretic, decreases the intensity of breathlessness provoked by a variety of respiratory stimuli in healthy adults (*e.g.* breath holding, hypercapnia with inspiratory resistive loading, and hypercapnia with and without constrained V'_E) [158–160]; at rest in patients with advanced cancer [161, 162]; and during cycle exercise testing in adults with COPD [163, 164].

Although the mechanisms underlying the relief of breathlessness with inhaled furosemide remain unclear, changes in the activity of sensory afferent receptors innervated by the vagus nerve are likely contributory (figure 2) [157]. To this end, SANT'AMBROGIO *et al.* [165] showed that inhaled furosemide inhibited the activity of laryngeal irritant receptors to stimulation by low-chloride solutions in anaesthetised dogs. In addition, SUDO *et al.* [166] reported that slowly adapting stretch receptors are sensitised and rapidly adapting stretch receptors are desensitised by inhaled, but not intravenous, furosemide in anaesthetised rats. Thus, inhaled furosemide may alleviate breathlessness by directly altering the activity of stretch-sensitive vagal afferent receptors.

It is possible that inhaled furosemide, by altering vagal afferent activity, may contribute to the relief of breathlessness *via* reflex inhibition of NRD [167–169]. However, the benefits of inhaled furosemide on breathlessness provoked by hypercapnia in healthy adults and by cycle exercise testing in patients with COPD could not be easily explained by concomitant reductions in the V'_E response to either of these stimuli [158, 160, 163, 164].

Relief of breathlessness with inhaled furosemide may also be because of, at least in part, improved static and dynamic airway function (*i.e.* bronchodilation) by mechanisms that are poorly understood. For example, an RCT by SHEIKH MOTAHAR VAHEDI *et al.* [170] reported that nebulised furosemide (40 mg) was superior to 0.9% saline placebo as an adjunct to conventional therapies for alleviating breathlessness and improving FEV_1 in older adults admitted to the ED with an acute exacerbation of COPD. Furthermore, JENSEN *et al.* [164] reported that alleviation of exertional breathlessness following single-dose inhalation of nebulised furosemide (40 mg) *versus* 0.9% saline placebo in patients with COPD was associated with modest but significant increases in IC, V_T and mean tidal expiratory flow rates during exercise.

Fan/cold air

As discussed in another chapter in this *Monograph* [107], cold air directed around the nose and mouth using a fan is an effective non-pharmacological treatment for breathlessness relief in cardiorespiratory and malignant disease. There is also evidence that breathlessness relief by supplemental oxygen is related, at least in part, to the sensation of airflow rather than normalisation of blood oxygen levels [131, 140].

Breathing cold air has been shown to alter the pattern of breathing and decrease the V'_E response to hypercapnia in healthy subjects [171, 172]. In COPD patients, cold air reduced end-exercise breathlessness associated with higher end-exercise P_{ETCO_2} compared to room air [173]. Thus, reduced NRD is one possible mechanism underlying the relief of breathlessness by facial airflow.

SCHWARTZSTEIN *et al.* [174] reported that cold air directed towards the face of normal subjects decreased the intensity ratings of breathlessness induced by the combination of hypercapnia and inspiratory resistive loading without decreasing either V'_E or the V'_E response to hypercapnia. SIMON *et al.* [175] similarly showed that, in normal subjects, stimulation of oral mucosal "flow receptors" modulated the intensity of breathlessness induced by hypercapnia and inspiratory resistive loading, independent of changes in V'_E and breathing pattern. NISHINO *et al.* [176] further demonstrated that stimulation of "cold receptors" in the upper airway of normal subjects with nasal inhalation of L-menthol decreased the intensity ratings of breathlessness caused by both resistive and elastic loading without a significant change in V'_E and breathing pattern. The collective results of these studies suggest that afferent information arising from the stimulation of facial receptors innervated by the trigeminal nerve, oral mucosal "flow receptors" and/or upper airway "cold receptors" is projected directly to sensory areas of the brain with attendant alterations of perceived breathlessness for any given level of increased NRD (figure 2).

Opioids

Opioids have profound effects on respiration and breathlessness when administered acutely (figure 2) [177], although their long-term clinical benefit in refractory breathlessness remains undetermined [178]. Studying opioid action in the brain with neuroimaging may provide new insights into the mechanisms of breathlessness and potential new avenues for its treatment. Opioid receptors are widely distributed throughout the brain, with particularly high densities in the insular cortex, thalamus, putamen, amygdala and PAG [179]. A study of healthy adults by PATTINSON *et al.* [180] reported that the μ-opioid agonist, remifentanil, depressed breath holding-related activity in the insular cortex, PAG, prefrontal cortex and anterior cingulate cortex, all areas identified in breathlessness. Remifentanil also decreased mean urge-to-breathe ratings by ~50% during the breath-holding manoeuvre [180]. Although this study did not investigate breathlessness *per se*, it demonstrated that higher cortical centres implicated in the perception of breathlessness in humans may influence brainstem respiratory control, and that opioids may affect this pathway at multiple points, even in the absence of changes in V'_E, breathing pattern and sensory feedback from pulmonary afferent receptors (figure 2).

Randomised, double blind, placebo-controlled, crossover studies by GIFFORD *et al.* [181] and MAHLER *et al.* [182] showed that blocking endogenous opioid receptor signalling by single-dose intravenous administration of naloxone, an opioid receptor antagonist, increased mean ratings of breathlessness throughout treadmill exercise and resistive load breathing in patients with COPD, despite no concurrent changes in V'_E, breathing pattern, gas exchange and/or cardiometabolic responses. The results of these studies suggest that neuromodulation of breathlessness by endogenous opioids, and presumably also exogenous opioids (*e.g.* morphine), is most likely mediated by binding to opioid receptors within the central nervous system, as previously discussed.

Conclusion

The mechanisms of breathlessness in health and disease are multifactorial and include a complex integration of efferent and afferent sensory information shaped by conscious and unconscious processes within cortical and subcortical neural networks. A growing body of evidence supports the hypothesis that higher breathlessness intensity at rest and during exercise in patients with obstructive and restrictive pulmonary disease compared with healthy individuals ultimately reflects the awareness of greater NRD needed to support V'_E in the face of increased intrinsic respiratory mechanical loading, reduced force-generating capacity of the respiratory muscles and/or increased ventilatory demand. It follows that any therapeutic intervention capable of reducing NRD by improving the load–capacity balance of the respiratory muscle pump and/or decreasing ventilatory demand has the potential to alleviate breathlessness in patients with pulmonary disease. Additionally, treatments targeting brain networks that mediate breathlessness may yield additional symptomatic benefits, particularly for those patients whose emotions exacerbate symptoms. Continued advances in physiological measurement, functional neuroimaging of the brain and individualised assessment of breathlessness will invariably enhance our fundamental understanding of the neurobiology of breathlessness across its sensory intensity, quality and affective domains, and help identify more effective pharmacological and non-pharmacological interventions targeted to relieving breathlessness in individual patients with pulmonary disease.

References

1. Parshall MB, Schwartzstein RM, Adams L, *et al.* An official American Thoracic Society statement: update on the mechanisms, assessment, and management of dyspnea. *Am J Respir Crit Care Med* 2012; 185: 435–452.
2. Lansing RW, Gracely RH, Banzett RB. The multiple dimensions of dyspnea: review and hypotheses. *Respir Physiol Neurobiol* 2009; 167: 53–60.
3. Jolley CJ, Luo YM, Steier J, *et al.* Neural respiratory drive in healthy subjects and in COPD. *Eur Respir J* 2009; 33: 289–297.
4. Reilly CC, Ward K, Jolley CJ, *et al.* Neural respiratory drive, pulmonary mechanics and breathlessness in patients with cystic fibrosis. *Thorax* 2011; 66: 240–246.
5. Faisal A, Alghamdi BJ, Ciavaglia CE, *et al.* Common mechanisms of dyspnea in chronic interstitial and obstructive lung disorders. *Am J Respir Crit Care Med* 2016; 193: 299–309.
6. Qin YY, Steier J, Jolley C, *et al.* Efficiency of neural drive during exercise in patients with COPD and healthy subjects. *Chest* 2010; 138: 1309–1315.
7. Sinderby C, Beck J, Spahija J, *et al.* Voluntary activation of the human diaphragm in health and disease. *J Appl Physiol* 1998; 85: 2146–2158.
8. McKenzie DK, Butler JE, Gandevia SC. Respiratory muscle function and activation in chronic obstructive pulmonary disease. *J Appl Physiol* 2009; 107: 621–629.
9. Jolley CJ, Moxham J. A physiological model of patient-reported breathlessness during daily activities in COPD. *Eur Respir Rev* 2009; 18: 66–79.
10. Flume PA, Eldridge FL, Edwards LJ, *et al.* The Fowler breathholding study revisited: continuous rating of respiratory sensation. *Respir Physiol* 1994; 95: 53–66.
11. Fowler WS. Breaking point of breath-holding. *J Appl Physiol* 1954; 6: 539–545.
12. Manning HL, Shea SA, Schwartzstein RM, *et al.* Reduced tidal volume increases 'air hunger' at fixed P_{CO_2} in ventilated quadriplegics. *Respir Physiol* 1992; 90: 19–30.
13. Widdicombe J. Lung afferent activity: implications for respiratory sensation. *Respir Physiol Neurobiol* 2009; 167: 2–8.
14. Buchanan GF, Richerson GB. Role of chemoreceptors in mediating dyspnea. *Respir Physiol Neurobiol* 2009; 167: 9–19.
15. Lee LY. Respiratory sensations evoked by activation of bronchopulmonary C-fibers. *Respir Physiol Neurobiol* 2009; 167: 26–35.
16. Burki NK, Lee LY. Mechanisms of dyspnea. *Chest* 2010; 138: 1196–1201.
17. Lee L-Y, Yu J. Sensory nerves in lung and airways. *Compr Physiol* 2014; 4: 287–324.
18. von Leupoldt A, Dahme B. Cortical substrates for the perception of dyspnea. *Chest* 2005; 128: 345–354.
19. Davenport PW, Vovk A. Cortical and subcortical central neural pathways in respiratory sensations. *Respir Physiol Neurobiol* 2009; 167: 72–86.
20. Chen Z, Eldridge FL, Wagner PG. Respiratory-associated rhythmic firing of midbrain neurones in cats: relation to level of respiratory drive. *J Physiol* 1991; 437: 305–325.
21. Chen Z, Eldridge FL, Wagner PG. Respiratory-associated thalamic activity is related to level of respiratory drive. *Respir Physiol* 1992; 90: 99–113.

22. Gandevia SC, Killian K, McKenzie DK, *et al.* Respiratory sensations, cardiovascular control, kinaesthesia and transcranial stimulation during paralysis in humans. *J Physiol* 1993; 470: 85–107.
23. Banzett RB, Pedersen SH, Schwartzstein RM, *et al.* The affective dimension of laboratory dyspnea: air hunger is more unpleasant than work/effort. *Am J Respir Crit Care Med* 2008; 177: 1384–1390.
24. Banzett RB, Lansing RW, Reid MB, *et al.* 'Air hunger' arising from increased P_{CO_2} in mechanically ventilated quadriplegics. *Respir Physiol* 1989; 76: 53–67.
25. Banzett RB, Lansing RW, Brown R, *et al.* 'Air hunger' from increased P_{CO_2} persists after complete neuromuscular block in humans. *Respir Physiol* 1990; 81: 1–17.
26. Banzett RB, O'Donnell CR, Guilfoyle TE, *et al.* Multidimensional Dyspnea Profile: an instrument for clinical and laboratory research. *Eur Respir J* 2015; 45: 1681–1691.
27. Demediuk BH, Manning H, Lilly J, *et al.* Dissociation between dyspnea and respiratory effort. *Am Rev Respir Dis* 1992; 146: 1222–1225.
28. Lansing RW, Im BS, Thwing JI, *et al.* The perception of respiratory work and effort can be independent of the perception of air hunger. *Am J Respir Crit Care Med* 2000; 162: 1690–1696.
29. Pattinson K. Functional brain imaging in respiratory medicine. *Thorax* 2015; 70: 598–600.
30. Pattinson KT. Functional magnetic resonance imaging in anaesthesia research. *Br J Anaesth* 2013; 111: 872–876.
31. Brannan S, Liotti M, Egan G, *et al.* Neuroimaging of cerebral activations and deactivations associated with hypercapnia and hunger for air. *Proc Natl Acad Sci USA* 2001; 98: 2029–2034.
32. Liotti M, Brannan S, Egan G, *et al.* Brain responses associated with consciousness of breathlessness (air hunger). *Proc Natl Acad Sci USA* 2001; 98: 2035–2040.
33. Parsons LM, Egan G, Liotti M, *et al.* Neuroimaging evidence implicating cerebellum in the experience of hypercapnia and hunger for air. *Proc Natl Acad Sci USA* 2001; 98: 2041–2046.
34. Banzett RB, Mulnier HE, Murphy K, *et al.* Breathlessness in humans activates insular cortex. *Neuroreport* 2000; 11: 2117–2120.
35. Peiffer C, Costes N, Hervé P, *et al.* Relief of dyspnea involves a characteristic brain activation and a specific quality of sensation. *Am J Respir Crit Care Med* 2008; 177: 440–449.
36. Peiffer C, Poline JB, Thivard L, *et al.* Neural substrates for the perception of acutely induced dyspnea. *Am J Respir Crit Care Med* 2001; 163: 951–957.
37. Evans KC, Banzett RB, Adams L, *et al.* BOLD fMRI identifies limbic, paralimbic, and cerebellar activation during air hunger. *J Neurophysiol* 2002; 88: 1500–1511.
38. Binks AP, Evans KC, Reed JD, *et al.* The time-course of cortico-limbic neural responses to air hunger. *Respir Physiol Neurobiol* 2014; 204: 78–85.
39. von Leupoldt A, Sommer T, Kegat S, *et al.* The unpleasantness of perceived dyspnea is processed in the anterior insula and amygdala. *Am J Respir Crit Care Med* 2008; 177: 1026–1032.
40. von Leupoldt A, Sommer T, Kegat S, *et al.* Dyspnea and pain share emotion-related brain network. *Neuroimage* 2009; 48: 200–206.
41. von Leupoldt A, Sommer T, Kegat S, *et al.* Down-regulation of insular cortex responses to dyspnea and pain in asthma. *Am J Respir Crit Care Med* 2009; 180: 232–238.
42. Hayen A, Herigstad M, Kelly M, *et al.* The effects of altered intrathoracic pressure on resting cerebral blood flow and its response to visual stimulation. *Neuroimage* 2013; 66: 479–488.
43. Craig AD. How do you feel? Interoception: the sense of the physiological condition of the body. *Nat Rev Neurosci* 2002; 3: 655–666.
44. Craig AD. How do you feel – now? The anterior insula and human awareness. *Nat Rev Neurosci* 2009; 10: 59–70.
45. Chalif JI, Sitsapesan HA, Pattinson KT, *et al.* Dyspnea as a side effect of subthalamic nucleus deep brain stimulation for Parkinson's disease. *Respir Physiol Neurobiol* 2014; 192: 128–133.
46. Hayen A, Herigstad M, Pattinson KT. Understanding dyspnea as a complex individual experience. *Maturitas* 2013; 76: 45–50.
47. Herigstad M, Hayen A, Reinecke R, *et al.* Development of a dyspnoea word cue set for studies of emotional processing in COPD. *Respir Physiol Neurobiol* 2016; 223: 37–42.
48. Herigstad M, Hayen A, Evans E, *et al.* Dyspnea-related cues engage the prefrontal cortex: evidence from functional brain imaging in COPD. *Chest* 2015; 148: 953–961.
49. Herigstad M, Hayen A, Wiech K, *et al.* Dyspnoea and the brain. *Respir Med* 2011; 105: 809–817.
50. Schön D, Rosenkranz M, Regelsberger J, *et al.* Reduced perception of dyspnea and pain after right insular cortex lesions. *Am J Respir Crit Care Med* 2008; 178: 1173–1179.
51. von Leupoldt A, Brassen S, Baumann HJ, *et al.* Structural brain changes related to disease duration in patients with asthma. *PLoS One* 2011; 6: e23739.
52. Evans KC, Shea SA, Saykin AJ. Functional MRI localisation of central nervous system regions associated with volitional inspiration in humans. *J Physiol* 1999; 520: 383–392.
53. von Leupoldt A, Dahme B. Psychological aspects in the perception of dyspnea in obstructive pulmonary diseases. *Respir Med* 2007; 101: 411–422.

54. Ploner M, Lee MC, Wiech K, *et al.* Prestimulus functional connectivity determines pain perception in humans. *Proc Natl Acad Sci USA* 2010; 107: 355–360.
55. Ploghaus A, Tracey I, Gati JS, *et al.* Dissociating pain from its anticipation in the human brain. *Science* 1999; 284: 1979–1981.
56. Faull OK, Jenkinson M, Ezra M, *et al.* Conditioned respiratory threat in the subdivisions of the human periaqueductal gray. *Elife* 2016; 5: e12047.
57. Berna C, Leknes S, Holmes EA, *et al.* Induction of depressed mood disrupts emotion regulation neurocircuitry and enhances pain unpleasantness. *Biol Psychiatry* 2010; 67: 1083–1090.
58. Farmer DG, Bautista TG, Jones SE, *et al.* The midbrain periaqueductal grey has no role in the generation of the respiratory motor pattern, but provides command function for the modulation of respiratory activity. *Respir Physiol Neurobiol* 2014; 204: 14–20.
59. von Leupoldt A, Kenn K. The psychology of chronic obstructive pulmonary disease. *Curr Opin Psychiatry* 2013; 26: 458–463.
60. Pattinson KT, Johnson MJ. Neuroimaging of central breathlessness mechanisms. *Curr Opin Support Palliat Care* 2014; 8: 225–233.
61. Johnson MJ, Simpson MI, Currow DC, *et al.* Magnetoencephalography to investigate central perception of exercise-induced breathlessness in people with chronic lung disease: a feasibility pilot. *BMJ Open* 2015; 5: e007535.
62. Guenette JA, Chin RC, Cheng S, *et al.* Mechanisms of exercise intolerance in global initiative for chronic obstructive lung disease grade 1 COPD. *Eur Respir J* 2014; 44: 1177–1187.
63. Wagner PD, Danzker DR, Dueck R. Ventilation-perfusion inequality in chronic obstructive pulmonary disease. *J Clin Invest* 1977; 59: 203–216.
64. Casaburi R, Patessio A, Ioli F, *et al.* Reductions in exercise lactic acidosis and ventilation as a result of exercise training in patients with obstructive lung disease. *Am Rev Respir Dis* 1991; 143: 9–18.
65. O'Donnell DE, D'Arsigny C, Fitzpatrick M, *et al.* Exercise hypercapnia in advanced chronic obstructive pulmonary disease: the role of lung hyperinflation. *Am J Respir Crit Care Med* 2002; 166: 663–668.
66. O'Donnell DE, Guenette JA, Maltais F, *et al.* Decline of resting inspiratory capacity in COPD: the impact on breathing pattern, dyspnea, and ventilatory capacity during exercise. *Chest* 2012; 141: 753–762.
67. Sinderby C, Spahija J, Beck J, *et al.* Diaphragm activation during exercise in chronic obstructive pulmonary disease. *Am J Respir Crit Care Med* 2001; 163: 1637–1641.
68. Leblanc P, Summers E, Inman MD, *et al.* Inspiratory muscles during exercise: a problem of supply and demand. *J Appl Physiol* 1988; 64: 2482–2489.
69. Byrd RB, Hyatt RE. Maximal respiratory pressures in chronic obstructive lung disease. *Am Rev Respir Dis* 1968; 98: 848–856.
70. Polkey MI, Kyroussis D, Hamnegard CH, *et al.* Diaphragm strength in chronic obstructive pulmonary disease. *Am J Respir Crit Care Med* 1996; 154: 1310–1317.
71. O'Donnell DE, Bertley JC, Chau LK, *et al.* Qualitative aspects of exertional breathlessness in chronic airflow limitation: pathophysiologic mechanisms. *Am J Respir Crit Care Med* 1997; 155: 109–115.
72. Jolley CJ, Luo YM, Steier J, *et al.* Neural respiratory drive and breathlessness in COPD. *Eur Respir J* 2015; 45: 355–364.
73. Murphy PB, Kumar A, Reilly C, *et al.* Neural respiratory drive as a physiological biomarker to monitor change during acute exacerbations of COPD. *Thorax* 2011; 66: 602–608.
74. Walterspacher S, Schlager D, Walker DJ, *et al.* Respiratory muscle function in interstitial lung disease. *Eur Respir J* 2013; 42: 211–219.
75. Gorini M, Spinelli A, Ginanni R, *et al.* Neural respiratory drive and neuromuscular coupling during CO_2 rebreathing in patients with chronic interstitial lung disease. *Chest* 1989; 96: 824–830.
76. Van Meerhaeghe A, Scano G, Sergysels R, *et al.* Respiratory drive and ventilatory pattern during exercise in interstitial lung disease. *Bull Eur Physiopathol Respir* 1981; 17: 15–26.
77. Baydur A, Alsalek M, Louie SG, *et al.* Respiratory muscle strength, lung function, and dyspnea in patients with sarcoidosis. *Chest* 2001; 120: 102–108.
78. Panagiotou M, Polychronopoulos V, Strange C. Respiratory and lower limb muscle function in interstitial lung disease. *Chron Respir Dis* 2016; 13: 162–172.
79. Kabitz HJ, Lang F, Walterspacher S, *et al.* Impact of impaired inspiratory muscle strength on dyspnea and walking capacity in sarcoidosis. *Chest* 2006; 130: 1496–1502.
80. Teixeira A, Cherin P, Demoule A, *et al.* Diaphragmatic dysfunction in patients with idiopathic inflammatory myopathies. *Neuromuscul Disord* 2005; 15: 32–39.
81. Gibson GJ, Pride NB. Pulmonary mechanics in fibrosing alveolitis: the effects of lung shrinkage. *Am Rev Respir Dis* 1977; 116: 637–647.
82. O'Donnell DE, Chau LK, Webb KA. Qualitative aspects of exertional dyspnea in patients with interstitial lung disease. *J Appl Physiol* 1998; 84: 2000–2009.

83. Aduen JF, Zisman DA, Mobin SI, *et al.* Retrospective study of pulmonary function tests in patients presenting with isolated reduction in single-breath diffusion capacity: implications for the diagnosis of combined obstructive and restrictive lung disease. *Mayo Clin Proc* 2007; 82: 48–54.
84. Agustí AG, Roca J, Gea J, *et al.* Mechanisms of gas-exchange impairment in idiopathic pulmonary fibrosis. *Am Rev Respir Dis* 1991; 143: 219–225.
85. Laveneziana P, Webb KA, Ora J, *et al.* Evolution of dyspnea during exercise in chronic obstructive pulmonary disease: impact of critical volume constraints. *Am J Respir Crit Care Med* 2011; 184: 1367–1373.
86. Laveneziana P, Webb KA, Wadell K, *et al.* Does expiratory muscle activity influence dynamic hyperinflation and exertional dyspnea in COPD? *Respir Physiol Neurobiol* 2014; 199: 24–33.
87. Spinelli A, Marconi G, Gorini M, *et al.* Control of breathing in patients with myasthenia gravis. *Am Rev Respir Dis* 1992; 145: 1359–1366.
88. García Río F, Prados C, Díez Tejedor E, *et al.* Breathing pattern and central ventilatory drive in mild and moderate generalised myasthenia gravis. *Thorax* 1994; 49: 703–706.
89. Georges M, Moraviec E, Raux M, *et al.* Cortical drive to breathe in amyotrophic lateral sclerosis: a dyspnoea-worsening defence? *Eur Respir J* 2016; 47:1818–1828.
90. Attali V, Mehiri S, Straus C, *et al.* Influence of neck muscles on mouth pressure response to cervical magnetic stimulation. *Am J Respir Crit Care Med* 1997; 156: 509–514.
91. Belman MJ, Botnick WC, Shin JW. Inhaled bronchodilators reduce dynamic hyperinflation during exercise in patients with chronic obstructive pulmonary disease. *Am J Respir Crit Care Med* 1996; 153: 967–975.
92. O'Donnell DE, Hamilton AL, Webb KA. Sensory-mechanical relationships during high-intensity, constant-work-rate exercise in COPD. *J Appl Physiol* 2006; 101: 1025–1035.
93. Man WD, Mustfa N, Nikoletou D, *et al.* Effect of salmeterol on respiratory muscle activity during exercise in poorly reversible COPD. *Thorax* 2004; 59: 471–476.
94. Duranti R, Misuri G, Gorini M, *et al.* Mechanical loading and control of breathing in patients with severe chronic obstructive pulmonary disease. *Thorax* 1995; 50: 127–133.
95. Easton PA, Hawes HG, Doig CJ, *et al.* Parasternal muscle activity decreases in severe COPD with salmeterol-fluticasone propionate. *Chest* 2010; 137: 558–565.
96. Gatta D, Fredi M, Aliprandi G, *et al.* Inspiratory drive is related to dynamic pulmonary hyperinflation in COPD patients. *Int J Chron Obstruct Pulmon Dis* 2013; 8: 169–173.
97. Pino-García JM, García-Río F, Gómez L, *et al.* Short-term effects of inhaled beta-adrenergic agonist on breathlessness and central inspiratory drive in patients with nonreversible COPD. *Chest* 1996; 110: 637–641.
98. Li Y, Li YH, Li S, *et al.* Efficiency of neural respiratory drive for the assessment of bronchodilator responsiveness in patients with chronic obstructive pulmonary disease: an exploratory study. *J Thorac Dis* 2016; 8: 958–965.
99. Qin YY, Li RF, Wu GF, *et al.* Effect of tiotropium on neural respiratory drive during exercise in severe COPD. *Pulmon Pharmacol Ther* 2015; 30: 51–56.
100. Hopkinson NS, Toma TP, Hansell DM, *et al.* Effect of bronchoscopic lung volume reduction on dynamic hyperinflation and exercise in emphysema. *Am J Respir Crit Care Med* 2005; 171: 453–460.
101. O'Donnell DE, Webb KA, Bertley JC, *et al.* Mechanisms of relief of exertional breathlessness following unilateral bullectomy and lung volume reduction surgery in emphysema. *Chest* 1996; 110: 18–27.
102. Celli BR, Montes de Oca M, Mendez R, *et al.* Lung reduction surgery in severe COPD decreases central drive and ventilatory response to CO_2. *Chest* 1997; 112: 902–906.
103. Gorman RB, McKenzie DK, Butler JE, *et al.* Diaphragm length and neural drive after lung volume reduction surgery. *Am J Respir Crit Care Med* 2005; 172: 1259–1266.
104. Lahrmann H, Wild M, Wanke T, *et al.* Neural drive to the diaphragm after lung volume reduction surgery. *Chest* 1999; 116: 1593–1600.
105. Martinez FJ, de Oca MM, Whyte RI, *et al.* Lung-volume reduction improves dyspnea, dynamic hyperinflation, and respiratory muscle function. *Am J Respir Crit Care Med* 1997; 155: 1984–1990.
106. Teschler H, Stamatis G, el-Raouf Farhat AA, *et al.* Effect of surgical lung volume reduction on respiratory muscle function in pulmonary emphysema. *Eur Respir J* 1996; 9: 1779–1784.
107. Johnson MJ, Barbetta C, Currow DC, *et al.* Management of chronic breathlessness. *In*: Bausewein C, Currow DC, Johnson MJ, eds. Palliative Care in Respiratory Disease (ERS Monograph). Sheffield, European Respiratory Society, 2016, pp. 153–171.
108. van't Hul A, Kwakkel G, Gosselink R. The acute effects of noninvasive ventilatory support during exercise on exercise endurance and dyspnea in patients with chronic obstructive pulmonary disease: a systematic review. *J Cardiopulm Rehabil* 2002; 22: 290–297.
109. Hernandez P, Maltais F, Gursahaney A, *et al.* Proportional assist ventilation may improve exercise performance in severe chronic obstructive pulmonary disease. *J Cardiopulm Rehabil* 2001; 21: 135–142.
110. Maltais F, Reissmann H, Gottfried SB. Pressure support reduces inspiratory effort and dyspnea during exercise in chronic airflow obstruction. *Am J Respir Crit Care Med* 1995; 151: 1027–1033.

111. O'Donnell DE, Sanii R, Younes M. Improvement in exercise endurance in patients with chronic airflow limitation using continuous positive airway pressure. *Am Rev Respir Dis* 1988; 138: 1510–1514.
112. van't Hul A, Gosselink R, Hollander P, *et al.* Acute effects of inspiratory pressure support during exercise in patients with COPD. *Eur Respir J* 2004; 23: 34–40.
113. Porszasz J, Cao R, Morishige R, *et al.* Physiologic effects of an ambulatory ventilation system in chronic obstructive pulmonary disease. *Am J Respir Crit Care Med* 2013; 188: 334–342.
114. Moran F, Bradley JM, Piper AJ. Non-invasive ventilation for cystic fibrosis. *Cochrane Database Syst Rev* 2013; 4: CD002769.
115. Henke KG, Regnis JA, Bye PT. Benefits of continuous positive airway pressure during exercise in cystic fibrosis and relationship to disease severity. *Am Rev Respir Dis* 1993; 148: 1272–1276.
116. Tsuboi T, Ohi M, Chin K, *et al.* Ventilatory support during exercise in patients with pulmonary tuberculosis sequelae. *Chest* 1997; 112: 1000–1007.
117. Moderno EV, Yamaguti WP, Schettino GP, *et al.* Effects of proportional assisted ventilation on exercise performance in idiopathic pulmonary fibrosis patients. *Respir Med* 2010; 104: 134–141.
118. Nava S, Ferrer M, Esquinas A, *et al.* Palliative use of non-invasive ventilation in end-of-life patients with solid tumours: a randomised feasibility trial. *Lancet Oncol* 2013; 14: 219–227.
119. Tripodoro VA, De Vito EL. Management of dyspnea in advanced motor neuron diseases. *Curr Opin Support Palliat Care* 2008; 2: 173–179.
120. Toussaint M, Soudon P, Kinnear W. Effect of non-invasive ventilation on respiratory muscle loading and endurance in patients with Duchenne muscular dystrophy. *Thorax* 2008; 63: 430–434.
121. Petrof BJ, Calderini E, Gottfried SB. Effect of CPAP on respiratory effort and dyspnea during exercise in severe COPD. *J Appl Physiol* 1990; 69: 179–188.
122. Kyroussis D, Polkey MI, Hamnegård CH, *et al.* Respiratory muscle activity in patients with COPD walking to exhaustion with and without pressure support. *Eur Respir J* 2000; 15: 649–655.
123. Menadue C, Piper AJ, van 't Hul AJ, *et al.* Non-invasive ventilation during exercise training for people with chronic obstructive pulmonary disease. *Cochrane Database Syst Rev* 2014; 5: CD007714.
124. Uronis HE, Ekström MP, Currow DC, *et al.* Oxygen for relief of dyspnoea in people with chronic obstructive pulmonary disease who would not qualify for home oxygen: a systematic review and meta-analysis. *Thorax* 2015; 70: 492–494.
125. Uronis H, McCrory DC, Samsa G, *et al.* Symptomatic oxygen for non-hypoxaemic chronic obstructive pulmonary disease. *Cochrane Database Syst Rev* 2011; 6: CD006429.
126. Bajwah S, Ross JR, Peacock JL, *et al.* Interventions to improve symptoms and quality of life of patients with fibrotic interstitial lung disease: a systematic review of the literature. *Thorax* 2013; 68: 867–879.
127. Snider GL. Enhancement of exercise performance in COPD patients by hyperoxia: a call for research. *Chest* 2002; 122: 1830–1836.
128. Ameer F, Carson KV, Usmani ZA, *et al.* Ambulatory oxygen for people with chronic obstructive pulmonary disease who are not hypoxaemic at rest. *Cochrane Database Syst Rev* 2014; 6: CD000238.
129. Hardinge M, Annandale J, Bourne S, *et al.* BTS guidelines for home oxygen use in adults. *Thorax* 2015; 70: Suppl. 1, i1–i43.
130. Clemens KE, Quednau I, Klaschik E. Use of oxygen and opioids in the palliation of dyspnoea in hypoxic and non-hypoxic palliative care patients: a prospective study. *Support Care Cancer* 2009; 17: 367–377.
131. Abernethy AP, McDonald CF, Frith PA, *et al.* Effect of palliative oxygen *versus* room air in relief of breathlessness in patients with refractory dyspnoea: a double-blind, randomised controlled trial. *Lancet* 2010; 376: 784–793.
132. Stein DA, Bradley BL, Miller WC. Mechanisms of oxygen effects on exercise in patients with chronic obstructive pulmonary disease. *Chest* 1982; 81: 6–10.
133. Swinburn CR, Wakefield JM, Jones PW. Relationship between ventilation and breathlessness during exercise in chronic obstructive airways disease is not altered by prevention of hypoxaemia. *Clin Sci (Lond)* 1984; 67: 515–519.
134. Peters MM, Webb KA, O'Donnell DE. Combined physiological effects of bronchodilators and hyperoxia on exertional dyspnoea in normoxic COPD. *Thorax* 2006; 61: 559–567.
135. O'Donnell DE, Bain DJ, Webb KA. Factors contributing to relief of exertional breathlessness during hyperoxia in chronic airflow limitation. *Am J Respir Crit Care Med* 1997; 155: 530–535.
136. O'Donnell DE, D'Arsigny C, Webb KA. Effects of hyperoxia on ventilatory limitation during exercise in advanced chronic obstructive pulmonary disease. *Am J Respir Crit Care Med* 2001; 163: 892–898.
137. Somfay A, Porszasz J, Lee SM, *et al.* Dose-response effect of oxygen on hyperinflation and exercise endurance in nonhypoxaemic COPD patients. *Eur Respir J* 2001; 18: 77–84.
138. Maltais F, Simon M, Jobin J, *et al.* Effects of oxygen on lower limb blood flow and O_2 uptake during exercise in COPD. *Med Sci Sports Exerc* 2001; 33: 916–922.
139. Dean NC, Brown JK, Himelman RB, *et al.* Oxygen may improve dyspnea and endurance in patients with chronic obstructive pulmonary disease and only mild hypoxemia. *Am Rev Respir Dis* 1992; 146: 941–945.
140. Booth S, Kelly MJ, Cox NP, *et al.* Does oxygen help dyspnea in patients with cancer? *Am J Respir Crit Care Med* 1996; 153: 1515–1518.

141. Dowman L, Hill CJ, Holland AE. Pulmonary rehabilitation for interstitial lung disease. *Cochrane Database Syst Rev* 2014; 10: CD006322.
142. McCarthy B, Casey D, Devane D, *et al.* Pulmonary rehabilitation for chronic obstructive pulmonary disease. *Cochrane Database Syst Rev* 2015; 2: CD003793.
143. Maltais F, Decramer M, Casaburi R, *et al.* An official American Thoracic Society/European Respiratory Society statement: update on limb muscle dysfunction in chronic obstructive pulmonary disease. *Am J Respir Crit Care Med* 2014; 189: e15–e62.
144. O'Donnell DE, McGuire M, Samis L, *et al.* General exercise training improves ventilatory and peripheral muscle strength and endurance in chronic airflow limitation. *Am J Respir Crit Care Med* 1998; 157: 1489–1497.
145. O'Donnell DE, McGuire M, Samis L, *et al.* The impact of exercise reconditioning on breathlessness in severe chronic airflow limitation. *Am J Respir Crit Care Med* 1995; 152: 2005–2013.
146. Gigliotti F, Coli C, Bianchi R, *et al.* Exercise training improves exertional dyspnea in patients with COPD: evidence of the role of mechanical factors. *Chest* 2003; 123: 1794–1802.
147. Gagnon P, Bussières JS, Ribeiro F, *et al.* Influences of spinal anesthesia on exercise tolerance in patients with chronic obstructive pulmonary disease. *Am J Respir Crit Care Med* 2012; 186: 606–615.
148. Carrieri-Kohlman V, Gormley JM, Eiser S, *et al.* Dyspnea and the affective response during exercise training in obstructive pulmonary disease. *Nurs Res* 2001; 50: 136–146.
149. Wadell K, Webb KA, Preston ME, *et al.* Impact of pulmonary rehabilitation on the major dimensions of dyspnea in COPD. *COPD* 2013; 10: 425–435.
150. Hallas CN, Howard C, Theadom A, *et al.* Negative beliefs about breathlessness increases panic for patients with chronic respiratory disease. *Psychol Health Med* 2012; 17: 467–477.
151. Norweg A, Collins EG. Evidence for cognitive-behavioral strategies improving dyspnea and related distress in COPD. *Int J Chron Obstruct Pulmon Dis* 2013; 8: 439–451.
152. Livermore N, Dimitri A, Sharpe L, *et al.* Cognitive behaviour therapy reduces dyspnoea ratings in patients with chronic obstructive pulmonary disease (COPD). *Respir Physiol Neurobiol* 2015; 216: 35–42.
153. Livermore N, Sharpe L, McKenzie D. Panic attacks and panic disorder in chronic obstructive pulmonary disease: a cognitive behavioral perspective. *Respir Med* 2010; 104: 1246–1253.
154. Baliki MN, Chialvo DR, Geha PY, *et al.* Chronic pain and the emotional brain: specific brain activity associated with spontaneous fluctuations of intensity of chronic back pain. *J Neurosci* 2006; 26: 12165–12173.
155. Apkarian AV, Hashmi JA, Baliki MN. Pain and the brain: specificity and plasticity of the brain in clinical chronic pain. *Pain* 2011; 152: Suppl. 3, S49–S64.
156. Boyden JY, Connor SR, Otolorin L, *et al.* Nebulized medications for the treatment of dyspnea: a literature review. *J Aerosol Med Pulm Drug Deliv* 2015; 28: 1–19.
157. Nishino T. Pathophysiology of dyspnea evaluated by breath-holding test: studies of furosemide treatment. *Respir Physiol Neurobiol* 2009; 167: 20–25.
158. Minowa Y, Ide T, Nishino T. Effects of inhaled furosemide on CO_2 ventilatory responsiveness in humans. *Pulm Pharmacol Ther* 2002; 15: 363–368.
159. Nishino T, Ide T, Sudo T, *et al.* Inhaled furosemide greatly alleviates the sensation of experimentally induced dyspnea. *Am J Respir Crit Care Med* 2000; 161: 1963–1967.
160. Moosavi SH, Binks AP, Lansing RW, *et al.* Effect of inhaled furosemide on air hunger induced in healthy humans. *Respir Physiol Neurobiol* 2007; 156: 1–8.
161. Shimoyama N, Shimoyama M. Nebulized furosemide as a novel treatment for dyspnea in terminal cancer patients. *J Pain Symptom Manage* 2002; 23: 73–76.
162. Kohara H, Ueoka H, Aoe K, *et al.* Effect of nebulized furosemide in terminally ill cancer patients with dyspnea. *J Pain Symptom Manage* 2003; 26: 962–967.
163. Ong KC, Kor AC, Chong WF, *et al.* Effects of inhaled furosemide on exertional dyspnea in chronic obstructive pulmonary disease. *Am J Respir Crit Care Med* 2004; 169: 1028–1033.
164. Jensen D, Amjadi K, Harris-McAllister V, *et al.* Mechanisms of dyspnoea relief and improved exercise endurance after furosemide inhalation in COPD. *Thorax* 2008; 63: 606–613.
165. Sant'Ambrogio FB, Sant'Ambrogio G, Anderson JW. Effect of furosemide on the response of laryngeal receptors to low-chloride solutions. *Eur Respir J* 1993; 6: 1151–1155.
166. Sudo T, Hayashi F, Nishino T. Responses of tracheobronchial receptors to inhaled furosemide in anesthetized rats. *Am J Respir Crit Care Med* 2000; 162: 971–975.
167. Eldridge FL, Chen Z. Respiratory-associated rhythmic firing of midbrain neurons is modulated by vagal input. *Respir Physiol* 1992; 90: 31–46.
168. Sant'Ambrogio G, Widdicombe JG. Respiratory reflexes acting on the diaphragm and inspiratory intercostal muscle of the rabbit. *J Physiol* 1965; 180: 766–779.
169. Dallak MA, Pirie LJ, Davies A. The influence of pulmonary receptors on respiratory drive in a rabbit model of pulmonary emphysema. *Respir Physiol Neurobiol* 2007; 156: 33–39.
170. Sheikh Motahar Vahedi H, Mahshidfar B, Rabiee H, *et al.* The adjunctive effect of nebulized furosemide in COPD exacerbation: a randomized controlled clinical trial. *Respir Care* 2013; 58: 1873–1877.

171. Burgess KR, Whitelaw WA. Reducing ventilatory response to carbon dioxide by breathing cold air. *Am Rev Respir Dis* 1984; 129: 687–690.
172. Burgess KR, Whitelaw WA. Effects of nasal cold receptors on pattern of breathing. *J Appl Physiol* 1988; 64: 371–376.
173. Wanigasekera V, Lee MC, Rogers R, *et al.* Neural correlates of an injury-free model of central sensitization induced by opioid withdrawal in humans. *J Neurosci* 2011; 31: 2835–2842.
174. Schwartzstein RM, Lahive K, Pope A, *et al.* Cold facial stimulation reduces breathlessness induced in normal subjects. *Am Rev Respir Dis* 1987; 136: 58–61.
175. Simon PM, Basner RC, Weinberger SE, *et al.* Oral mucosal stimulation modulates intensity of breathlessness induced in normal subjects. *Am Rev Respir Dis* 1991; 144: 419–422.
176. Nishino T, Tagaito Y, Sakurai Y. Nasal inhalation of L-menthol reduces respiratory discomfort associated with loaded breathing. *Am J Respir Crit Care Med* 1997; 156: 309–313.
177. Pattinson KT. Opioids and the control of respiration. *Br J Anaesth* 2008; 100: 747–758.
178. Barnes H, McDonald J, Smallwood N, *et al.* Opioids for the palliation of refractory breathlessness in adults with advanced disease and terminal illness. *Cochrane Database Syst Rev* 2016; 3: CD011008.
179. Baumgärtner U, Buchholz HG, Bellosevich A, *et al.* High opiate receptor binding potential in the human lateral pain system. *Neuroimage* 2006; 30: 692–699.
180. Pattinson KT, Governo RJ, MacIntosh BJ, *et al.* Opioids depress cortical centers responsible for the volitional control of respiration. *J Neurosci* 2009; 29: 8177–8186.
181. Gifford AH, Mahler DA, Waterman LA, *et al.* Neuromodulatory effect of endogenous opioids on the intensity and unpleasantness of breathlessness during resistive load breathing in COPD. *COPD* 2011; 8: 160–166.
182. Mahler DA, Murray JA, Waterman LA, *et al.* Endogenous opioids modify dyspnoea during treadmill exercise in patients with COPD. *Eur Respir J* 2009; 33: 771–777.

Disclosures: D. Jensen has received grants from Boehringer Ingelheim and AstraZeneca, for work outside the subject of this chapter.

Chapter 9

Measurement of breathlessness

Mark B. Parshall[1] and Janelle Yorke[2]

There are many measurement approaches and instruments for assessing the sensory-perceptual experience of breathlessness, the associated affective distress and how breathlessness impacts an individual's functioning and quality of life. Choices of which measures to use should be driven by the relevance of the measured construct(s) to the context(s) of use, and, in palliative care, by the responsiveness of measures to clinical change and by their ease of administration and scoring. Evidence of adequate psychometric performance characteristics can be viewed as necessary but not sufficient for preferring one measurement approach or instrument to another in palliative care.

Guidelines for research with and care of patients with advanced cardiopulmonary disease [1–6] or palliative care [7–10] generally recommend routine measurement of patient-reported outcomes, particularly breathlessness and its impact on quality of life (QoL) [1–4, 11–14]. When it is feasible to do so, breathlessness should be measured by self-report [11, 14, 15]. Poor agreement between breathlessness ratings of patients, physicians and nurses has been reported in mechanically ventilated patients undergoing spontaneous breathing trials [16]. In palliative care, agreement between health professionals and patients is stronger for the presence of breathlessness than for its severity [17]. Self-report is preferred for QoL measurement, but proxy estimation by family members can be reliable in situations in which self-report is infeasible or would be excessively burdensome for the patient.

Many instruments have been developed for measuring various aspects of breathlessness [3, 11, 13, 18, 19]. Relatively few have been rigorously evaluated for research [13] or clinical use [10] in palliative care settings where, ideally, breathlessness measures should be simple to administer, responsive to clinical change, and relevant across diagnoses and contexts of care [8, 15, 20]. QoL has always been an overarching concern in palliative care, and in this context, the focus for measurement of breathlessness is often the impact of the symptom on functioning, daily activities and QoL, rather than how breathing feels. It is also common for ratings of breathlessness to be embedded in an inventory of QoL concerns or multiple symptoms (such as pain or fatigue) [21–27]. However, as disease becomes more advanced and the focus of care is on EOL, scales that require linking breathlessness to usual activities become less appropriate and useful.

[1]College of Nursing, University of New Mexico, Albuquerque, NM, USA. [2]University of Manchester and The Christie NHS Foundation Trust, Manchester, UK.

Correspondence: Mark B. Parshall, College of Nursing, MSC07 4380, Box 9, 1 University of New Mexico, Albuquerque, NM 87131-0001, USA. E-mail: MParshall@salud.unm.edu

 Print ISBN: 978-1-84984-071-2. Online ISBN: 978-1-84984-072-9. Print ISSN: 2312-508X. Online ISSN: 2312-5098.

The multidimensional nature of breathlessness is emphasised in conceptual models of the symptom [9, 15, 28–32] and in frameworks and models for its measurement [11, 33–37]. According to a framework proposed by the American Thoracic Society [11], measures of breathlessness can be categorised as pertaining to domains of sensory-perceptual experience (what breathing feels like), affective distress (how unpleasant or distressing it is or how it makes one feel), or symptom impact or burden (how it affects QoL and psychosocial or physical functioning). The domains are not mutually exclusive, and many measures tap into more than one domain. Conceptual clarity about measurement domains and their potential relevance to clinical or research purposes should guide the choice and timing of measurement approaches. In clinical palliative care, there is a close correspondence between these measurement domains and "operational levels in the experience of breathlessness" proposed by Ryan *et al.* [29]: breathlessness perception, emotional–behavioural response and functional impact. The choice of measures can be guided by which of these levels is of greatest concern to the patient [15].

Several systematic reviews focused on measurement of breathlessness or QoL in advanced disease have been published [18, 19, 38, 39]. For this chapter, multiple PubMed searches were conducted using combinations of the search terms shown in table 1, plus names and acronyms of various instruments. Choices of which measures to include in this chapter were based on considerations such as ease of use, responsiveness, relevance across diagnoses and availability of published data on use in palliative care.

Measuring sensory-perceptual and affective distress domains of breathlessness

Breathlessness measures can be single-item ratings or multi-item scales that can be either unidimensional or multidimensional. Measured aspects of breathlessness include: intensity of overall breathing discomfort or unpleasantness; severity of overall or breathlessness-related distress; presence/absence or intensity of various sensory qualities (*e.g.* effort, air hunger, tightness); frequency of episodes of breathlessness or of related distress or impairment; or the extent of activity limitation or level of task or activity at which breathlessness typically occurs. Time frames commonly include: right now or some recent point in time (*e.g.* last minute of an exercise stimulus; when someone sought unscheduled care), elapsed time (*e.g.* last week or month; worst episode in past 24 h), how things usually are, or the time of day when breathlessness episodes typically occur.

Table 1. Search terms used in PubMed

("dyspnea"[All Fields] OR "dyspnoea"[All Fields] OR "breathlessness"[All Fields])
AND
("surveys and questionnaires"[MeSH Terms] OR "reproducibility of results"[MeSH Terms] OR "psychometrics"[MeSH Terms] OR "questionnaire"[All Fields] OR "psychometrics"[All Fields] OR "psychometric"[All Fields] OR "patient reported outcome"[All Fields] OR "reliability"[All Fields])
AND
("pulmonary disease, chronic obstructive"[MeSH Terms] OR "COPD"[All Fields] OR "COPD"[All Fields] OR "heart failure"[MeSH Terms] OR "heart failure"[All Fields] OR "neoplasms"[MeSH Terms] OR "cancer"[All Fields])
AND
("palliative care" [MeSH Terms] OR "palliative care"[All Fields] OR "advanced disease"[TIAB] OR "advanced disease"[TW])

Unidimensional measures

Self-report scales

Single-item ratings of breathlessness include VASs or NRSs [40–42] and the modified Borg category-ratio scale [43, 44]. Given their relative ease of completion and the fact that they are not necessarily linked to an activity, such scales can be useful in the palliative care setting. Breathlessness can be quantified by asking the patient and/or carer to point to or say the number reflecting their shortness of breath. No compelling evidence exists to indicate superiority of any of these scale types over any other; rather, one or another may be preferred according to practical or contextual considerations (table 2). For example, the modified Borg scale was derived from an earlier Rating of Perceived Exertion [53], and is often preferred by researchers using cardiopulmonary exercise testing as a stimulus for eliciting breathlessness [32]. However, in relatively uncontrolled clinical settings, some evidence indicates that patients may be less likely to choose modified Borg numerical ratings that are not coupled with categorical labels (*i.e.* 6 or 8) [49], which may make it less useful in a palliative care setting compared with an NRS. Minimum clinically important differences (MCIDs; *i.e.* the threshold score difference that patients associate with beneficial change) are similar for the modified Borg scale and NRS for breathlessness (approximately 1 point in both cases [45, 46, 54]) and proportionate for the VAS (~10–12 mm for a moderate effect size [46, 47] or relative 10% change [48]). In a distribution-based secondary analysis of VAS breathlessness ratings from clinical trials of opioids for refractory, chronic breathlessness, decreases of 5.5 mm, 11.3 mm and 18.2 mm corresponded to standardised effect sizes of 0.25, 0.5 and 0.8 SD, respectively, and an anchor-based decrease of 9 mm was identified as clinically meaningful in relation to masked preference ratings from participants [47].

In clinical practice, if only a single rating is used, it may not matter whether the anchor statements emphasise the intensity of sensation (*e.g.* "maximum breathlessness") or affect (*e.g.* "unbearable"), as long as the rating and instructions are consistent across administrations. Evidence from pain research shows that patients may not make much distinction between various anchoring statements [55]. Conflicting findings exist with respect to whether single ratings tend to capture distress to a greater degree than sensory intensity [56], or *vice versa* [57]. It is not clear to what extent differences in language/culture or diagnosis influence how patients or research subjects construe anchor statements [56, 57].

A limitation of a single-item rating is that it represents only one dimension at a time. With VASs or NRSs, anchors commonly refer to the intensity of sensation or severity of unpleasantness, distress or bother [58–61]. It is not unusual for multiple single-item ratings to be used together to capture different time points or intervals (*e.g.* right now, worst in past 24 h and on average over last 24 h) [60–62] or multiple symptoms [63]. If practitioners or researchers are using multiple unidimensional ratings to capture more than one measurement domain, it is important to instruct patients or subjects clearly and consistently about each rating and how to distinguish between them [33, 64]. In addition, the practicality of using multiple single-item scales in the palliative care setting requires careful consideration. For example, BOOTH *et al.* [15, p. 27] recommend assessing clinical breathlessness in a palliative care setting with three 0–10 NRSs: for severity of breathlessness (0=not breathless, 10=worst breathlessness you can imagine), severity of anxiety (0=not anxious at all, 10=worst anxiety you can imagine) and confidence in one's ability to self-manage breathlessness (0=not confident at all, 10=extremely confident). They also recommend asking whether activity has increased, decreased or remained about the same since the initial or most recent evaluation [15].

Table 2. Unidimensional measures of sensory-perceptual and affective distress measurement domains

Scale [refs]	Construct(s) and time frame(s)	Responsiveness	Ease of use	Clinically important difference	Limitations
NRS or VAS [40–42]	Intensity or distress at present ("now") or recall of recent past event (*e.g.* decision to seek emergency care), or interval (*e.g.* past 24 h)	Generally high in a variety of clinical and experimental contexts	Simple to use	1 point (0–10 NRS) [45]; 9–12 mm (100 mm VAS) [46, 47] or relative score change of ~10% of scale range [48]	Reliability indeterminate for single-item ratings
Modified Borg category-ratio scale [43, 44]	Perceived exertion/effort at present ("now") or immediate past time point (*e.g.* end or peak of exercise test) or interval (*e.g.* past 24 h)	Generally high in a variety of clinical and experimental contexts	Scaling may require some explanation (*e.g.* meaning of a 0.5 rating or ratings without verbal categories)	1 point [45, 46]	Potential response bias against numerical levels with no corresponding verbal category [49]
RDOS [50, 51]	Respiratory distress at a specific point in time or serial time points	Responsive to treatment with opioids [51]	Need to train observers and ascertain inter-rater agreement	RDOS $\leqslant 2$ consistent with minimal to no distress; $\geqslant 3$ moderate to severe distress [52]	To date, concurrent validation against self-reported breathlessness ratings [52, 51]

RDOS: Respiratory Distress Observation Scale.

In addition, equivalence across single-item ratings with different levels of measurement cannot be assumed, despite what may seem like semantic similarity. For example, in a recent study with neurologically and cognitively intact adult patients with cardiopulmonary disease or lung cancer, participants were asked the binary question "Are you short of breath? (Yes/No)" and were also asked to categorise current breathing distress as none, mild, moderate or severe [52]. Approximately 53% (72 out of 136) answered no to the binary shortness-of-breath question, whereas only half as many (36 out of 136) used none as the ordinal breathing distress rating. Over half of those who answered no to the binary question about shortness of breath (38 out of 72) applied an ordinal rating of at least mild to breathing distress [52]. However, a recent analysis among patients with refractory breathlessness due to life-limiting illness found an equivalence between a 0–10 NRS and a four-level categorical rating (0=none, 1–4=mild, 5–8=moderate, 9–10=severe) based on concurrent administrations [65].

Unable to self-report

The Respiratory Distress Observation Scale (RDOS) is an observational rating designed for use with patients unable to self-report [50, 51, 66, 67]. Eight signs associated with respiratory distress are each scored from 0 to 2: fearful facial expression, restlessness, accessory muscle use, paradoxical breathing, nasal flaring, end-expiratory grunting, heart rate and respiratory rate. Total scores can range from 0 to 16, with higher scores indicating greater respiratory distress [51].

A common approach to validation involves concurrent administration of other measures of the same (or a similar) construct. To the extent that this involves concurrent self-reports of breathlessness by patients capable of providing them [50, 51, 68], validation to date has involved populations other than those for whom clinical use is intended. This, in turn, can create a ceiling effect attenuating the correlation of RDOS scores with self-reports of breathlessness [52], which have been on the order of r≈0.4, regardless of scale type (NRS or VAS) or population (advanced lung disease with hypoxaemia [50], palliative care consultation [51], cancer inpatients [69] or intensive care patients [68]), or whether the concurrent rating ostensibly pertained to breathing difficulty [50], breathing distress [51], shortness of breath [69] or breathing discomfort [68]. These findings would seem to support a hypothesis that, regardless of anchors, patients tend to construe a single breathlessness rating as a self-report of affective distress [56] and that the RDOS should, in keeping with its name, be referred to as a rating of respiratory distress rather than breathlessness *per se* (table 2). Campbell and Templin [52] recommended that an RDOS of ≤2 in a patient whose initial score was ≥3 might be considered consistent with achieving reasonable relief from respiratory distress. However, this conclusion was based on a study with adult inpatients with lung cancer, heart failure, pneumonia or COPD. Therefore, further validation is needed, ideally with palliative care patients unable to self-report.

A study of ICU patients found that a modification of signs and scoring correlated more strongly with a concurrent breathlessness VAS in a validation cohort (r=0.54, 95% CI 0.39–0.70; n=100) than the original RDOS had in a derivation cohort (r=0.43, 95% CI 0.29–0.58; n=120) [68]. The scoring modification was based on heart rate, inspiratory use of neck muscles, inspiratory abdominal paradox, fear expression and supplemental oxygen use (*i.e.* it did not include respiratory rate, restlessness, grunting or nasal flaring, which may be affected by sedation or intubation and thus are less appropriate for assessment in this setting) [68].

Multidimensional measures

The experience of breathlessness is multidimensional [2, 11, 13, 28, 31, 70–72], but, with respect to sensory-perceptual and affective measurement domains (as opposed to, for example, impacts on QoL or functional ability), relatively few breathlessness measures have been developed with this explicitly in mind. In PEOLC, it is often the case that treatment may not alter the underlying pathophysiology or breathing mechanics. Therefore, in clinical practice and research in such settings, it is potentially important to distinguish between the intensity of breathlessness sensation(s) and the intensity of the emotional response to breathlessness, because the latter may be more responsive to treatment. Multidimensional measures that incorporate sensory-perceptual and affective domains of breathlessness include the Cancer Dyspnoea Scale (CDS) [73, 74], the Dyspnoea-12 (D-12) [37, 75] and the MDP [33] (table 3).

The CDS comprises 12 items related to "breathlessness or difficulty in breathing... during the past few days" among patients with advanced cancer [76]. It has three subscales: sense of effort (five items; scale range 0–20; *e.g.* "Do you feel as if you are panting?"), anxiety (four items; scale range 0–16; *e.g.* "Do you feel as if you are drowning?") and discomfort (three reverse-scored items; scale range 0–12; *e.g.* "Can you inhale easily?"). A higher score indicates a worse status. In patients with lung cancer, the subscales have adequate internal consistency reliability (Cronbach's alpha=0.8–0.9), with moderate correlations across factors [76, 85]. For the total score (range 0–48), a cut-point of ⩾8 *versus* ⩽7 points had approximately 62% sensitivity and 78% specificity for dyspnoea interference with any daily activity [74]. The CDS was originally created in Japanese [73, 74, 76]. Translations have been validated in Swedish [78, 86, 87] and English [85]; however, minor inconsistencies of factor structure have been found across different languages (*e.g.* one item in the English translation and a different item in the Swedish translation loaded primarily to a different factor from the original CDS [76, 78, 85], and, in the English translation, several items had more ambiguous loadings across factors [85]). The developers of the English version proposed a "reduced" scale with just three items per subscale to minimise these discrepancies and simplify scoring [85].

The D-12 [37, 79, 80, 88] was developed using Rasch modelling [36]. Rasch analysis (a one-parameter variant of item-response analysis) locates items and respondents along the same continuum of "item difficulty" (which, in a symptom measure, can be construed as symptom severity). The 12 items represent sensory-perceptual (*e.g.* "I have difficulty catching my breath") and affective distress (*e.g.* "My breathing makes me feel miserable") domains of breathlessness. Each item is scored using a four-point numerical scale (0=none, 1=mild, 2=moderate, 3=severe); total scores range from 0 to 36. The instrument can also be scored for physical and emotional components comprising seven and five items, respectively, for component scores ranging from 0 to 21 for the physical component items and from 0 to 15 for the emotional component items. The time frame for items is "these days", rather than a specific interval or activity; the less-specific time frame may be useful in a palliative care context. Based on data from a randomised, controlled feasibility trial of a non-pharmacological intervention for self-managing the breathlessness–cough–fatigue symptom cluster in patients with lung cancer, an MCID of 3 points in the total D-12 score has been recommended [81].

The D-12 has been validated in patients with COPD [37, 89, 90], ILD [37, 75, 80], heart failure [37], asthma [79] and pulmonary arterial hypertension [88]. In addition to English, psychometric data on an Arabic version have been published [90]. Translations into a number of other languages are available (J. Yorke, unpublished data).

Table 3. Multidimensional measures of sensory-perceptual and affective distress measurement domains

Scale [refs]	Construct(s) and time frame(s)	Responsiveness	Ease of use	Clinically important difference	Limitations
Cancer Dyspnoea Scale [74, 76]	Severity of sense of effort, anxiety and discomfort related to breathing difficulty, over the past few days	Responsive to nebulised furosemide [77]	$\leqslant$2.5 min to complete [76, 78]	Not determined	Validated for advanced cancer only
Dyspnoea-12 [37, 79, 80]	Overall dyspnoea severity or severity of physical (sensory-perceptual) affective aspects of breathlessness, which occurs "these days"	Score change over 2 weeks parallels transition scores for general health in adults with asthma [79]	Rated by patients with COPD, ILD and heart failure as easily understood and easy to use [37]	3 points recommended for sample size estimation purposes [81]	Needs further validation in palliative care
MDP [33, 34, 82]	Unpleasantness/discomfort in breathing, severity of sensory qualities (immediate perception) and affective distress (emotional response), "now" or referred to a particular event or time point	Responsive to nonspecific ED treatment [34, 82] and to inspiratory muscle training in pulmonary rehabilitation [83]	Requires some training to administer; takes <5 min on initial administration and ~2 min subsequently [33, 34, 84]	Not determined for immediate perception or emotional response domains; unpleasantness rating likely to be similar to other NRSs (see table 2)	Needs validation in patients with advanced cancer and in palliative care

The MDP is based on a conceptual model of sensory-perceptual and affective processing with origins in pain research [28, 33]. It was developed to be used in either laboratory experiments [33, 91] or in clinical studies of patients with a variety of cardiopulmonary diseases in acute care settings [34, 82]. Recently, extensive validation was published pertaining to use with community-residing persons with COPD [84]. As yet, no studies have been published on its use in palliative care, although it has been used with patients with amyotrophic lateral sclerosis comparing spontaneous breathing with NIV [92]. The MDP has one item pertaining to overall unpleasantness or discomfort of breathing ("how bad your breathing feels/felt"), five sensory quality (SQ) items (based on factor analytic studies of dyspnoea descriptors [35, 93]; *e.g.* "I am not getting enough air, I am smothering or I feel hunger for air") and five emotion items (*e.g.* frustrated). The unpleasantness and emotional response items are rated using 0–10 NRSs with appropriate anchors (0=neutral, 10=unbearable for unpleasantness; 0=none, 10=the most I can imagine for negative emotions). The SQ items are rated first for whether a given grouping does or does not apply and which most accurately describes the individual's breathlessness. The intensity of each SQ grouping is then rated on a 0–10 NRS (0=none, 10=as intense as I can imagine). The time frame for ratings can be "right now", a specific time point (*e.g.* last minute of an experimental stimulus) or event (*e.g.* when someone decided to seek emergency care), or is potentially customisable to a particular context of use (*e.g.* worst episode in the past 2 weeks [84]).

The MDP has been used in patients with a variety of cardiopulmonary conditions, in particular COPD, heart failure and pneumonia [34, 82, 84], as well as in healthy subjects exposed to experimental stimuli [91]. It is published in English and French versions [33], and translations into other languages are being developed.

Complete versions of the D-12 [88] and MDP [33] have been published, and extensive psychometric data are available in the publications cited for each. A comparison of the items in both instruments is also available [33]. Neither is diagnosis specific, which is a potential advantage for palliative care, but so far only the D-12 has been validated in lung cancer [81], and further research is needed to support their use in a palliative care setting.

Measuring breathlessness impact or burden

Measures of the impact of breathlessness are commonly focused on functional impact (*e.g.* activity limitation or disability) or impact on QoL. Symptom burden does not have a consistent theoretical definition but is typically assessed with inventories of multiple symptoms [21, 23].

Functional impact

Unidimensional

In palliative care, most unidimensional functional impact measures related to breathlessness have only limited validation or have issues related to responsiveness (table 4). The three shortness-of-breath items (at rest, walking and climbing stairs) from the European Organisation for Research and Treatment of Cancer (EORTC) Quality of Life Questionnaire Lung Cancer 13 module (QLQ-LC13) [27, 106] have been used as a functional impact scale [104]. The developers recommend that all three shortness-of-breath items must have valid responses to be treated as a scale; if any have missing values, the others can be used separately, as single items [104].

Table 4. Unidimensional measures of functional impact

Scale [refs]	Construct(s) and time frame(s)	Responsiveness	Ease of use	Clinically important difference	Limitations
mMRC Scale [94, 95]	Activity limitation/ disability attributable to breathlessness. Time frame not specified	Poorly responsive to small or short-term changes that may be clinically meaningful in palliative care	Simple to use	Not determined	In palliative care, it may be used to categorise patients, but is likely to be range restricted and not as sensitive as outcome assessment in palliative care
Dyspnea Exertion Scale [13, 60, 96]	First-person self-report version of mMRC	Same as mMRC, except that a change in distribution (n or %) across categories has been noted in the palliative care setting [60]	Same as mMRC	Not determined	Same as mMRC
Oxygen-cost diagram [97–99]	Exercise tolerance; time frame not specified	Not associated with change in pulmonary function, P_{aO_2}, P_{aCO_2}, 6MWD or resting Borg after 1 year of home NIV [100]	Similar to VAS but with verbal descriptors representing putative oxygen demand of common activities	Not determined	Only one published study in patients with advanced cancer; only weakly correlated with ESAS shortness-of-breath rating [99]
LCADL Scale [101, 102]	Breathlessness during activities of daily living	Responsive to 6 weeks of pulmonary rehabilitation in COPD [102], but not to 6 weeks of breathlessness support intervention for refractory chronic breathlessness [103]	Relatively simple to administer	Not determined	Originally developed with patients with severe COPD, but only one published study in palliative care of breathlessness [103]

Continued

Table 4. Continued

Scale [refs]	Construct(s) and time frame(s)	Responsiveness	Ease of use	Clinically important difference	Limitations
Numbers reading test [61, 96]	Proxy for exercise limitation in patients with advanced cancer for whom exercise testing is not feasible	Responsive to drainage of malignant pleural effusion [61]	Requires repeated, timed administration and counting of breaths while numbers are read	25% change in numbers read or 50% change in numbers read per breath have been suggested, but there is limited evidence [61]	Scoring is somewhat complex (greatest number of numbers read in 60 s and numbers per breath over 60 s from best of five attempts)
Three shortness-of-breath items from EORTC QLQ-LC13 module [87, 104, 105]	Activity-related breathlessness (at rest, walking, climbing stairs)	Not determined	Simple to administer	Not determined	Extensive validation for the entire LC-13 module [106], but very limited for use as a three-item breathlessness measure

mMRC: modified Medical Research Council; LCADL: London Chest Activities of Daily Living; P_{aO_2}: arterial oxygen tension; P_{aCO_2}: arterial carbon dioxide tension; 6MWD: 6-min walk distance; ESAS: Edmonton Symptom Assessment System; EORTC QLQ-LC13: European Organisation for Research and Treatment of Cancer Quality of Life Questionnaire Lung Cancer 13 module.

Multidimensional

Commonly used multidimensional breathlessness functional impact measures include the Baseline Dyspnea Index (BDI) and Transition Dyspnea Index (TDI) [44, 95, 107] and the Functional Assessment of Chronic Illness Therapy (FACIT)–Dyspnea and Functional Limitations scales [108–111].

The BDI measures the extent of functional impairment due to breathlessness and the magnitude of activity and magnitude of effort inducing breathlessness; the TDI measures the extent of change in these three dimensions from a previous measurement with the BDI. The MCID for the TDI is 1 point [112, 113]. The BDI and TDI are commonly used in clinical trials of pulmonary rehabilitation and pharmacotherapy of COPD but infrequently in a palliative care context [114]. However, they have been used as criterion measures for validating other instruments included in this chapter [111, 115].

The FACIT–Dyspnea 10-item short forms were derived from an item bank of 33 activity-related items. (An item bank is a database of items developed through expert consensus and pilot-testing or derived from extant measures; items are calibrated using either Rasch or item-response theory modelling methods to locate them along a continuum, such as symptom severity. Item banks can be used to develop short, valid questionnaires or as the basis for computerised, adaptive testing.) Respondents rate FACIT–Dyspnea items for how short of breath they became over the past 7 days with a given activity (no shortness of breath; mildly, moderately, or severely short of breath; and I did not do this in the past 7 days) and for how difficult a given activity was due to shortness of breath (no difficulty, a little difficulty, some difficulty or much difficulty) [108, 111]. For those who mark "I did not do…", branching logic is used to differentiate between those who stopped doing "because I have stopped trying, or knew I could not do… because of my shortness of breath" (scored as severe) *versus* those who did not do "for some other reason", including not having the opportunity or due to other health issues (scored as missing). The same item bank and short-form items have been adopted by the Patient Reported Outcomes Measurement Information Systems (PROMIS) initiative [116, 117]. In either case, raw scores are converted to a standardised (T-score) metric with persons with self-reported COPD as the reference population [109]. The FACIT–Dyspnea and FACIT–Dyspnea Functional Limitation short forms correlate very strongly with each other and with their respective full item banks [108], moderately to strongly with the Modified Medical Research Council Scale (mMRC) [108, 109, 118], and moderately with Borg CR-10 scores at rest and during a 6-min walk test [118]. Both short forms correlate strongly and significantly with the St George's Respiratory Questionnaire (SGRQ) total score [109] and Chronic Respiratory Questionnaire Dyspnea Subscale [108] and more strongly with the SF-36 Health Survey physical functioning and physical component scores than with other SF-36 domain scores [108].

QoL impact

QoL measurement tends to be more comprehensive in palliative care research (*e.g.* as a patient-reported outcome or end-point assessment in clinical trials) than in clinical practice, where time and resources are often more limited. Most generic and disease-specific health status or QoL instruments are multidimensional. However, the EuroQol EQ-5D [119–121] includes a global health state VAS (EQ-VAS: 0=worst imaginable health state, 100=best imaginable health state) and the 30-item EORTC Core QLQ (QLQ-C30) [26] includes overall health and QoL items (How would you rate your overall health/quality of life during the past week? 1=very poor, 7=excellent) that potentially can be used as single-item [122] or two-item composite [123] global assessments.

Multidimensional health status instruments commonly used in patients with advanced pulmonary disease include various versions of the Chronic Respiratory Disease Questionnaire (CRQ) [124], the SGRQ [125] and the Clinical COPD Questionnaire (CCQ) [126, 127]. For patients with cancer, the 30-item or 15-item palliative care versions of the EORTC Quality of Life Questionnaire (QLQ-C30 or QLQ-C15 PAL) are commonly used with or without the lung cancer module (QLQ-LC13) [27, 106, 128–130]. Generic health status is commonly assessed using the EuroQol EQ-5D [131]. In addition, General Health profiles from the PROMIS initiative [116] have been used in patients with COPD [118], pulmonary fibrosis [117] or systemic sclerosis [109, 110].

The CRQ has subscales for dyspnoea, fatigue, emotional function and mastery. In its original form, it was interviewer administered, and the dyspnoea domain was individualised (the five activities or situations associated with dyspnoea that a respondent believed had the greatest day-to-day importance over the previous 2 weeks); the remaining 15 items were standardised [124]. A modification was developed for patients with heart failure [132]. Subsequent iterations include versions for self-report [133] and with standardised items [134]. Scores on each scale are standardised to a 1 (maximum impairment) to 7 (no impairment) range, and a 0.5 point change is considered clinically meaningful. A short-form version has also been developed (eight items, two per domain) [135]. In palliative care, the mastery subscale has been used by itself as an end-point measure in a clinical trial of a breathlessness intervention service [103].

The SGRQ is often used as an end-point measure in clinical trials of pharmacological therapy or pulmonary rehabilitation for patients with obstructive lung disease. The SGRQ can be reported as a total score or by subscales for symptoms, activities and impacts. A higher score indicates a worse health status. The length (50 items) and scoring of the SGRQ make it somewhat impractical for routine use in a palliative care context, but it is commonly used as a criterion measure for validation of newer, shorter measures [127, 136–139]. A difference of 4 points is commonly used as the MCID [140]; however, it was recently recommended that a larger difference (7–8 points) would be more appropriate for sample size determination for clinical trials for patients with severe COPD [141].

The CCQ [126, 127] is a 10-item disease-specific health status questionnaire that has three subdomains: symptoms (frequency of shortness of breath at rest and during physical activity, cough and phlegm), functional limitation (with strenuous or moderate physical activities, during activities of daily living and during social activities) and mental state (depression and concern). All items are rated on a 0–6 ordinal scale, with a frequency rating for symptom and mental state items (0=never, 6=almost all the time) and degree of limitation for functional items (0=not limited at all, 6=totally limited or unable to do). Scores can be reported as the mean score for all items (total CCQ score) or for each subdomain. The CCQ is available in daily (past 24 h) or weekly (past 7 days) time frames and has been translated into many languages/dialects. For the daily and weekly versions, a decrease of 0.4 points has been reported as an anchor-based MCID [138, 139, 142]. The total CCQ score is one of two recommended symptom severity assessments for the Global Initiative for Chronic Obstructive Lung Disease (GOLD) staging scheme [6]. (The other tool recommended for this purpose is the COPD Assessment Test (CAT), an eight-item, unidimensional scale of the current impact of COPD on well-being that is commonly used for initial and periodic follow-up evaluation [137].)

The EORTC QLQ-30 [26] has been in use for over 20 years in a wide variety of cancer populations. It covers common symptoms, physical and social functioning, and well-being [143], with subscales for: global QoL and health status (two items); physical functioning (five items); emotional functioning (four items); role, cognitive and social functioning (two items each); fatigue (three items); nausea and vomiting (two items); pain (two items); and dyspnoea, insomnia, constipation, diarrhoea, appetite loss and financial difficulties (one item each). For multi-item scales, the raw score is the mean of item scores standardised to a 0–100 range, with higher scores representing higher functioning or a worse symptom level [144]. A 15-item version is available to reduce respondent burden for palliative care populations [129]. Disease-specific modules (intended for co-administration with the QLQ-30) are available for various primary and metastatic cancers, including a 13-item module for lung cancer (QLQ-LC13), which, as noted above, includes three items for the extent of shortness of breath (rest, walking and stairs). In addition, it includes three items for pain (in the chest, upper extremities and other body parts), two pertaining to pain medication (whether any was taken and, if so, how much it helped), plus single items pertaining to coughing, haemoptysis, sore mouth/tongue, dysphagia, neuropathy and hair loss [27, 104]. The QLQ-LC13 symptom items have four response categories (not at all, a little, quite a bit and very much). For the QLQ-30, five items do not have a specific time frame, while the others pertain to the past week. All QLQ-LC13 items refer to the past week. The QLQ-LC13 has been used extensively in clinical trials, more often as a secondary than as a primary end-point [106].

The EuroQol EQ-5D in any of several versions covers five domains (mobility, self-care, usual activities, pain/discomfort and anxiety/depression), as well as a global health state VAS (EQ-VAS; 0=worst health you can imagine, 100=best health you can imagine) [120, 121, 131, 145, 146]. It is available in versions with three or five ordinal levels (EQ-5D-3L and EQ-5D-5L) per domain [120, 121]. The results can be summarised by domain, or, for cost–utility comparisons, can be transformed to an overall 0–1.0 index score using country-specific value sets. The EQ-5D is much shorter, with a considerably lower respondent burden than the SF-36 as a generic health status measure. A recent study found that the EQ-VAS discriminated reasonably well in a pulmonary rehabilitation setting between those who improved (a TDI improvement ⩾1 point) *versus* those who did not (receiver operating characteristic area under the curve=0.85, p<0.001) with an optimal cut-off point for improvement at 8 points on the EQ-VAS (sensitivity=0.78, specificity=0.81) [115]. For patients with COPD, mean EQ-5D-5L index and EQ-VAS scores as well relative category proportions for the mobility, self-care and usual activity domains discriminate GOLD 1 or 2 from GOLD 3 or 4 patients [118].

The PROMIS family of profiles for adult self-reported health encompass domains of physical, mental and social health. Profile domains for physical health include physical function, pain intensity, pain interference, fatigue and sleep disturbance. Profile domains for mental health include anxiety and depression. The social health domain pertains to participation in social activities and roles [116]. Item banks for these domains were developed using item-response theory analysis to enable computerised adaptive testing. In addition, profile instruments are available as 29-, 43- and 57-item questionnaires. Scores are standardised as T-scores, with healthy adults as the reference population. The physical function, fatigue, depression and social role domains of the PROMIS-43 profile demonstrated significant associations with

GOLD stage in patients with COPD, whereas the pain interference and intensity, anxiety and sleep disturbance domain scores did not; however, only the physical functioning and social role domains showed a monotonically decreasing association with GOLD stage [118]. In patients with IPF, all PROMIS-29 domains except sleep disturbance showed significant score differences by mMRC grade [117]. In patients with systemic sclerosis, the PROMIS-29 physical functioning score discriminated significantly, with large effect sizes for differences between mMRC levels 0 and 1 and between mMRC level 1 and levels 2–4; it also correlated strongly with the physical component score of the SF-36 [109] and performed similarly to the SF-36 physical functioning, role-physical and physical component scores with respect to discriminating levels of disease severity [110]; the anxiety and depression scores correlated moderately with the SF-36 mental component score [109]. Thresholds for clinically important differences need further investigation, but a T-score metric at least facilitates the provisional use of effect size conventions referenced to SDs.

In addition to the foregoing measures, disease-specific QoL measures are in varying stages of development for use with patients with ILD (King's Brief ILD questionnaire (K-BILD)) [147, 148] and lymphangioleiomyomatosis (A Tool to Assess Quality of Life in LAM (ATAQ-LAM)) [149].

Conclusion

There is no one-size-fits-all approach to measuring breathlessness or its impact. Decisions to adopt a particular approach involve optimising among concerns for overall purpose (*e.g.* description, classification or outcome assessment), construct relevance to the population and setting, responsiveness, and pragmatic considerations, such as ease and consistency of administration, simplicity of scoring and minimising respondent burden [8, 9, 13, 15, 19, 20]. When feasible, self-report is generally preferable on theoretical grounds [11] and because it can open up possibilities for improved communication between the patient and the provider [15]. After all, if no attempt is made to measure breathlessness or its impact, patients may be led to believe that nothing can be done to change it. As with clinical measurement of pain, routine measurement of breathlessness or its impact communicates to patients that what they are feeling and how it affects them are problems that are important to their healthcare providers and are potentially treatable.

References

1. Lanken PN, Terry PB, DeLisser HM, *et al.* An official American Thoracic Society clinical policy statement: palliative care for patients with respiratory diseases and critical illnesses. *Am J Respir Crit Care Med* 2008; 177: 912–927.
2. Mahler DA, Selecky PA, Harrod CG, *et al.* American College of Chest Physicians consensus statement on the management of dyspnea in patients with advanced lung or heart disease. *Chest* 2010; 137: 674–691.
3. Mularski RA, Campbell ML, Asch SM, *et al.* A review of quality of care evaluation for the palliation of dyspnea. *Am J Respir Crit Care Med* 2010; 181: 534–538.
4. Marciniuk DD, Goodridge D, Hernandez P, *et al.* Managing dyspnea in patients with advanced chronic obstructive pulmonary disease: a Canadian Thoracic Society clinical practice guideline. *Can Respir J* 2011; 18: 69–78.
5. IMPRESS Breathlessness Working Party. Breathlessness IMPRESS tips: responding effectively to people with long term breathlessness 2014. www.impressresp.com/index.php?option=com_docman&Itemid=82 Date last updated: December 2, 2013. Date last accessed: July 11, 2016.
6. Global Initiative for Chronic Obstructive Lung Disease (GOLD). Global Strategy for the Diagnosis, Management, and Prevention of COPD. 2016. Available from: www.goldcopd.org/

7. Qaseem A, Snow V, Shekelle P, *et al.* Evidence-based interventions to improve the palliative care of pain, dyspnea, and depression at the end of life: a clinical practice guideline from the American College of Physicians. *Ann Intern Med* 2008; 148: 141–146.
8. Evans CJ, Benalia H, Preston NJ, *et al.* The selection and use of outcome measures in palliative and end-of-life care research: the MORECare international consensus workshop. *J Pain Symptom Manage* 2013; 46: 925–937.
9. Currow DC, Higginson IJ, Johnson MJ. Breathlessness – current and emerging mechanisms, measurement and management: a discussion from an European Association of Palliative Care workshop. *Palliat Med* 2013; 27: 932–938.
10. Bausewein C, Booth S, Higginson IJ. Measurement of dyspnoea in the clinical rather than the research setting. *Curr Opin Support Palliat Care* 2008; 2: 95–99.
11. Parshall MB, Schwartzstein RM, Adams L, *et al.* An official American Thoracic Society statement: update on the mechanisms, assessment, and management of dyspnea. *Am J Respir Crit Care Med* 2012; 185: 435–452.
12. Ekström MP, Abernethy AP, Currow DC. The management of chronic breathlessness in patients with advanced and terminal illness. *BMJ* 2015; 349: g7617.
13. Dorman S, Jolley C, Abernethy A, *et al.* Researching breathlessness in palliative care: consensus statement of the National Cancer Research Institute Palliative Care Breathlessness Subgroup. *Palliat Med* 2009; 23: 213–227.
14. Reeve BB, Mitchell SA, Dueck AC, *et al.* Recommended patient-reported core set of symptoms to measure in adult cancer treatment trials. *J Nat Cancer Inst* 2014; 106: dju129.
15. Booth S, Burkin J, Moffat C, *et al.* Managing Breathlessness in Clinical Practice. London, Springer, 2014.
16. Haugdahl HS, Storli SL, Meland B, *et al.* Underestimation of patient breathlessness by nurses and physicians during a spontaneous breathing trial. *Am J Respir Crit Care Med* 2015; 192: 1440–1448.
17. Simon ST, Altfelder N, Alt-Epping B, *et al.* Is breathlessness what the professional says it is? Analysis of patient and professionals' assessments from a German nationwide register. *Support Care Cancer* 2014; 22: 1825–1832.
18. Bausewein C, Farquhar M, Booth S, *et al.* Measurement of breathlessness in advanced disease: a systematic review. *Respir Med* 2007; 101: 399–410.
19. Dorman S, Byrne A, Edwards A. Which measurement scales should we use to measure breathlessness in palliative care? A systematic review. *Palliat Med* 2007; 21: 177–191.
20. Bausewein C, Daveson BA, Currow DC, *et al.* EAPC White Paper on outcome measurement in palliative care: improving practice, attaining outcomes and delivering quality services – recommendations from the European Association for Palliative Care (EAPC) Task Force on Outcome Measurement. *Palliat Med* 2016; 30: 6–22.
21. Bruera E, Kuehn N, Miller MJ, *et al.* The Edmonton Symptom Assessment System (ESAS): a simple method for the assessment of palliative care patients. *J Palliat Care* 1991; 7: 6–9.
22. Watanabe SM, Nekolaichuk C, Beaumont C, *et al.* A multicenter study comparing two numerical versions of the Edmonton Symptom Assessment System in palliative care patients. *J Pain Symptom Manage* 2011; 41: 456–468.
23. Portenoy RK, Thaler HT, Kornblith AB, *et al.* The Memorial Symptom Assessment Scale: an instrument for the evaluation of symptom prevalence, characteristics and distress. *Eur J Cancer* 1994; 30A: 1326–1336.
24. Zambroski CH, Moser DK, Bhat G, *et al.* Impact of symptom prevalence and symptom burden on quality of life in patients with heart failure. *Eur J Cardiovasc Nurs* 2005; 4: 198–206.
25. Masel EK, Berghoff AS, Schur S, *et al.* The PERS^2 ON score for systemic assessment of symptomatology in palliative care: a pilot study. *Eur J Canc Care* 2016; 25: 544–550.
26. Aaronson NK, Ahmedzai S, Bergman B, *et al.* The European Organization for Research and Treatment of Cancer QLQ-C30: a quality-of-life instrument for use in international clinical trials in oncology. *J Nat Cancer Inst* 1993; 85: 365–376.
27. Bergman B, Aaronson NK, Ahmedazi S, *et al.* The EORTC QLQ-LC13: a modular supplement to the EORTC Core Quality of Life Questionnaire (QLQ-C30) for use in lung cancer clinical trials. EORTC Study Group on Quality of Life. *Eur J Cancer* 1994; 30A: 635–642.
28. Lansing RW, Gracely RH, Banzett RB. The multiple dimensions of dyspnea: review and hypotheses. *Respir Physiol Neurobiol* 2009; 167: 53–60.
29. Ryan R, Spathis A, Booth S. Correlates between basic science and therapeutic interventions: the theory and the practice. *Curr Opin Support Palliat Care* 2014; 8: 200–207.
30. Thomas S, Bausewein C, Higginson I, *et al.* Breathlessness in cancer patients – implications, management and challenges. *Eur J Oncol Nurs* 2011; 15: 459–469.
31. Mahler DA, O'Donnell DE. Recent advances in dyspnea. *Chest* 2015; 147: 232–241.
32. O'Donnell DE, Ora J, Webb KA, *et al.* Mechanisms of activity-related dyspnea in pulmonary diseases. *Respir Physiol Neurobiol* 2009; 167: 116–132.
33. Banzett RB, O'Donnell CR, Guilfoyle TE, *et al.* Multidimensional Dyspnea Profile: an instrument for clinical and laboratory research. *Eur Respir J* 2015; 45: 1681–1691.
34. Meek PM, Banzett R, Parshall MB, *et al.* Reliability and validity of the Multidimensional Dyspnea Profile. *Chest* 2012; 141: 1546–1553.
35. Parshall MB, Carle AC, Ice U, *et al.* Validation of a 3-factor measurement model of dyspnea in hospitalized adults with heart failure. *Heart Lung* 2012; 41: 44–56.

36. Yorke J, Horton M, Jones PW. A critique of Rasch analysis using the Dyspnoea-12 as an illustrative example. *J Adv Nurs* 2012; 68: 191–198.
37. Yorke J, Moosavi SH, Shuldham C, *et al.* Quantification of dyspnoea using descriptors: development and initial testing of the Dyspnoea-12. *Thorax* 2010; 65: 21–26.
38. Johnson MJ, Oxberry SG, Cleland JGF, *et al.* Measurement of breathlessness in clinical trials in patients with chronic heart failure: the need for a standardized approach: a systematic review. *Eur J Heart Fail* 2010; 12: 137–147.
39. Weldam SW, Schuurmans MJ, Liu R, *et al.* Evaluation of Quality of Life instruments for use in COPD care and research: a systematic review. *Int J Nurs Stud* 2013; 50: 688–707.
40. Aitken RCB. Measurement of feelings using visual analogue scales. *Proc R Soc Med* 1969; 62: 989–993.
41. Gift AG. Validation of a vertical visual analogue scale as a measure of clinical dyspnea. *Rehabil Nurs* 1989; 14: 323–325.
42. Gift AG, Narsavage G. Validity of the numeric rating scale as a measure of dyspnea. *Am J Crit Care* 1998; 7: 200–204.
43. Borg GA. Psychophysical bases of perceived exertion. *Med Sci Sports Exerc* 1982; 14: 377–381.
44. Mahler DA, Rosiello RA, Harver A, *et al.* Comparison of clinical dyspnea ratings and psychophysical measurements of respiratory sensation in obstructive airway disease. *Am Rev Respir Dis* 1987; 135: 1229–1233.
45. Oxberry SG, Bland JM, Clark AL, *et al.* Minimally clinically important difference in chronic breathlessness: Every little helps. *Am Heart J* 2012; 164: 229–235.
46. Ries AL. Minimally clinically important difference for the UCSD Shortness of Breath Questionnaire, Borg Scale, and Visual Analog Scale. *COPD* 2005; 2: 105–110.
47. Johnson MJ, Bland JM, Oxberry SG, *et al.* Clinically important differences in the intensity of chronic refractory breathlessness. *J Pain Symptom Manage* 2013; 46: 957–963.
48. Johnson MJ, Bland JM, Oxberry SG, *et al.* Opioids for chronic refractory breathlessness: patient predictors of beneficial response. *Eur Respir J* 2013; 42: 758–766.
49. Johnson MJ, Close L, Gillon SC, *et al.* Use of the modified Borg scale and numerical rating scale to measure chronic breathlessness: a pooled data analysis. *Eur Respir J* 2016.
50. Campbell ML. Psychometric testing of a respiratory distress observation scale. *J Palliat Med* 2008; 11: 44–50.
51. Campbell ML, Templin T, Walch J. A Respiratory Distress Observation Scale for patients unable to self-report dyspnea. *J Palliat Med* 2010; 13: 285–290.
52. Campbell ML, Templin TN. Intensity cut-points for the Respiratory Distress Observation Scale. *Palliat Med* 2015; 29: 436–442.
53. Borg G. Perceived exertion as an indicator of somatic stress. *Scand J Rehab Med* 1970; 2: 92–98.
54. Khair RM, Nwaneri C, Damico RL, *et al.* The minimal important difference in Borg dyspnea score in pulmonary arterial hypertension. *Ann Am Thorac Soc* 2016; 13: 842–849.
55. Seymour RA, Simpson JM, Ed Charlton J, *et al.* An evaluation of length and end-phrase of visual analogue scales in dental pain. *Pain* 1985; 21: 177–185.
56. Clark WC, Yang JC, Tsui S-L, *et al.* Unidimensional pain rating scales: a multidimensional affect and pain survey (MAPS) analysis of what they really measure. *Pain* 2002; 98: 241–247.
57. Huber A, Suman AL, Rendo CA, *et al.* Dimensions of "unidimensional" ratings of pain and emotions in patients with chronic musculoskeletal pain. *Pain* 2007; 130: 216–224.
58. Corner J, Plant H, A'Hern R, *et al.* Non-pharmacological intervention for breathlessness in lung cancer. *Palliat Med* 1996; 10: 299–305.
59. Stulbarg MS, Carrieri-Kohlman V, Gormley JM, *et al.* Accuracy of recall of dyspnea after exercise training sessions. *J Cardiopulm Rehabil* 1999; 19: 242–248.
60. Hately J, Laurence V, Scott A, *et al.* Breathlessness clinics within specialist palliative care settings can improve quality of life and functional capacity in patients with cancer. *Palliat Med* 2003; 17: 410–417.
61. Wilcock A, Crosby V, Clarke D, *et al.* Reading numbers aloud: a measure of the limiting effect of breathlessness in patients with cancer. *Thorax* 1999; 54: 1099–1103.
62. Abernethy AP, McDonald CF, Frith PA, *et al.* Effect of palliative oxygen *versus* room air in relief of breathlessness in patients with refractory dyspnoea: a double-blind, randomised controlled trial. *Lancet* 2010; 376: 784–793.
63. Hoekstra J, Vernooij-Dassen MJFJ, de Vos R, *et al.* The added value of assessing the 'most troublesome' symptom among patients with cancer in the palliative phase. *Patient Educ Couns* 2007; 65: 223–229.
64. Price DD, McGrath PA, Rafii A, *et al.* The validation of visual analogue scales as ratio scale measures for chronic and experimental pain. *Pain* 1983; 17: 45–56.
65. Wysham NG, Miriovsky BJ, Currow DC, *et al.* Practical dyspnea assessment: relationship between the 0–10 Numerical Rating Scale and the four-level categorical Verbal Descriptor Scale of dyspnea intensity. *J Pain Symptom Manage* 2015; 50: 480–487.
66. Campbell ML, Templin T, Walch J. Patients who are near death are frequently unable to self-report dyspnea. *J Palliat Med* 2009; 12: 881–884.
67. van der Maaden T, van der Steen JT, de Vet HCW, *et al.* Prospective observations of discomfort, pain, and dyspnea in nursing home residents with dementia and pneumonia. *J Am Med Dir Assoc* 2016; 17: 128–135.

68. Persichini R, Gay F, Schmidt M, *et al.* Diagnostic accuracy of respiratory distress observation scales as surrogates of dyspnea self-report in intensive care unit patients. *Anesthesiology* 2015; 123: 830–837.
69. Hui D, Morgado M, Vidal M, *et al.* Dyspnea in hospitalized advanced cancer patients: subjective and physiologic correlates. *J Palliat Med* 2013; 16: 274–280.
70. American Thoracic Society. Dyspnea. Mechanisms, assessment, and management: a consensus statement. *Am J Respir Crit Care Med* 1999; 159: 321–340.
71. Laviolette L, Laveneziana P, on behalf of the ERS Research Seminar Faculty. Dyspnoea: a multidimensional and multidisciplinary approach. *Eur Respir J* 2014; 43: 1750–1762.
72. Mularski RA, Reinke LF, Carrieri-Kohlman V, *et al.* An official American Thoracic Society workshop report: assessment and palliative management of dyspnea crisis. *Ann Am Thoracic Soc* 2013; 10: S98–S106.
73. Tanaka K, Akechi T, Okuyama T, *et al.* Factors correlated with dyspnea in advanced lung cancer patients: organic causes and what else? *J Pain Symptom Manage* 2002; 23: 490–500.
74. Tanaka K, Akechi T, Okuyama T, *et al.* Prevalence and screening of dyspnea interfering with daily life activities in ambulatory patients with advanced lung cancer. *J Pain Symptom Manage* 2002; 23: 484–489.
75. Swigris JJ, Yorke J, Sprunger DB, *et al.* Assessing dyspnea and its impact on patients with connective tissue disease-related interstitial lung disease. *Respir Med* 2010; 104: 1350–1355.
76. Tanaka K, Akechi T, Okuyama T, *et al.* Development and validation of the Cancer Dyspnoea Scale: a multidimensional, brief, self-rating scale. *Br J Cancer* 2000; 82: 800–805.
77. Kohara H, Ueoka H, Aoe K, *et al.* Effect of nebulized furosemide in terminally ill cancer patients with dyspnea. *J Pain Symptom Manage* 2003; 26: 962–967.
78. Henoch I, Bergman B, Gaston-Johansson F. Validation of a Swedish version of the Cancer Dyspnea Scale. *J Pain Symptom Manage* 2006; 31: 353–361.
79. Yorke J, Russell AM, Swigris J, *et al.* Assessment of dyspnea in asthma: validation of the Dyspnea-12. *J Asthma* 2011; 48: 602–608.
80. Yorke J, Swigris J, Russell AM, *et al.* Dyspnea-12 is a valid and reliable measure of breathlessness in patients with interstitial lung disease. *Chest* 2011; 139: 159–164.
81. Yorke J, Lloyd-Williams M, Smith J, *et al.* Management of the respiratory distress symptom cluster in lung cancer: a randomised controlled feasibility trial. *Support Care Cancer* 2015; 23: 3373–3384.
82. Parshall MB, Meek PM, Sklar D, *et al.* Test-retest reliability of Multidimensional Dyspnea Profile recall ratings in the emergency department: a prospective, longitudinal study. *BMC Emerg Med* 2012; 12: 6.
83. Beaumont M, Mialon P, Ber-Moy CL, *et al.* Inspiratory muscle training during pulmonary rehabilitation in chronic obstructive pulmonary disease: a randomized trial. *Chronic Respir Dis* 2015; 12: 305–312.
84. Morélot-Panzini C, Gilet H, Aguilaniu B, *et al.* Real-life assessment of the multidimensional nature of dyspnoea in COPD outpatients. *Eur Respir J* 2016; 47: 1668–1679.
85. Uronis HE, Shelby RA, Currow DC, *et al.* Assessment of the psychometric properties of an English version of the Cancer Dyspnea Scale in people with advanced lung cancer. *J Pain Symptom Manage* 2012; 44: 741–749.
86. Henoch I, Bergman B, Gustafsson M, *et al.* The impact of symptoms, coping capacity, and social support on quality of life experience over time in patients with lung cancer. *J Pain Symptom Manage* 2007; 34: 370–379.
87. Henoch I, Bergman B, Gustafsson M, *et al.* Dyspnea experience in patients with lung cancer in palliative care. *Eur J Oncol Nurs* 2008; 12: 86–96.
88. Yorke J, Armstrong I. The assessment of breathlessness in pulmonary arterial hypertension: reliability and validity of the Dyspnoea-12. *Eur J Cardiovasc Nurs* 2014; 13: 506–514.
89. Al-Gamal E, Yorke J. Perceived breathlessness and psychological distress among patients with chronic obstructive pulmonary disease and their spouses. *Nurs Health Sci* 2014; 16: 103–111.
90. Al-Gamal E, Yorke J, Al-Shwaiyat MKEA. Dyspnea-12-Arabic: testing of an instrument to measure breathlessness in Arabic patients with chronic obstructive pulmonary disease. *Heart Lung* 2014; 43: 244–248.
91. Banzett RB, Pedersen SH, Schwartzstein RM, *et al.* The affective dimension of laboratory dyspnea: air hunger is more unpleasant than work/effort. *Am J Respir Crit Care Med* 2008; 177: 1384–1390.
92. Georges M, Moraviec E, Raux M, *et al.* Cortical drive to breathe in amyotrophic lateral sclerosis: a dyspnoea-worsening defence? *Eur Respir J* 2016; 47: 1818–1828.
93. Parshall MB. Psychometric characteristics of dyspnea descriptor ratings in emergency department patients with exacerbated chronic obstructive pulmonary disease. *Res Nurs Health* 2002; 25: 331–344.
94. Fletcher CM. The clinical diagnosis of pulmonary emphysema: an experimental study. *Proc R Soc Med* 1952; 45: 577–584.
95. Mahler DA, Wells CK. Evaluation of clinical methods for rating dyspnea. *Chest* 1988; 93: 580–586.
96. Wilcock A, Walton A, Manderson C, *et al.* Randomised, placebo controlled trial of nebulised furosemide for breathlessness in patients with cancer. *Thorax* 2008; 63: 872–875.
97. Cancer Care Ontario, Action Cancer Ontario. Symptom Management Pocket Guidelines: Dyspnea 2010. www.cancercare.on.ca/CCO_DrugFormulary/Pages/FileContent.aspx?fileId=97467 Date last updated: March 8, 2016.

98. McGavin CR, Artvinli M, Naoe H, *et al.* Dyspnoea, disability, and distance walked: comparison of estimates of exercise performance in respiratory disease. *BMJ* 1978; 2: 241–243.
99. Reddy SK, Parsons HA, Elsayem A, *et al.* Characteristics and correlates of dyspnea in patients with advanced cancer. *J Palliat Med* 2009; 12: 29–36.
100. Janssens JP, Breitenstein E, Rochat T, *et al.* Does the 'oxygen cost diagram' reflect changes in six minute walking distance in follow up studies? *Respir Med* 1999; 93: 810–815.
101. Garrod R, Bestall JC, Paul EA, *et al.* Development and validation of a standardized measure of activity of daily living in patients with severe COPD: the London Chest Activity of Daily Living scale (LCADL). *Respir Med* 2000; 94: 589–596.
102. Garrod R, Paul EA, Wedzicha JA. An evaluation of the reliability and sensitivity of the London Chest Activity of Daily Living Scale (LCADL). *Respir Med* 2002; 96: 725–730.
103. Higginson IJ, Bausewein C, Reilly CC, *et al.* An integrated palliative and respiratory care service for patients with advanced disease and refractory breathlessness: a randomised controlled trial. *Lancet Respir Med* 2014; 2: 979–987.
104. European Organisation for Research and Treatment of Cancer (EORTC). Lung cancer module: QLQ-LC13. www.eortc.be/qol/files/ScoringInstructions/LC13_summary.pdf Date last updated: 1994. Date last accessed: July 11, 2016.
105. Mohan A, Singh P, Singh S, *et al.* Quality of life in lung cancer patients: impact of baseline clinical profile and respiratory status. *Eur J Cancer Care* 2007; 16: 268–276.
106. Koller M, Warncke S, Hjermstad MJ, *et al.* Use of the lung cancer-specific Quality of Life Questionnaire EORTC QLQ-LC13 in clinical trials: a systematic review of the literature 20 years after its development. *Cancer* 2015; 121: 4300–4323.
107. Mahler DA, Weinberg DH, Wells CK, *et al.* The measurement of dyspnea. Contents, interobserver agreement, and physiologic correlates of two new clinical indexes. *Chest* 1984; 85: 751–758.
108. Choi SW, Victorson DE, Yount S, *et al.* Development of a conceptual framework and calibrated item banks to measure patient-reported dyspnea severity and related functional limitations. *Value Health* 2011; 14: 291–306.
109. Hinchcliff M, Beaumont JL, Thavarajah K, *et al.* Validity of two new patient-reported outcome measures in systemic sclerosis: patient-reported outcomes measurement information system 29-item health profile and functional assessment of chronic illness therapy–dyspnea short form. *Arthritis Care Res* 2011; 63: 1620–1628.
110. Hinchcliff ME, Beaumont JL, Carns MA, *et al.* Longitudinal evaluation of PROMIS-29 and FACIT-dyspnea short forms in systemic sclerosis. *J Rheumatol* 2015; 42: 64–72.
111. Yount SE, Choi SW, Victorson D, *et al.* Brief, valid measures of dyspnea and related functional limitations in chronic obstructive pulmonary disease (COPD). *Value Health* 2011; 14: 307–315.
112. Witek TJ Jr, Mahler DA. Meaningful effect size and patterns of response of the transition dyspnea index. *J Clin Epidemiol* 2003; 56: 248–255.
113. Witek TJ, Mahler DA. Minimal important difference of the transition dyspnoea index in a multinational clinical trial. *Eur Respir J* 2003; 21: 267–272.
114. Wong BC, Cake L, Kachuik L, *et al.* Indwelling peritoneal catheters for managing malignancy-associated ascites. *J Palliat Care* 2015; 31: 243–249.
115. Zanini A, Aiello M, Adamo D, *et al.* Estimation of minimal clinically important difference in EQ-5D visual analog scale score after pulmonary rehabilitation in subjects with COPD. *Respir Care* 2015; 60: 88–95.
116. Health Measures. Intro to PROMIS®: PROMIS adult self-reported health 2016. www.healthmeasures.net/explore-measurement-systems/promis/intro-to-promis Date last updated: 2016. Date last accessed: July 11, 2016.
117. Yount SE, Beaumont JL, Chen SY, *et al.* Health-related quality of life in patients with idiopathic pulmonary fibrosis. *Lung* 2016; 194: 227–234.
118. Lin F-J, Pickard AS, Krishnan JA, *et al.* Measuring health-related quality of life in chronic obstructive pulmonary disease: properties of the EQ-5D-5L and PROMIS-43 short form. *BMC Med Res Methodol* 2014; 14: 1–12.
119. EuroQol Group. What is EQ-5D? www.euroqol.org/home.html Date last updated: 2016. Date last accessed: July 11, 2016.
120. van Reenen M, Janssen B. EQ-5D-5L User Guide: Basic Information on How to Use the EQ-5D-5L Instrument. Version 2.1. Rotterdam, EuroQol Research Foundation, 2015. www.euroqol.org/fileadmin/user_upload/Documenten/PDF/Folders_Flyers/EQ-5D-5L_UserGuide_2015.pdf
121. van Reenen M, Oppe M. EQ-5D-3L User Guide: Basic Information on How to Use the EQ-5D-3L Instrument. Version 5.1. Rotterdam, EuroQol Research Foundation, 2015. www.euroqol.org/fileadmin/user_upload/Documenten/PDF/Folders_Flyers/EQ-5D-3L_UserGuide_2015.pdf
122. Cramarossa G, Chow E, Zhang L, *et al.* Predictive factors for overall quality of life in patients with advanced cancer. *Support Care Cancer* 2013; 21: 1709–1716.
123. Janse M, Sprangers MAG, Ranchor AV, *et al.* Long-term effects of goal disturbance and adjustment on well-being in cancer patients. *Qual Life Res* 2015: 1–11.
124. Guyatt GH, Berman LB, Townsend M, *et al.* A measure of quality of life for clinical trials in chronic lung disease. *Thorax* 1987; 42: 773–778.

125. Jones PW, Quirk FH, Baveystock CM, *et al.* A self-complete measure of health status for chronic airflow limitation. The St. George's Respiratory Questionnaire. *Am Rev Respir Dis* 1992; 145: 1321–1327.
126. van der Molen T. CCQ: Clinical COPD Questionnaire. http://ccq.nl/ Date last updated: 1999. Date last accessed: July 11, 2016.
127. van der Molen T, Willemse BW, Schokker S, *et al.* Development, validity and responsiveness of the Clinical COPD Questionnaire. *Health Qual Life Outcomes* 2003; 1: 13.
128. Grande GE, Farquhar MC, Barclay SIG, *et al.* Quality of life measures (EORTC QLQ-C30 and SF-36) as predictors of survival in palliative colorectal and lung cancer patients. *Palliat Support Care* 2009; 7: 289–297.
129. Groenvold M, Petersen MA, Aaronson NK, *et al.* The development of the EORTC QLQ-C15-PAL: a shortened questionnaire for cancer patients in palliative care. *Eur J Cancer* 2006; 42: 55–64.
130. Suarez-del-Real Y, Allende-Perez S, Alferez-Mancera A, *et al.* Validation of the Mexican-Spanish version of the EORTC QLQ-C15-PAL questionnaire for the evaluation of health-related quality of life in patients on palliative care. *Psychooncology* 2011; 20: 889–896.
131. EuroQol Group. EuroQoL – a new facility for the measurement of health-related quality of life. *Health Policy* 1990; 16: 199–208.
132. Guyatt GH, Nogradi S, Halcrow S, *et al.* Development and testing of a new measure of health status for clinical trials in heart failure. *J Gen Intern Med* 1989; 4: 101–107.
133. Williams JEA, Singh SJ, Sewell L, *et al.* Development of a self-reported Chronic Respiratory Questionnaire (CRQ-SR). *Thorax* 2001; 56: 954–959.
134. Schünemann HJ, Griffith L, Jaeschke R, *et al.* A comparison of the original Chronic Respiratory Questionnaire with a standardized version. *Chest* 2003; 124: 1421–1429.
135. Tsai C-L, Hodder RV, Page JH, *et al.* The short-form Chronic Respiratory Disease Questionnaire was a valid, reliable, and responsive quality-of-life instrument in acute exacerbations of chronic obstructive pulmonary disease. *J Clin Epidemiol* 2008; 61: 489–497.
136. Jones PW, Harding G, Berry P, *et al.* Development and first validation of the COPD Assessment Test. *Eur Respir J* 2009; 34: 648–654.
137. Kon SSC, Canavan JL, Jones SE, *et al.* Minimum clinically important difference for the COPD Assessment Test: a prospective analysis. *Lancet Respir Med* 2014; 2: 195–203.
138. Tsiligianni IG, van der Molen T, Moraitaki D, *et al.* Assessing health status in COPD. A head-to-head comparison between the COPD assessment test (CAT) and the clinical COPD questionnaire (CCQ). *BMC Pulm Med* 2012; 12: 1–9.
139. Kon SSC, Dilaver D, Mittal M, *et al.* The Clinical COPD Questionnaire: response to pulmonary rehabilitation and minimal clinically important difference. *Thorax* 2014; 69: 793–798.
140. Jones PW, Beeh KM, Chapman KR, *et al.* Minimal clinically important differences in pharmacological trials. *Am J Respir Crit Care Med* 2014; 189: 250–255.
141. Welling JBA, Hartman JE, Ten Hacken NHT, *et al.* The minimal important difference for the St George's Respiratory Questionnaire in patients with severe COPD. *Eur Respir J* 2015; 46: 1598–1604.
142. Kocks JW, Tuinenga MG, Uil SM, *et al.* Health status measurement in COPD: the minimal clinically important difference of the clinical COPD questionnaire. *Respir Res* 2006; 7: 62.
143. European Organization for Research and Treatment of Cancer. EORTC quality of life. http://groups.eortc.be/qol/ Date last accessed: July 11, 2016.
144. Fayers PM, Aaronson NK, Bjordal K, *et al.* The EORTC QLQ-C30 scoring manual. 3rd Edn. Brussels, European Organisation for Research and Treatment of Cancer, 2001.
145. Brooks R. EuroQol: the current state of play. *Health Policy* 1996; 37: 53–72.
146. Herdman M, Gudex C, Lloyd A, *et al.* Development and preliminary testing of the new five-level version of EQ-5D (EQ-5D-5L). *Qual Life Res* 2011; 20: 1727–1736.
147. Patel AS, Siegert RJ, Bajwah S, *et al.* Rasch analysis and impact factor methods both yield valid and comparable measures of health status in interstitial lung disease. *J Clin Epidemiol* 2015; 68: 1019–1027.
148. Bajwah S, Ross JR, Wells AU, *et al.* Palliative care for patients with advanced fibrotic lung disease: a randomised controlled phase II and feasibility trial of a community case conference intervention. *Thorax* 2015; 70: 830–839.
149. Walker TD, Desserich J, Albright K, *et al.* Development of ATAQ-LAM: a tool to assess quality of life in lymphangioleiomyomatosis. *Health Qual Life Outcomes* 2015; 13: 112.

Acknowledgements: The authors wish to thank Douglas Mapel for helpful comments on a preliminary draft, and Anne Mattarella for assistance with technical editing (both Health Services Research Division, Lovelace Clinic Foundation, Albuquerque, NM, USA).

Disclosures: None declared.

Chapter 10

Management of chronic breathlessness

Miriam J. Johnson[1], Carlo Barbetta[2], David C. Currow[3], Matthew Maddocks[4], Vanessa McDonald[5], Ravi Mahadeva[6] and Martina Mason[7]

Effective interventions for chronic breathlessness exist and are distinct from interventions directed at the pathophysiology of the medical condition causing the breathlessness. Some, like pulmonary rehabilitation, have been accepted by the clinical community and are integrated into respiratory care, at least in part and for people with COPD. Others, such as breathlessness clinics, are less well recognised but have strong evidence to support their use. A better understanding of the ways that can be used to integrate breathlessness management systematically alongside disease management should drive further implementation research. Low-dose, steady-state oral morphine has a developing evidence base in support of a net benefit. However, not all people tolerate opioids and further research into alternative drug options is needed to help this distressing symptom.

When a patient presents with breathlessness, it is fundamental that a careful search for the underlying cause of the symptom is conducted, a diagnosis of the medical condition is made, and treatment directed at that condition or conditions is initiated, optimised and monitored. Despite this, with many causes of breathlessness, patients will continue to experience breathlessness to a degree, or intermittently, especially if their disease progresses. If breathlessness itself is not seen by the patient as a legitimate concern to present to the clinician, and the clinician does not recognise the breathlessness as a potential therapeutic target in its own right even though the physiological measure may not alter, then the patient may be unable to access a range of evidence-based breathlessness interventions. Pulmonary rehabilitation is one such intervention. It has a strong evidence base and is accepted as part of management alongside disease-directed treatment, although this is not systematically provided or accessed. Further, other less well-known interventions, of which clinicians may be less aware, can improve this difficult symptom. This chapter summarises the current evidence base for breathlessness-directed interventions.

[1]Wolfson Palliative Care Research Centre, Hull York Medical School, University of Hull, Hull, UK. [2]Respiratory Medicine, S. Anna University Hospital, Ferrara, Italy. [3]Palliative and Supportive Services, Flinders University, Adelaide, Australia. [4]Palliative Care, Policy and Rehabilitation, King's College London, London, UK. [5]Respiratory and Sleep Medicine, Hunter Medical Research Institute, Newcastle, Australia. [6]Dept of Medicine, University of Cambridge, Cambridge, UK. [7]Respiratory Medicine, Addenbrooke's and Papworth Hospitals, Cambridge, UK.

Correspondence: Miriam J. Johnson, Wolfson Palliative Care Research Centre, Hull York Medical School, Hertford Building, University of Hull, Hull, HU6 7RX, UK. E-mail: Miriam.johnson@hyms.ac.uk

 Print ISBN: 978-1-84984-071-2. Online ISBN: 978-1-84984-072-9. Print ISSN: 2312-508X. Online ISSN: 2312-5098.

Non-pharmacological interventions

Complex interventions

Non-pharmacological treatments provide a foundation to manage breathlessness and address how the patient breathes (sensory-perceptive domain), thinks (affective domain) and functions (impact domain) (table 1) [1–3].

Physical inactivity is a major consequence of breathlessness. This can precipitate a downward spiral of disease and reduced function [4]. A rehabilitation approach is recommended to counter this spiral. Pulmonary rehabilitation represents the gold standard [5, 6] and should be provided for patients who can tolerate the course. Programmes can address the distress and burden related to breathlessness, provide education in self-management and a supportive environment for patients to retain or regain control of their health behaviour [5]. Pulmonary rehabilitation provides a benchmark against which to compare the effects of other treatments. Breathlessness and mastery scores on the Chronic Respiratory Questionnaire improve by 0.79 (95% CI 0.56–1.03) and 0.71 (95% CI 0.47–0.95) points respectively, and in the majority of patients exercise performance improves beyond the minimally important clinical difference (MCID) for any given test [6]. The affective and impact domains of breathlessness can improve even in the absence of physiological change [7]; a patient's perceived inability to physically train should not prevent programme referral. It can be challenging to encourage patients to start a programme, particularly in the presence of advanced disease when prognosis can be uncertain, practical issues such as attending the venue when frail, and fears about the ability to comply with the required level of exercise. The assurance that breathlessness *per se* is not dangerous, and will often settle with rest, is a prerequisite to encouraging exercise in people with refractory breathlessness. Even when exercising to a symptom-limited maximum, the intensity of breathlessness will recover rapidly (<5 min) [8]. Physical activity should be promoted and where relevant supported by the provision of appropriate mobility aids [9] and/or assistive equipment [10]. These can enhance functional exercise performance through increased ventilatory capacity and/or walking efficiency [11]. Where upper limb tasks, such as cooking or dressing, are limited by breathlessness [12], arm exercise training can also be used to good effect [13].

Table 1. Examples of non-pharmacological interventions according to breathlessness domain

Patient focus	Breathing	Thinking	Functioning
Breathlessness domain	Sensory-perceptive experience	Affective distress	Symptom impact or burden
Treatments (by primary target or mechanism of effect)	Breathing retraining Positioning Fan/facial cooling Chest wall vibration Acupressure	Relaxation Distraction Mindfulness therapies Cognitive therapies Music	Physical exercise Mobility aids Neuromuscular electrical stimulation
Complex services (multiple treatment)	Pulmonary rehabilitation Breathlessness support services or clinics Self-management programmes		

People who cannot tolerate a full programme of pulmonary rehabilitation because of advanced disease may benefit from chronic breathlessness intervention services that provide many of the same components, but in an individually tailored manner, and in fewer sessions. Three phase 3 RCTs have confirmed the benefit for breathlessness and such approaches should be considered [14–16]. A subprotocol [17] of the trial by FARQUHAR *et al.* [15] tested the intervention in people with non-malignant disease. Unlike the trial in cancer patients, although a beneficial trend was seen, this was not statistically significant. This mixed-methods study, however, reported clear narrative from the qualitative interviews of value to the participants, including value of the study interview itself. The authors discussed whether the therapeutic benefit of the interviews diluted the quantitatively measured primary outcome (distress due to breathlessness), especially in view of the different experience of people with cancer who often have had less time to find their own ways of managing breathlessness, but who typically have better access to supportive services [17]. A trial evaluating delivery of a breathing retraining intervention in patients with malignant lung disease compared a combination intervention (breathing training, anxiety management, relaxation, pacing, and prioritisation) delivered over three sessions compared to one training session. In both groups, there was a clinically significant improvement in breathlessness intensity; however, there was no difference between groups [18], suggesting a single training session was as effective. Furthermore, the distress due to breathlessness in the three-session group was worse ($p=0.01$). This is an important consideration for patients suffering a high symptom burden and impaired health status, such as those with lung cancer, where significant breathlessness is often a sign of poor prognosis.

Other non-pharmacological intervention components to relieve breathlessness have been studied, including: breathing retraining; handheld fans; chest wall vibration (CWV); neuromuscular electrical stimulation (NMES); and acupuncture and acupressure.

Breathing retraining involving pursed-lip breathing and diaphragmatic breathing can be delivered as a single or multidimensional intervention. Pursed-lip breathing may reduce respiratory rate and dynamic hyperinflation and may therefore be more effective in certain conditions than others, for example, COPD rather than interstitial fibrosis. Systematic reviews report moderate quality evidence to support the use of pursed-lip breathing in reducing breathlessness [2, 3].

Handheld fans have received an increasing amount of attention in the last few years, as a simple and cheap intervention for the relief of refractory breathlessness by directing cool air across the face [19–24]; they are discussed more fully in the next section.

CWV to relieve breathlessness in COPD patients is supported by strong evidence from five RCTs representing 97 participants with motor neuron disease or COPD [2]. While the mechanism is not completely understood, it is likely to involve activation of muscle spindles in the intercostal muscles [3].

NMES for the relief of breathlessness is supported by evidence from three studies representing 50 participants with COPD who used NMES over 4–6 weeks [2, 3, 25, 26]. NMES of the quadriceps also improves muscle strength and physical performance and can be used in conjunction with pulmonary rehabilitation or as an alternative for patients with severe COPD [2, 3].

Other non-pharmacological methods include acupuncture and acupressure, relaxation, distractive auditory stimuli and counselling; however, their evidence base remains inadequate [2, 3]. There is an urgent need for further well-designed trials in this field [27].

Summary
Non-pharmacological interventions for patients with refractory breathlessness are an important consideration for management. Multiple interventions are effective in relieving symptoms and improving health status and these interventions can be combined to deliver multidimensional strategies, tailored for individuals, even those with advanced disease.

The role of oxygen and airflow for the relief of chronic breathlessness

The role of oxygen therapy and facial airflow in relieving breathlessness in mildly hypoxaemic or normoxaemic patients is an interesting study area. There is emerging evidence to support the efficacy of airflow in chronic breathlessness; the mechanism of action may be the modulation of central perception [28] and reduction of central ventilator drive by airflow stimulation [29]. Airflow can be delivered from a cylinder of compressed medical air *via* a face mask, nasal cannulae, or handheld fan.

The use of oxygen in chronic breathlessness in patients with COPD was reviewed in a recent Cochrane systematic review and meta-analysis [30]. This review included 18 RCTs where a total of 427 participants with moderate-to-severe COPD and a mean P_{aO_2} ⩾7.3 kPa were randomised to supplemental oxygen or medical air delivered through a nasal cannula, mouthpiece or mask. Oxygen therapy led to significant reduction in breathlessness in mildly or non-hypoxaemic COPD patients, with a standardised mean difference (SMD) of −0.37 (95% CI −0.5–−0.24) compared to medical air. On further analysis, the significant reduction in breathlessness was only confirmed in 14 RCTs using continuous oxygen (SMD −0.46; 95% CI −0.59–0.33; clinically meaningful reduction of 12 mm (0–100 mm VAS)). Meta-analysis of secondary outcomes could not be performed due to heterogeneity in data presentation and outcome measures. Because of the heterogeneity of the included studies and small sample sizes, these data must be interpreted with caution. Two double-blind RCTs were published after this review. In contrast to the Cochrane review, they showed no significant reduction in breathlessness with palliative or ambulatory oxygen, compared to medical air [31, 32]. A systematic literature review examining the effect of oxygen in relieving dyspnoea in patients with advanced cancer or cardiac disease also failed to show significant benefit [33]. To date, the largest international, multicentre RCT examining the role of oxygen in mildly hypoxaemic or normoxaemic patients randomised 239 participants (63% COPD) to oxygen delivered *via* home oxygen concentrator for at least 15 h per day for 7 days during everyday general activity or to medical air [31]. A significant reduction in breathlessness intensity was observed in both study arms. Similarly, the other double-blind RCT tested ambulatory oxygen during general activity in 143 patients with COPD without resting hypoxaemia and showed significant benefit in both oxygen and medical air groups during the 12-week study period [32]. This latest evidence suggests that medical airflow may represent an active intervention rather than a placebo comparator.

The role of airflow delivered *via* a handheld fan was examined in three RCTs [20, 21, 24]. In an adequately powered crossover study, 50 inpatients with an advanced disease were randomised to handheld fan directed to their face or leg for 5 min at rest [20]. They reported a significant, 7-mm reduction in VAS (95% CI 2.5–11.7 mm; p=0.003) in the fan directed to face group. A feasibility study of 70 outpatients with COPD or cancer with a 2-month follow-up found no difference in breathlessness intensity (Modified Borg Dyspnoea Scale) with general activity. After 2 months, 48% of the handheld fan group still reported intervention use compared to 20% of the wristband group [24]. This did not reach statistical significance but the study was not designed to detect effectiveness. More recently, a feasibility cohort study of 31 patients using a handheld fan showed a mean±SD difference of −12.8±20.7 mm in VAS breathlessness following 5 min of airflow to the face while at rest [22]. These results support the benefit of handheld fans at rest, but their effectiveness and potential use in relieving dyspnoea in everyday general activity remains unconfirmed. However, change in breathlessness may not be the most appropriate primary outcome when assessing the effect of airflow on breathlessness in everyday activity, as patients' level of breathlessness may increase or remain the same as their exercise tolerance increases. Appropriate outcome measures to reflect breathlessness improvement related to changes in exercise tolerance must, therefore, be identified.

A feasibility mixed-methods trial of the handheld fan [21] indicated that because the fan was cheap, had no side-effects, and was clearly used by patients as part of a complex intervention, which was consistent with other qualitative work [23], then further trials of the fan as a single component would not provide value of information.

Summary

The role of oxygen in relieving refractory breathlessness in patients with COPD with mild hypoxaemia and normoxaemia remains questionable; however, there is limited evidence that continuous exertional oxygen relieves breathlessness. Further research is needed to examine whether the benefit of oxygen therapy in normoxaemic patients outweighs any harm, and whether it is cost-effective. Understanding the mechanisms of breathlessness in specific COPD subgroups, *e.g.* major hyperinflation, airway obstruction, skeletal muscle deconditioning, obesity, and significant oxygen desaturation on exercise, would allow personalised therapies and would aid further research in this area.

The handheld fan should be considered as a component of complex intervention in the management of patients with refractory breathlessness. Future research should focus on implementing its use in clinical practice and further elucidating its mechanism of action [21].

Assisted ventilation and relief of breathlessness

NPPV refers to the application of positive pressure to the upper airway using a mask or similar device to augment ventilation. While the evidence base for NPPV is strong in certain clinical conditions, in others, it remains uncertain.

Ventilatory failure develops when there is an imbalance between the capacity of the respiratory muscle pump, the load placed on it and an inadequate ventilatory drive. Although the mechanism of ventilatory failure is not fully understood, in physiological studies NPPV improves lung mechanics, respiratory muscle strength and respiratory drive, and reduces ventilation–perfusion mismatch in patients with neuromuscular/restrictive extrathoracic respiratory disorders and hypercapnic COPD [34, 35]. The main areas of clinical use are in management of chronic ventilatory failure in extrapulmonary restrictive disease, neuromuscular disorders and COPD. NPPV is also used to manage acute ventilatory failure, particularly in exacerbations of COPD and acute cardiogenic pulmonary oedema, to reduce the requirement for intubation and support patients for whom intubation is considered inappropriate.

There is a strong evidence for NPPV use in acute ventilatory failure in COPD exacerbation; multiple RCTs have demonstrated reduced intubation, hospital length of stay and mortality rates [36]. No RCT has assessed the benefit of NPPV in patients with restrictive extrathoracic disease but case series indicate survival benefit in patients treated with NPPV [37–39]. A systematic literature review of people with neuromuscular and extrathoracic restrictive lung disease confirmed improved survival, quality of life (QoL) and gas exchange with ventilation [40, 41].

Although the effect of NPPV in patients with chronic, stable COPD has been examined in numerous RCTs, systematic reviews have showed no significant improvement in respiratory function [42, 43]. A recent meta-analysis provided no evidence of efficacy for NPPV in patients with stable hypercapnic COPD [44] but definite conclusions could not be drawn because of small study sample sizes.

The sensation of breathlessness strongly correlates with inspiratory load [45]. NPPV reduces inspiratory effort [33], which is possibly the mechanism by which it relieves breathlessness. RCTs examining the effect of NPPV have mainly focused on respiratory function with breathlessness assessed as a secondary outcome. The heterogeneity in assessment tools used has rendered comparison and generation of pooled outcomes impossible.

Four RCTs assessed NPPV in relieving breathlessness in acute exacerbations of COPD. Three studies reported clinically and statistically significant improvement in subjective breathlessness. Plant *et al.* [46] reported more rapid relief in breathlessness in the NIV group but used unvalidated breathlessness scales with unknown MCID, making interpretation difficult. Bott *et al.* [47] showed a significant difference (22 mm VAS) between groups. VAS breathlessness was assessed daily until day 3 and on the day of discharge. The median of the 3-day mean scores between the groups was significantly lower in the NIV group. Breathlessness data were presented graphically without any statistical analysis, thereby limiting interpretation. In addition, four patients could not tolerate NIV and were excluded from the analysis, making the conclusions questionable. Keenan *et al.* [48] reported greater than MCID improvement in Borg score with NPPV, compared to the usual care group. Breathlessness was assessed at randomisation, 1 h after randomisation and then daily for the rest of the hospital stay. No significant difference in baseline Borg score between the NIV (5.8) and control (6.2) groups was noted. The Borg index between the groups was significantly lower at 1 h and day 2; however, breathlessness data were again only presented graphically. Nonetheless, visual comparison of the plotted data suggested clinically significant improvement in breathlessness in the NPPV group. This study was underpowered for the primary outcome and poor adherence in the NIV group led to possible underestimation of the NIV effect on breathlessness. Kolodziej *et al.* [42] assessed the benefits of domiciliary NPPV on relieving breathlessness in patients with stable COPD. In this systematic review, four out of six RCTs demonstrated an improvement in breathlessness score in patients treated with nocturnal NPPV. Renston *et al.* [49] showed a 66.3% reduction in breathlessness (Borg) in 17 patients treated with NPPV *versus* a nonsignificant 27% reduction in the sham-treated NPPV group following 5 days of treatment. There was no significant difference between the NPPV and sham-treated NPPV group with regard to the modified Medical Research Council (MRC) dyspnoea scale or oxygen cost scales after 5 days of treatment. Casanova *et al.* [50] showed a significant reduction in breathlessness (Borg) in the NIV plus standard care group (96% long-term oxygen therapy (LTOT)), compared to the standard care group (93% LTOT) at 3 and 6 months ($p=0.03$). Using the MRC dyspnoea scale, Clini *et al.* [51] reported significant reduction in breathlessness in 43 patients randomised to NPPV and LTOT, compared to LTOT at both 12 months (treatment effect 0.4; 95% CI 0.02–0.78) and 24 months (treatment effect 0.6; 95% CI 0.15–1.05). In the RCT by GARROD *et al.* [52], the breathlessness portion of the Chronic Respiratory Disease Questionnaire improved more in the NPPV and exercise group than in the exercise alone group after 12 weeks of follow-up, but this difference did not reach statistical significance (mean difference 3.29, 95% CI −1.26–7.84; p=0.15). However, exercise tolerance improved significantly better in the intervention group at 12 weeks, with a mean end study difference in shuttle walk distance of 65.8 m (95% CI 17.1–114 m). None of the trials in this review used breathlessness as a primary outcome measure; because of different outcome measures, data could not be pooled. Current consensus recommends initiation of long-term NPPV in people with obstructive lung disease and symptoms associated with ventilatory failure, including breathlessness, and those who develop significant gas exchange abnormality and fail to respond to optimal medical therapy [53].

The current consensus of professional societies on palliative NPPV for acute respiratory failure recognises its use in people for whom endotracheal intubation is inappropriate, provided the cause is reversible and NPPV improves patient comfort [54].

Summary

NPPV is not routinely recommended for use in non-hypercapnic individuals. However, the data to date support more research into the mechanisms of breathlessness and NPPV to identify the subgroups of people with intractable breathlessness most likely to receive palliation from NPPV. The current work on breathlessness phenotypes could facilitate a focused study with detailed breathlessness measures as a primary outcome.

Pharmacological interventions

Non-opioid drugs

Many drugs have been used empirically for breathlessness in clinical practice with the rationale that they may modulate the central perception and peripheral genesis of the symptom. Some are being investigated systematically with an emerging evidence base (*e.g.* opioids), but others have not, thus illustrating the need for systematic research in the field of chronic breathlessness [27]. A summary of studies is shown in table 2, which illustrates the paucity of phase 3 RCTs evaluating non-opioid drugs for breathlessness.

Anxiolytics

The close relationship between breathlessness, anxiety, panic and distress has led to the common use of anxiolytics, such as benzodiazepines, for breathlessness. A 2010 Cochrane review [55] failed to show evidence to support or refute their use. Since this meta-analysis, RCTs have mainly aimed to explore the safety of benzodiazepines because of concerns about respiratory depression. No significant changes in respiratory parameters were found [56, 57]. A small prospective [58], and a larger retrospective analysis of benzodiazepines in combination with opioids was associated with a greater benefit [59]. However, findings from a longitudinal cohort study of 2249 people with COPD on LTOT found that benzodiazepines were associated with increased mortality with a dose–response trend (hazard ratio 1.21, 95% CI 1.05–1.39), either when used alone, or in combination with opioids [60]. Despite the common clinical use of such a combination, no adequately powered clinical trial evidence exists that supports its use. Care should be taken given the lack of robust evidence that benzodiazepines improve breathlessness.

Table 2. Non-opioid drugs for breathlessness: benzodiazepines

First author [ref.]	Type of study	Drug tested	Patients enrolled	Breathlessness measure	Statistically significant benefit	Notes
Simon [55]	Cochrane systematic review	Diazepam Midazolam Alprazolam Lorazepam	COPD Cancer	VAS Breathlessness Grade scale[#] Borg scale	No	Small heterogeneous studies
Stege [56]	RCT	Temazepam	14 severe normocapnic COPD	VAS	No	Safety[¶] in normocapnic COPD
Clemens [57]	Prospective, non-randomised	Lorazepam 1 mg and morphine as needed	26 patients admitted to a palliative care unit	Numerical scale (0–10)	No	Safety[¶] of co-administration
Allcroft [58]	Open-label trial	Clonazepam 0.5 mg nocte and sustained-release morphine 10 mg	11 COPD with modified MRC breathlessness scale >2	VAS	5 patients reported benefit	Safety[¶] of co-administration
Gomutbutra [59]	Retrospective analysis of clinical records	Lorazepam Clonazepam Diazepam alone or combined with opioids	115 between cancer, heart failure, COPD	4-point dyspnoea scale	Yes, when opioids were co-administered with BDZ	Safety[¶] of co-administration

MRC: Medical Research Council; BDZ: benzodiazepine. #: grades breathlessness from 1 (little breathlessness) to 6 (extreme breathlessness); ¶: effect of benzodiazepines on breathing, ventilation and gas exchange.

Buspirone, an azapirone drug used for anxiety disorders, has been suggested as a useful alternative since it does not suppress respiration. However, a recent adequately powered phase 3 trial failed to show benefit for breathlessness in patients with cancer and there is no evidence to support its use in COPD [61–63].

There is no current evidence to support the use of anxiolytics as first-line breathlessness management. Benzodiazepine use should be limited to treat associated anxiety/panic if this is a significant driver for breathlessness. Patients should be monitored carefully given the association with increased mortality.

Antidepressants

Antidepressants, such as selective serotonin re-uptake inhibitors and tricyclic antidepressants, have been investigated, since serotonin affects the modulation of central respiratory control and sensitivity to carbon dioxide [64]. Furthermore, there is an independent association between depression and breathlessness [65, 66]. One prospective cohort study did not show an association between depression and breathlessness at baseline but did so at follow-up, indicating that breathlessness may play a causative role in depression [67].

Preliminary small studies in COPD patients [68–73], show potential benefit for anxiety symptoms, breathlessness and QoL. A systematic review, however, could not demonstrate clear benefit for breathlessness in COPD patients with anxiety disorder, although there were improvements in other patient-centred outcomes with paroxetine [74]. Most studies have been conducted in patients undergoing rehabilitation programmes; improvement in breathlessness could therefore also be due to an incremental benefit from these two interventions [75, 76]. Teasing out benefit from treating anxiety and depression is difficult, although some studies included people who had neither. However, it does seem appropriate that COPD patients with concomitant depression should be actively screened and treated. Results from a phase 3 RCT of sertraline *versus* placebo (Efficacy of sertraline for palliative management of refractory breathlessness; trial number: ACTRN12610000464066) with breathlessness as a primary outcome measure are expected in 2017.

Antihistamines

The antihistamine agents (H1 antagonists) promethazine and chlorpromazine have been investigated alone or in association with benzodiazepines and morphine; however, no phase 3 trials have been conducted [77–79]. These drugs have antimuscarinic and antiserotonergic activity leading to sedative and antipsychotic effects [80]. Promethazine showed improvement in exercise tolerance [81–83], but only in association to morphine at larger doses than those acceptable in contemporary practice [84]. No long-term data are available, and given their side-effect profile, current evidence does not support their use for breathlessness.

Nebulised inhaled furosemide

Nebulised inhaled furosemide shows potential (table 3) [85–96]. A possible mechanism is because of a depressant effect on C-fibres and vagal irritant receptors, such as pulmonary stretch receptors [94]. Reduction of dyspnoea does not seem to be related to a change in the carbon dioxide ventilatory drive [86], or secondary to a cardiovascular effect, although a diuresis was seen in one study [95].

In COPD patients, 40 mg of nebulised inhaled furosemide were effective in reducing dyspnoea intensity and improving lung volumes and levels of arterial oxygen saturation measured by pulse oximetry, with no apparent diuretic effect [88, 89]. A larger clinical trial

Table 3. Non-opioid drugs for breathlessness: nebulised inhaled furosemide

First author [ref.]	Type of study	Nebulised furosemide dose mg	Patients enrolled	Breathlessness measure	Statistically significant benefit
Nishino [85]	RCT crossover	40	12 healthy	VAS	Yes
Minowa [86]	RCT	40	10 healthy	VAS	Yes
Moosavi [87]	RCT crossover	40	10 healthy	Effective in relieving air hunger	Yes
Ong [88]	RCT crossover	40	19 COPD	VAS	Yes
Jensen [89]	RCT crossover	40	20 COPD	Borg	Yes
Sheikh Motahar Vahedi [90]	RCT	40	100 COPD during exacerbation	VAS	Yes
Stone [91]	RCT crossover	20	7 terminal lung cancer	VAS	No
Kohara [92]	Open-label cohort	20	15 terminal lung cancer	Cancer dyspnoea scale	Yes
Wilcock [93]	RCT	40	15 cancer	Borg	No

suggested a potential role in the management of exacerbation as an adjunct treatment for breathlessness [90].

Nebulised inhaled furosemide has also been tested to relieve dyspnoea in lung cancer patients, but a series of small studies have not found benefit [91–93, 96].

It is worth noting that all studies used nebulised normal saline as the placebo comparator. However, an RCT comparing nebulised saline administered using an efficient nebuliser or an inefficient one, showed that participants allocated to efficiently delivered saline improved breathlessness scores and sputum clearance. Therefore, normal saline should not be considered an inactive comparator [97].

Further evaluation is needed to identify the potential role of inhaled furosemide and those most likely to benefit.

Herbal-based treatments

A secondary subset analysis of 136 patients (>65 years old) from an open-label RCT enrolling 352 COPD patients showed that those taking Bu-Fei Jian-Pi granules, Bu-Fei Yi-Shen granules and Yi-Qi Zi-Shen granules, in addition to COPD inhaled therapies prescribed according to the Global Initiative for Chronic Obstructive Lung Disease guidelines, reported a reduction in breathlessness and COPD-related symptoms [98, 99]. Herbal/traditional products represent a US billion-dollar market; these are mostly sold as over-the-counter remedies [100, 101]. Further research based on placebo-controlled RCTs designed to test safety and efficacy is needed.

So far, no role has been detected for cannabis-related medications [102, 103].

Summary

A number of non-opioid options are being investigated, but they currently do not have a robust evidence base. Their current place is therefore as second- and third-line agents, and they should be monitored for benefit and any potential harms. However, as not everyone tolerates opioid medication, further research is needed to develop alternative options (see next section).

Opioid drugs

Chronic breathlessness, defined as breathlessness that persists despite the optimal treatment of underlying causes and results in negative consequences for the person concerned, requires a staged approach to care. This includes ensuring that any reversible causes are adequately treated and that non-pharmacological measures have been optimised before opioids are introduced [3].

Opioids have a role to play in safely and predictably reducing chronic breathlessness, with the strongest evidence in people with chronic obstructive disease [3, 60, 104, 105]. Clinical studies have used oral morphine, with the larger studies using extended-release preparations [84, 106].

The relationship between opioids and respiratory depression was made very early after the isolation of morphine from opium by Sertürner in an experiment that included self-administration of the drug [107]. Although opioids have been available and identified for millennia, the real observations of the effect on respiration were made in the middle of the 20th century and respiratory compromise was seen as an (almost) absolute contraindication to the use of opioids [108]. More recently, the respiratory effects have been confirmed to be the result of the agonist effect on μ-opioid receptors in knockout mice models [109].

The science of opioids in breathlessness

Using functional magnetic resonance imaging, the perceptions associated with breathlessness are processed in the insular cortex, dorsal anterior cingulate cortex, amygdala and medial thalamus, areas shared with processing the perception of pain [110]. These are areas of the brain richly innervated with opioid receptors [111].

Much of the early laboratory work looking at the impact of opioids on breathlessness was done to see whether or not opioids could improve exercise tolerance. As an end-point, this was important in laboratory-based work but did not relate to the symptomatic benefits that opioids may generate for people with chronic breathlessness. As such, much of the work in the 1980s and 1990s had less relevance to symptom control and much more to functional status. These same studies were often single-dose studies and therefore did not reflect opioids in steady state. As shown by contemporary pain studies, extrapolating from single-dose opioid studies does not necessarily equate with the symptomatic benefit that people may ultimately achieve.

Laboratory testing of the *in vivo* impact of opioids is more recent. A study established that endogenous opioids reduce breathlessness: when opioid receptors are blocked by an opioid antagonist, such as naloxone, which acts centrally and peripherally, the perceived work of breathlessness on a treadmill in people with moderate-to-severe COPD increases while the same workload can be achieved [112]. This was reproduced in a model with resistive load breathing in a similar population [113]. In healthy volunteers, the addition of exogenous opioids at a standardised dose also generated symptomatic benefit in this patient population [114].

A study of pathways and receptors known to modulate the effects of opioids was done on a large cross-sectional cohort of people on opioids for pain [115]. One single nucleotide polymorphism was identified that, when present, required much higher doses of morphine to achieve the same (reduction of) breathlessness. The same effect was not seen with oxycodone or fentanyl. This observation is awaiting confirmation in other prospective studies.

Clinical studies

The evidence base for the net beneficial effects of opioids on breathlessness has been built up over the last 35 years. This allows confidence in the process of prescribing opioids for people with chronic breathlessness.

The first meta-analysis bringing together the work of the 1980s and 1990s was published in 2002. The study was a meta-analysis of 116 participants in nine studies, which demonstrated a symptomatic benefit of opioids in reducing breathlessness [116], although the benefit was for systemic but not nebulised opioids.

A randomised, double-blind, crossover phase 2 study of 48 participants, the majority of whom had COPD (88%) and were on LTOT (71%), was published in 2003 [106]. This study was conducted with a 20-mg sustained-release morphine preparation administered once daily in a typical population of people with chronic, refractory breathlessness. Benefit was demonstrated in both morning and evening measures of breathlessness on a 100-mm VAS. This study demonstrated that regular oral administration of low-dose, extended-release morphine was effective and safe in a population with COPD. Most people tolerated this therapy and experienced a reduction in their symptomatic breathlessness. Constipation had to be treated actively from the time morphine was initiated and a small proportion of people experienced transient drowsiness as the medication was commenced.

A systematic review of people with COPD where breathlessness was the outcome, clearly demonstrated again that morphine in this setting is safe [105]. There were no reported cases of respiratory depression or obtundation. Importantly, those on systemic opioids derived benefit from them. The benefit was most marked in people in steady state, as would be expected. This is significant in light of widespread practice that uses small doses of immediate-release morphine at widely spaced dosing intervals for up to several weeks before considering a change to sustained-release preparations, for fear of adverse events. This meta-analysis again demonstrated that there is symptomatic benefit in this patient population and that symptomatic benefit can be achieved safely even in people with COPD. No benefit was seen for exercise capacity in this review, but this is an area of interest, and a phase 2 trial of opioids during pulmonary rehabilitation is ongoing (Effect of opioids on outcomes of pulmonary rehabilitation; trial number: ACTRN12615000121561). For the first time, it appears that benefit can be obtained from the use of nebulised opioids, but this requires further work [105].

The recent Cochrane review update by Barnes *et al.* [117] concluded that there was only low-level evidence to support the use of oral opioids to manage breathlessness. However, there are identifiable subgroups likely to benefit [105, 118]. The inclusion of all studies in the review conducted by Barnes *et al.* [117] is likely to have diluted the significance of benefit and the level of evidence was categorised as low because of an arbitrary sample size cut-off of 50 patients rather than an assessment of statistical power.

Dosing and dose titration

A phase 2 dose-ranging study was conducted when a lower-dose daily capsule of extended-release morphine became available and with a view to studying longer-term effects [84]. People were commenced on 10 mg daily for a week and if they had a response (>10% reduction over baseline breathlessness), they went to the extension phase at that dose. If they received no benefit at that dose, the dose was escalated to 20 mg for a week and that algorithm was repeated up to 30 mg as necessary. In all, 83 people were enrolled of whom two out of three derived symptomatic benefit. 70% of those people derived benefit at 10 mg per 24 h, 20% at 20 mg per 24 h and 8% at 30 mg per 24 h. There were a few people who had no toxicity but had still not experienced a symptomatic benefit at 30 mg. Patients were followed for up to 22 months after commencing extended-release morphine. There was no evidence of tachyphylaxis in this cohort and no admissions to hospital for obtundation or respiratory depression. Once again, most participants had COPD.

A secondary analysis of this dose-ranging study looked at people who successfully had reductions in breathlessness after a successful titration from either 10–20 mg or 20–30 mg [119]. Notably, when people derived benefit, they experienced a marked improvement in the first 24 h and that initial benefit continued to increase over the ensuing 6 days. As such, in people taking extended-release morphine, when a symptomatic benefit is achieved it will be marked, but the maximal benefit occurs several days later; hence, upward titration should not occur within that time window.

Only one study has addressed the issue of how opioids for breathlessness should be titrated for people who are already taking opioids for pain [120]. This randomised, double-blind study showed that people who had a 25% increase in opioid dose taken for pain derived benefit for breathlessness, but a dose increment of 50% delivered no further symptomatic benefit.

Safety

Safety has been measured in a number of ways. Some single-dose studies looked at changes in oxygenation and carbon dioxide retention and showed no untoward effects [121]. An updated review concluded that regular, low-dose systemic morphine does not affect oxygenation nor does it worsen carbon dioxide retention in a clinically meaningful way [122].

The largest longer-term studies have been conducted as observational consecutive cohort studies looking at outcomes after opioids are started. At doses ⩽30 mg oral morphine equivalents a day, the large consecutive COPD and LTOT cohort of EKSTRÖM *et al.* [60] showed no increase in hospital admissions or mortality.

Summary

Data from imaging and *in vivo* studies support the role of opioids in modulating breathlessness. These observations are supported by studies of exogenous opioids in healthy volunteers experiencing induced breathlessness. Clinical studies of efficacy and safety, even in people with advanced COPD, continue to build a strong evidence base of net benefit from opioids for the management of chronic breathlessness.

Conclusions

Systematic assessment of chronic breathlessness in the clinic should identify people with this difficult symptom and improve access to effective interventions. Some, like pulmonary rehabilitation, have been accepted by the clinical community and are integrated into respiratory care, at least in part and for people with COPD. Others are less well recognised but strong evidence supports their use, such as breathlessness clinics. Low-dose, oral steady-state morphine has a developing evidence base to support its benefit and safety. There is a need for further research into alternative drug options to help this distressing symptom.

References

1. Parshall MB, Schwartzstein RM, Adams L, *et al.* An official American Thoracic Society statement: update on the mechanisms, assessment, and management of dyspnea. *Am J Respir Crit Care Med* 2012; 185: 435–452.
2. Bausewein C, Booth S, Gysels M, *et al.* Non-pharmacological interventions for breathlessness in advanced stages of malignant and non-malignant diseases. *Cochrane Database Syst Rev* 2008; 2: CD005623.
3. Marciniuk DD, Goodridge D, Hernandez P, *et al.* Managing dyspnea in patients with advanced chronic obstructive pulmonary disease: a Canadian Thoracic Society clinical practice guideline. *Can Respir J* 2011; 18: 69–78.
4. Jolley CJ, Moxham J. A physiological model of patient-reported breathlessness during daily activities in COPD. *Eur Respir Rev* 2009; 18: 66–79.
5. Spruit MA, Singh SJ, Garvey C, *et al.* An official American Thoracic Society/European Respiratory Society statement: key concepts and advances in pulmonary rehabilitation. *Am J Respir Crit Care Med* 2013; 188: e13–e64.
6. McCarthy B, Casey D, Devane D, *et al.* Pulmonary rehabilitation for chronic obstructive pulmonary disease. *Cochrane Database Syst Rev* 2015; 2: CD003793.
7. Wadell K, Webb KA, Preston ME, *et al.* Impact of pulmonary rehabilitation on the major dimensions of dyspnea in COPD. *COPD* 2013; 10: 425–435.

8. Maddocks M, Taylor V, Klezlova R, *et al.* When will I get my breath back? Recovery time of exercise-induced breathlessness in patients with thoracic cancer. *Lung Cancer* 2012; 76: 128–129.
9. Gupta RB, Brooks D, Lacasse Y, *et al.* Effect of rollator use on health-related quality of life in individuals with COPD. *Chest* 2006; 130: 1089–1095.
10. Bentley R, Hussain A, Maddocks M, *et al.* Occupational therapy needs of patients with thoracic cancer at the time of diagnosis: findings of a dedicated rehabilitation service. *Suppor Care Cancer* 2013; 21: 1519–1524.
11. Probst VS, Troosters T, Coosemans I, *et al.* Mechanisms of improvement in exercise capacity using a rollator in patients with COPD. *Chest* 2004; 126: 1102–1107.
12. Wilcock A, Maddocks M, Lewis M, *et al.* Symptoms limiting activity in cancer patients with breathlessness on exertion: ask about muscle fatigue. *Thorax* 2008; 63: 91–92.
13. Pan L, Guo YZ, Yan JH, *et al.* Does upper extremity exercise improve dyspnea in patients with COPD? A meta-analysis. *Respir Med* 2012; 106: 1517–1525.
14. Bredin M, Corner J, Krishnasamy M, *et al.* Multicentre randomised controlled trial of nursing intervention for breathlessness in patients with lung cancer. *BMJ* 1999; 318: 901–904.
15. Farquhar MC, Prevost A, McCrone P, *et al.* Is a specialist breathlessness service more effective and cost-effective for patients with advanced cancer and their carers than standard care? Findings of a mixed-method randomised controlled trial. *BMC Med* 2014; 12: 194.
16. Higginson IJ, Bausewein C, Reilly C, *et al.* An integrated palliative and respiratory care service for patients with advanced disease and refractory breathlessness: a randomised controlled trial. *Lancet Respir Med* 2014; 2: 979–987.
17. Farquhar MC, Prevost AT, McCrone P, *et al.* The clinical and cost effectiveness of a Breathlessness Intervention Service for patients with advanced non-malignant disease and their informal carers: mixed findings of a mixed method randomised controlled trial. *Trials* 2016; 17: 185.
18. Johnson MJ, Kanaan M, Richardson G, *et al.* A randomised controlled trial of three or one breathing technique training sessions for breathlessness in people with malignant lung disease. *BMC Med* 2015; 13: 213.
19. Swan F, Booth S. The role of airflow for the relief of chronic refractory breathlessness. *Curr Opin Support Palliat Care* 2015; 9: 206–211.
20. Galbraith S, Fagan P, Perkins P, *et al.* Does the use of a handheld fan improve chronic dyspnea? A randomized, controlled, crossover trial. *J Pain Symptom Manage* 2010; 39: 831–838.
21. Johnson MJ, Booth S, Currow DC, *et al.* A mixed-methods, randomized, controlled feasibility trial to inform the design of a phase III trial to test the effect of the handheld fan on physical activity and carer anxiety in patients with refractory breathlessness. *J Pain Symptom Manage* 2016; 51: 807–815.
22. Booth S, Galbraith S, Ryan R, *et al.* The importance of the feasibility study: lessons from a study of the hand-held fan used to relieve dyspnea in people who are breathless at rest. *Palliat Med* 2015; 30: 504–509.
23. Booth S, Farquhar M, Gysels M, *et al.* The impact of a breathlessness intervention service (BIS) on the lives of patients with intractable dyspnea: a qualitative phase 1 study. *Palliat Support Care* 2006; 4: 287–293.
24. Bausewein C, Booth S, Gysels M, *et al.* Effectiveness of a hand-held fan for breathlessness: a randomised phase II trial. *BMC Palliat Care* 2010; 9: 22.
25. Bourjeily-Habr G, Rochester CL, Palermo F, *et al.* Randomised controlled trial of transcutaneous electrical muscle stimulation of the lower extremities in patients with chronic obstructive pulmonary disease. *Thorax* 2002; 57: 1045–1049.
26. Neder JA, Sword D, Ward SA, *et al.* Home based neuromuscular electrical stimulation as a new rehabilitative strategy for severely disabled patients with chronic obstructive pulmonary disease (COPD). *Thorax* 2002; 57: 333–337.
27. Currow DC, Abernethy AP, Allcroft P, *et al.* The need to research refractory breathlessness. *Eur Respir J* 2016; 47: 342–343.
28. Johnson MJ, Simpson MI, Currow DC, *et al.* Magnetoencephalography to investigate central perception of exercise-induced breathlessness in people with chronic lung disease: a feasibility pilot. *BMJ Open* 2015; 5: e007535.
29. Simon PM, Basner RC, Weinberger SE, *et al.* Oral mucosal stimulation modulates intensity of breathlessness induced in normal subjects. *Am Rev Respir Dis* 1991; 144: 419–422.
30. Uronis HE, Ekström MP, Currow DC, *et al.* Oxygen for relief of dyspnoea in people with chronic obstructive pulmonary disease who would not qualify for home oxygen: a systematic review and meta-analysis. *Thorax* 2015; 70: 492–494.
31. Abernethy AP, McDonald CF, Frith PA, *et al.* Effect of palliative oxygen versus room air in relief of breathlessness in patients with refractory dyspnoea: a double-blind, randomised controlled trial. *Lancet* 2010; 376: 784–793.
32. Moore RP, Berlowitz DJ, Denehy L, *et al.* A randomised trial of domiciliary, ambulatory oxygen in patients with COPD and dyspnoea but without resting hypoxaemia. *Thorax* 2011; 66: 32–37.
33. Uronis HE, Currow DC, McCrory DC, *et al.* Oxygen for relief of dyspnoea in mildly- or non-hypoxaemic patients with cancer: a systematic review and meta-analysis. *Br J Cancer* 2008; 98: 294–299.
34. Brochard L, Isabey D, Piquet J, *et al.* Reversal of acute exacerbations of chronic obstructive lung disease by inspiratory assistance with a face mask. *N Engl J Med* 1990; 323: 1523–1530.

35. Kallet RH, Diaz JV. The physiologic effects of noninvasive ventilation. *Respir Care* 2009; 54: 102–115.
36. Ram FS, Picot J, Lightowler J, *et al.* Non-invasive positive pressure ventilation for treatment of respiratory failure due to exacerbations of chronic obstructive pulmonary disease. *Cochrane Database Syst Rev* 2004; 1: CD004104.
37. Simonds AK, Elliott MW. Outcome of domiciliary nasal intermittent positive pressure ventilation in restrictive and obstructive disorders. *Thorax* 1995; 50: 604–609.
38. Leger P, Bedicam JM, Cornette A, *et al.* Nasal intermittent positive pressure ventilation. Long-term follow-up in patients with severe chronic respiratory insufficiency. *Chest* 1994; 105: 100–105.
39. Chailleux E, Fauroux B, Binet F, *et al.* Predictors of survival in patients receiving domiciliary oxygen therapy or mechanical ventilation. A 10-year analysis of ANTADIR Observatory. *Chest* 1996; 109: 741–749.
40. Annane D, Orlikowski D, Chevret S. Nocturnal mechanical ventilation for chronic hypoventilation in patients with neuromuscular and chest wall disorders. *Cochrane Database Syst Rev* 2014; 12: CD001941.
41. Radunovic A, Annane D, Rafiq MK, *et al.* Mechanical ventilation for amyotrophic lateral sclerosis/motor neuron disease. *Cochrane Database Syst Rev* 2013; 3: CD004427.
42. Kolodziej MA, Jensen L, Rowe B, *et al.* Systematic review of noninvasive positive pressure ventilation in severe stable COPD. *Eur Respir J* 2007; 30: 293–306.
43. Wijkstra PJ, Lacasse Y, Guyatt GH, *et al.* A meta-analysis of nocturnal noninvasive positive pressure ventilation in patients with stable COPD. *Chest* 2003; 124: 337–343.
44. Struik FM, Lacasse Y, Goldstein R, *et al.* Nocturnal non-invasive positive pressure ventilation for stable chronic obstructive pulmonary disease. *Cochrane Database Syst Rev* 2013; 6: CD002878.
45. Killian KJ, Bucens DD, Campbell EJ. Effect of breathing patterns on the perceived magnitude of added loads to breathing. *J Appl Physiol Respir Environ Exerc Physiol* 1982; 52: 578–584.
46. Plant PK, Owen JL, Elliott MW. Early use of non-invasive ventilation for acute exacerbations of chronic obstructive pulmonary disease on general respiratory wards: a multicentre randomised controlled trial. *Lancet* 2000; 355: 1931–1935.
47. Bott J, Carroll MP, Conway JH, *et al.* Randomised controlled trial of nasal ventilation in acute ventilatory failure due to chronic obstructive airways disease. *Lancet* 1993; 341: 1555–1557.
48. Keenan SP, Powers CE, McCormack DG. Noninvasive positive-pressure ventilation in patients with milder chronic obstructive pulmonary disease exacerbations: a randomized controlled trial. *Respir Care* 2005; 50: 610–616.
49. Renston JP, DiMarco AF, Supinski GS. Respiratory muscle rest using nasal BiPAP ventilation in patients with stable severe COPD. *Chest* 1994; 105: 1053–1060.
50. Casanova C, Celli BR, Tost L, *et al.* Long-term controlled trial of nocturnal nasal positive pressure ventilation in patients with severe COPD. *Chest* 2000; 118: 1582–1590.
51. Clini E, Sturani C, Rossi A, *et al.* The Italian multicentre study on noninvasive ventilation in chronic obstructive pulmonary disease patients. *Eur Respir J* 2002; 20: 529–538.
52. Garrod R, Mikelsons C, Paul EA, *et al.* Randomized controlled trial of domiciliary noninvasive positive pressure ventilation and physical training in severe chronic obstructive pulmonary disease. *Am J Respir Crit Care Med* 2000; 162: 1335–1341.
53. Mehta S, Hill NS. Noninvasive ventilation. *Am J Respir Crit Care Med* 2001; 163: 540–577.
54. Evans TW. International Consensus Conferences in Intensive Care Medicine: non-invasive positive pressure ventilation in acute respiratory failure. Organised jointly by the American Thoracic Society, the European Respiratory Society, the European Society of Intensive Care Medicine, and the Société de Réanimation de Langue Française, and approved by the ATS Board of Directors, December 2000. *Intensive Care Med* 2001; 27: 166–178.
55. Simon ST, Higginson IJ, Booth S, *et al.* Benzodiazepines for the relief of breathlessness in advanced malignant and non-malignant diseases in adults. *Cochrane Database Syst Rev* 2010; 1: CD007354.
56. Stege G, Heijdra YF, van den Elshout FJ, *et al.* Temazepam 10 mg does not affect breathing and gas exchange in patients with severe normocapnic COPD. *Respir Med* 2010; 104: 518–524.
57. Clemens KE, Klaschik E. Dyspnoea associated with anxiety—symptomatic therapy with opioids in combination with lorazepam and its effect on ventilation in palliative care patients. *Support Care Cancer* 2011; 19: 2027–2033.
58. Allcroft P, Margitanovic V, Greene A, *et al.* The role of benzodiazepines in breathlessness: a single site, open label pilot of sustained release morphine together with clonazepam. *J Palliat Med* 2013; 16: 741–744.
59. Gomutbutra P, O'Riordan DL, Pantilat SZ. Management of moderate-to-severe dyspnea in hospitalized patients receiving palliative care. *J Pain Symptom Manage* 2013; 45: 885–891.
60. Ekström MP, Bornefalk-Hermansson A, Abernethy AP, *et al.* Safety of benzodiazepines and opioids in very severe respiratory disease: national prospective study. *BMJ* 2014; 348: g445.
61. Argyropoulou P, Patakas D, Koukou A, *et al.* Buspirone effect on breathlessness and exercise performance in patients with chronic obstructive pulmonary disease. *Respiration* 1993; 60: 216–220.
62. Peoples AR, Bushunow PW, Garland SN, *et al.* Buspirone for management of dyspnea in cancer patients receiving chemotherapy: a randomized placebo-controlled URCC CCOP study. *Support Care Cancer* 2016; 24: 1339–1347.
63. Singh NP, Despars JA, Stansbury DW, *et al.* Effects of buspirone on anxiety levels and exercise tolerance in patients with chronic airflow obstruction and mild anxiety. *Chest* 1993; 103: 800–804.

64. Feldman JL, Mitchell GS, Nattie EE. Breathing: rhythmicity, plasticity, chemosensitivity. *Annu Rev Neurosci* 2003; 26: 239–266.
65. Miravitlles M, Molina J, Quintano JA, *et al.* Factors associated with depression and severe depression in patients with COPD. *Respir Med* 2014; 108: 1615–1625.
66. Borges-Santos E, Wada JT, da Silva CM, *et al.* Anxiety and depression are related to dyspnea and clinical control but not with thoracoabdominal mechanics in patients with COPD. *Respir Physiol Neurobiol* 2015; 210: 1–6.
67. Smoller JW, Pollack MH, Systrom D, *et al.* Sertraline effects on dyspnea in patients with obstructive airways disease. *Psychosomatics* 1998; 39: 24–29.
68. Gordon GH, Michiels TM, Mahutte CK, *et al.* Effect of desipramine on control of ventilation and depression scores in patients with severe chronic obstructive pulmonary disease. *Psychiatry Res* 1985; 15: 25–32.
69. Light RW, Merrill EJ, Despars J, *et al.* Doxepin treatment of depressed patients with chronic obstructive pulmonary disease. *Arch Intern Med* 1986; 146: 1377–1380.
70. Borson S, McDonald GJ, Gayle T, *et al.* Improvement in mood, physical symptoms, and function with nortriptyline for depression in patients with chronic obstructive pulmonary disease. *Psychosomatics* 1992; 33: 190–201.
71. Papp LA, Weiss JR, Greenberg HE, *et al.* Sertraline for chronic obstructive pulmonary disease and comorbid anxiety and mood disorders. *Am J Psychiatry* 1995; 152: 1531.
72. Lacasse Y, Beaudoin L, Rousseau L, *et al.* Randomized trial of paroxetine in end-stage COPD. *Monaldi Arch Chest Dis* 2004; 61: 140–147.
73. Eiser N, Harte R, Spiros K, *et al.* Effect of treating depression on quality-of-life and exercise tolerance in severe COPD. *COPD* 2005; 2: 233–241.
74. Usmani ZA, Carson KV, Cheng JN, *et al.* Pharmacological interventions for the treatment of anxiety disorders in chronic obstructive pulmonary disease. *Cochrane Database Syst Rev* 2011; 11: CD008483.
75. Momtaz OM, Rabei SM, Tawfike NR, *et al.* Effect of treatment of depression and anxiety on physiological state of severe COPD patients. *Egypt J Chest Dis Tuberc* 2015; 64: 29–34.
76. Alexopoulos GS, Kiosses DN, Sirey JA, *et al.* Untangling therapeutic ingredients of a personalized intervention for patients with depression and severe COPD. *Am J Geriatr Psychiatry* 2014; 22: 1316–1324.
77. Stark RD, Gambles SA, Lewis JA. Methods to assess breathlessness in healthy subjects: a critical evaluation and application to analyse the acute effects of diazepam and promethazine on breathlessness induced by exercise or by exposure to raised levels of carbon dioxide. *Clin Sci* 1981; 61: 429–439.
78. O'Neill PA, Morton PB, Stark RD. Chlorpromazine: a specific effect on breathlessness? *Br J Clin Pharmacol* 1985; 19: 793–797.
79. Fainsinger RL, Waller A, Bercovici M, *et al.* A multicentre international study of sedation for uncontrolled symptoms in terminally ill patients. *Palliat Med* 2000; 14: 257–265.
80. Church MK, Maurer M, Simons FE, *et al.* Risk of first-generation H_1-antihistamines: a GA^2LEN position paper. *Allergy* 2010; 65: 459–466.
81. Woodcock AA, Gross ER, Geddes DM. Drug treatment of breathlessness: contrasting effects of diazepam and promethazine in pink puffers. *Br Med J (Clin Res Ed)* 1981; 283: 343–346.
82. Rice KL, Kronenberg RS, Hedemark LL, *et al.* Effects of chronic administration of codeine and promethazine on breathlessness and exercise tolerance in patients with chronic airflow obstruction. *Br J Dis Chest* 1987; 81: 287–292.
83. Light RW, Stansbury DW, Webster JS. Effect of 30 mg of morphine alone or with promethazine or prochlorperazine on the exercise capacity of patients with COPD. *Chest* 1996; 109: 975–981.
84. Currow DC, McDonald C, Oaten S, *et al.* Once-daily opioids for chronic dyspnea: a dose increment and pharmacovigilance study. *J Pain Symptom Manage* 2011; 42: 388–399.
85. Nishino T, Tohru Ide, Sudo T, *et al.* Inhaled furosemide greatly alleviates the sensation of experimentally induced dyspnea. *Am J Respir Crit Care Med* 2000; 161: 1963–1967.
86. Minowa Y, Ide T, Nishino T. Effects of inhaled furosemide on CO_2 ventilatory responsiveness in humans. *Pulm Pharmacol Ther* 2002; 15: 363–368.
87. Moosavi SH, Binks AP, Lansinga RW, *et al.* Effect of inhaled furosemide on air hunger induced in healthy humans. *Respir Physiol Neurobiol* 2007; 156: 1–8.
88. Ong KC, Kor AC, Chong WF, *et al.* Effects of inhaled furosemide on exertional dyspnea in chronic obstructive pulmonary disease. *Am J Respir Crit Care Med* 2004; 169: 1028–1033.
89. Jensen D, Amjadi K, Harris-McAllister V, *et al.* Mechanisms of dyspnoea relief and improved exercise endurance after furosemide inhalation in COPD. *Thorax* 2008; 63: 606–613.
90. Sheikh Motahar Vahedi H, Mahshidfar B, Rabiee H, *et al.* The adjunctive effect of nebulized furosemide in COPD exacerbation: a randomized controlled clinical trial. *Respir Care* 2013; 58: 1873–1877.
91. Stone P, Rix E, Kurowska A, *et al.* Re: Nebulized furosemide for dyspnea in terminal cancer patients. *J Pain Symptom Manage* 2002; 24: 274–275.
92. Kohara H, Ueoka H, Aoe K, *et al.* Effect of nebulized furosemide in terminally ill cancer patients with dyspnea. *J Pain Symptom Manage* 2003; 26: 962–967.

93. Wilcock A, Walton A, Manderson C, *et al.* Randomised, placebo controlled trial of nebulised furosemide for breathlessness in patients with cancer. *Thorax* 2008; 63: 872–875.
94. Sudo T, Hayashi F, Nishino T. Responses of tracheobronchial receptors to inhaled furosemide in anesthetized rats. *Am J Respir Crit Care Med* 2000; 162: 971–975.
95. Newton PJ, Davidson PM, Krum H, *et al.* The acute haemodynamic effect of nebulised frusemide in stable, advanced heart failure. *Heart Lung Circ* 2012; 21: 260–266.
96. Shimoyama N, Shimoyama M. Nebulized furosemide as a novel treatment for dyspnea in terminal cancer patients. *J Pain Symptom Manage* 2002; 23: 73–76.
97. Khan SY, O'Driscoll BR. Is nebulized saline a placebo in COPD? *BMC Pulm Med* 2004; 4: 9.
98. Wang M, Li J, Li S, *et al.* Effects of comprehensive therapy based on traditional Chinese medicine patterns on older patients with chronic obstructive pulmonary disease: a subgroup analysis from a four-center, randomized, controlled study. *Front Med* 2014; 8: 368–375.
99. Li SY, Li JS, Wang MH, *et al.* Effects of comprehensive therapy based on traditional Chinese medicine patterns in stable chronic obstructive pulmonary disease: a four-center, open-label, randomized, controlled study. *BMC Complement Altern Med* 2012; 12: 197.
100. Euromonitor International. Herbal and traditional products. www.euromonitor.com/herbal-traditional-products Date last accessed: April 6, 2016.
101. Research and Markets. Herbal Supplements and Remedies – Global Strategic Business Report. www.researchandmarkets.com/reports/338400/herbal_supplements_and_remedies_global#pos-0 Date last updated: February 2015. Date last accessed: April 6, 2016.
102. Pickering EE, Semple SJ, Nazir MS, *et al.* Cannabinoid effects on ventilation and breathlessness: A pilot study of efficacy and safety. *Chron Respir Dis* 2011; 8: 109–118.
103. Whiting PF, Wolff RF, Deshpande S, *et al.* Cannabinoids for medical use: a systematic review and meta-analysis. *JAMA* 2015; 313: 2456–2473.
104. Mahler DA, Selecky PA, Harrod CG, *et al.* American College of Chest Physicians consensus statement on the management of dyspnea in patients with advanced lung or heart disease. *Chest* 2010; 137: 674–691.
105. Ekström M, Nilsson F, Abernethy AA, *et al.* Effects of opioids on breathlessness and exercise capacity in chronic obstructive pulmonary disease. A systematic review. *Ann Am Thorac Soc* 2015; 12: 1079–1092.
106. Abernethy AP, Currow DC, Frith P, *et al.* Randomised, double-blind, placebo-controlled crossover trial of sustained release morphine for the management of refractory dyspnoea. *BMJ* 2003; 327: 523–528.
107. Sertürner F. Über das Morphium, eine neue salzfähige Grundlage, und die Mekonsäure, als Hauptbestandtheile des Opiums [About morphine, a new salt-capable base and meconic acid as a principal component of opium]. *Annalen der Physik* 1817; 5: 56–75.
108. LeGrand SB, Khawam EA, Walsh D, *et al.* Opioids, respiratory function, and dyspnea. *Am J Hosp Palliat Care* 2003; 20: 57–61.
109. Dahan A, Sarton E, Teppema L, *et al.* Anesthetic potency and influence of morphine and sevoflurane on respiration in mu-opioid receptor knockout mice. *Anesthesiology* 2001; 94: 824–832.
110. von Leupoldt A, Sommer T, Kegat S, *et al.* Dyspnea and pain share emotion-related brain network. *Neuroimage* 2009; 48: 200–206.
111. Baumgärtner U, Buchholz HG, Bellosevich A, *et al.* High opiate receptor binding potential in the human lateral pain system. *Neuroimage* 2006; 30: 692–699.
112. Mahler DA, Murray JA, Waterman LA, *et al.* Endogenous opioids modify dyspnoea during treadmill exercise in patients with COPD. *Eur Respir J* 2009; 33: 771–777.
113. Gifford AH, Mahler DA, Waterman LA, *et al.* Neuromodulatory effect of endogenous opioids on the intensity and unpleasantness of breathlessness during resistive load breathing in COPD. *COPD* 2011; 8: 160–166.
114. Banzett RB, Adams L, O'Donnell CR, *et al.* Using laboratory models to test treatment: morphine reduces dyspnea and hypercapnic ventilatory response. *Am J Respir Crit Care Med* 2011; 184: 920–927.
115. Currow DC, Quinn S, Ekstrom M, *et al.* Can variability in the effect of opioids on refractory breathlessness be explained by genetic factors? *BMJ Open* 2015; 5: e006818.
116. Jennings AL, Davies AN, Higgins JP, *et al.* A systematic review of the use of opioids in the management of dyspnoea. *Thorax* 2002; 57: 939–944.
117. Barnes H, McDonald J, Smallwood N, *et al.* Opioids for the palliation of refractory breathlessness in adults with advanced disease and terminal illness. *Cochrane Database Syst Rev* 2016; 3: CD011008.
118. Johnson MJ, Bland JM, Oxberry SG, *et al.* Opioids for chronic refractory breathlessness: patient predictors of beneficial response. *Eur Respir J* 2013; 42: 758–766.
119. Currow DC, Quinn S, Greene A, *et al.* The longitudinal pattern of response when morphine is used to treat chronic refractory dyspnea. *J Palliat Med* 2013; 16: 881–886.
120. Allard P, Lamontagne C, Bernard P, *et al.* How effective are supplementary doses of opioids for dyspnea in terminally ill cancer patients? A randomized continuous sequential clinical trial. *J Pain Symptom Manage* 1999; 17: 256–265.

121. Clemens KE, Klaschik E. Symptomatic therapy of dyspnea with strong opioids and its effect on ventilation in palliative care patients. *J Pain Symptom Manage* 2007; 33: 473–481.
122. López-Saca JM, Centeno C. Opioids prescription for symptoms relief and the impact on respiratory function: updated evidence. *Curr Opin Support Palliat Care* 2014; 8: 383–390.

Disclosures: In relation to the subject of this chapter, M.J. Johnson has worked as a consultant to Mayne Pharma. D.C. Currow is an unpaid advisory board member for Helsinn Pharmaceuticals. He is also a paid consultant and received payment for intellectual property with Mayne Pharma, and is a consultant with Specialised Therapeutics Australia Pty Ltd. For work outside the subject of this chapter, V. McDonald has received personal fees as a member of advisory boards for AstraZeneca, GSK, Menarini and Novartis; and has received speaker fees from GSK, Menarini and Boehringer Ingelheim. R. Mahadeva has received honoraria for non-promotional advisory boards/educational lectures from Novartis, Boehringer Ingelheim, Chiesi, Pfizer, Teva, Pulmonx and Nutricia; and travel, accommodation and registration to international respiratory meetings from Boehringer Ingelheim, Chiesi and Pulmonx. He has been an unpaid specialist advisor on COPD and α_1-antitrypsin deficiency for the European Medicines Agency and the National Institute for Health and Care Excellence (scoping, horizon scanning, interventional pulmonology), and an unpaid Specialised Respiratory Clinical Reference Group member. He also performs contract research into COPD assessment and treatment, which is costed through standardised R&D costing (no personal income), for AstraZeneca, Cambridge Respiratory Innovations Limited and Talecris/Grifols; and has received investigator-led grants for α_1-antitrypsin deficiency from Grifols, the Wellcome Trust and the Alpha-1 Foundation (no personal income).

Chapter 11

Service planning and delivery for chronic adult breathlessness

Siân Williams[1] and Chiara De Poli[2]

The diagnosis and management of the symptom and underlying causes of chronic breathlessness challenge current health service organisation and delivery, as evidenced by late diagnosis or misdiagnosis, underuse of effective treatments and resource waste in times of health service austerity. A new approach that builds on the evidence and experience of managing complexity in healthcare is needed. This chapter summarises where we are now in terms of the scope and scale of the problem and offers some options to tackle it. It describes how to improve diagnosis and treatment in all settings by using a decision support tool derived from multidisciplinary case-based discussion and the literature on heart failure, COPD, asthma, obesity and anxiety interventions. It also describes how to set up specific cardiorespiratory services, and how to extend the learning from the best palliative care services for breathless patients. For the longer term, it offers the vision of a population-based approach, describing aims, objectives and criteria to evaluate the impact of a breathlessness system.

> It sounded an excellent plan, no doubt, and very neatly and simply arranged. The only difficulty was, she had not the smallest idea how to set about it.
>
> Lewis Carroll, *Alice in Wonderland.*

Why is a chapter on planning for breathlessness services necessary? After all, primary care physicians and respiratory specialists see and treat breathless patients every day. The simple answer is that the way current services are organised and delivered is unsatisfactory, and they do not provide value for the patient, the population or healthcare systems.

First, breathlessness is a problem with a high degree of complexity [1]. Chronic breathlessness has a gradual onset, leading to unpredictable presentation to health services, and may have multiple possible causes, which may be interrelated. The interactions between its causes create uncertainty in diagnosis, often requiring more than one consultation and multispecialist engagement. Research lags behind practice needs, formulaic approaches and disease-specific clinical guidelines have only a limited role, and healthcare professional expertise may not be enough.

[1]London Respiratory Network, NHS London Strategic Clinical Networks, London, UK. [2]London School of Economics and Political Science, London, UK.

Correspondence: Siân Williams, 30 Uplands Road, London, N8 9NL, UK. E-mail: sian.health@gmail.com

 Print ISBN: 978-1-84984-071-2. Online ISBN: 978-1-84984-072-9. Print ISSN: 2312-508X. Online ISSN: 2312-5098.

Secondly, breathlessness illustrates the substantial challenges to traditional health and care services of the increasing prevalence of people with multimorbidities. For example, only 18% of patients diagnosed with COPD have only COPD [2, 3], and by the time a patient with COPD and disabling daily breathlessness presents to a GP, they may have up to 13 other symptoms [4]. Health and care services that are not equipped to cope with this complexity have unintended consequences in terms of late diagnosis and misdiagnosis, under- and overtreatment, and waste. These compromise outcomes, some of which increase inequity [5] and all of which are costly and probably unaffordable in times of financial and health service austerity [6, 7].

Thirdly, there is a problem of scale. Breathless patients are frequent users of primary, secondary and emergency services, and this also has implications for care coordination.

This chapter argues that planning services for a breathless population presents real opportunities to create an innovative and sustainable response to 21st-century healthcare complexity. Aimed at clinicians, health service planners and policy makers, the chapter is organised into three parts. The first two sections summarise the complexity of breathlessness and why the current services fail to deal with this complexity. The next section then describes how ideal care for breathless patients would look. In the third part, three options for improving how breathlessness is assessed, managed and treated are discussed. The first option, which could be used in the short term, suggests the adoption of the IMPRESS (IMProving and Integrating RESpiratory Services in the NHS) decision support tool for the assessment of breathlessness. The tool has been designed to be used in a range of settings. In the medium term, specific breathlessness services could be developed, along the lines of those being set up in the English NHS (*e.g.* the Breathlessness Intervention Service in Cambridge, and cardiorespiratory assessment clinics). The ultimate option would be a population-based breathlessness system, where multiple providers, payers and health professionals work with patients to coordinate efforts and pool resources and knowledge in order to improve outcomes for a breathless population. The chapter concludes with five guiding principles for any stakeholders involved in designing, planning and implementing breathlessness services, together with some questions for reflection and review of local data for continuing professional development.

Chronic breathlessness is a complex and common problem

Chronic breathlessness is a common symptom, affecting up to 10% of adults [8, 9], and about 60% of older people experience some degree of breathlessness [10]. It is the feeling associated with impaired breathing, a subjective [11] and often frightening experience that may limit all aspects of life and can be associated with poor clinical outcomes [12, 13].

Patients use an array of terms to describe their breathing sensation, and the term breathlessness can represent a number of qualitatively distinct sensations [14–17]. These different sensations will depend on personally felt interactions between physiological, psychological, social and environmental factors [11]. Breathlessness can also be described by the individual in terms of time course, frequency and triggers [18], its intensity and the distress it evokes [19–21], its impact on function, and psychological and social well-being [22]. Qualitative studies on the experience of breathlessness show that the range of descriptors used by patients varies across the underlying conditions causing their breathlessness [16, 23–25].

There is no single test to objectively and conclusively diagnose its root cause or multiple causes. For the tests available, cut-off points can be controversial, and the several measures to assess it are not validated against each other. The New York Heart Association (NYHA) classification, developed by the cardiovascular community, is a functional classification that includes breathlessness, among other symptoms. The Medical Research Council (MRC) dyspnoea scale is also a functional classification, focusing exclusively on breathlessness, and is used by the respiratory community. The wording of this scale has altered over time, with consequences for clinical practice, as grade 3 in some pathways is the threshold for referral to pulmonary rehabilitation.

Breathlessness can be caused by a single underlying condition, or by the interaction of two or more underlying conditions (*e.g.* COPD, heart failure, anaemia, asthma and/or obesity). Two-thirds of the cases of breathlessness receive a cardiac or respiratory diagnosis [10, 26–28], and about 20–30% of cases receive more than one diagnosis [26, 28].

The diagnosis of breathlessness must take into account the individual's mental and psychological health, because their emotional reaction to their sense of breathlessness intensifies the perception of breathlessness [29]. It should also be contextualised with respect to their demographic characteristics and physical activity levels [30, 31]. It is a common symptom among older people and those in the last year of life because of the accumulation of long-term conditions [32]. It can be caused by obesity or tobacco dependence, which can partially explain why it is often underreported by patients who silently adapt to its limitations by doing less, assuming that it is part of the ageing process [33, 34], or attribute it to being overweight or generally unfit [35] or to smoking.

The subjective nature of the symptom, its potential multiple causes (physical, mental and behavioural), the lack of a single and objective test or measure to assess it, and the unpredictable reporting by patients can each explain why diagnosing breathlessness can be difficult [26, 28]. In some cases, the diagnosis or contribution of various components to the person's breathlessness remains uncertain, if not unexplained [36].

There is no consensus on the optimal pathway for the diagnosis of chronic breathlessness, or on how best to organise and deliver breathlessness services. Currently, experiences available in the English context represent local clinician-led improvements rather than whole-system changes [37].

Unsurprisingly in such a patchy context, breathlessness is often mis-, under- or overdiagnosed. Causes such as COPD, heart failure and anxiety are all underdiagnosed in primary care [38–40] and are often diagnosed late, sometimes after a first hospital admission, and therefore are suboptimally treated. Similarly, obesity is identified and referred inadequately [26, 28, 41]. These failures in diagnosis can result in poor-quality and therefore poor-value care, with increased costs, waste and harm to the person [42].

Where are the problems today?

Traditional health and care systems are not equipped for dealing with these complexities. Poor outcomes are almost inevitable and can be explained by a number of interrelated problems.

A first order of problems relates to how healthcare services are organised and delivered. Breathlessness triggers many primary care consultations [43–46], although the number of reported cases of breathlessness are substantially lower than expected from epidemiological studies. This mismatch between expected and reported data can be explained by a combination of poor or inconsistent coding practices by physicians and equivocal patient help-seeking behaviour. Acute episodes of breathlessness are a major cause of ambulance call-outs, hospital attendance and emergency admission [47–49], putting a great strain on hospital beds already under increasing pressure given the growing prevalence of long-term conditions and their exacerbations. However, routine analysis of admissions by International Classification of Diseases (ICD) 9 or 10 will miss this. Given the paucity of data, there has been little analysis of the impact of breathlessness on service use, despite its prevalence.

Similarly, little is known about the impact of chronic breathlessness on patient outcomes, which can be substantial. For example, in people living with COPD, their comorbid psychological difficulties are frequently associated with poorer outcomes (*e.g.* rates of exacerbation, hospitalisation and readmission, length of stay and treatment adherence, self-management and survival rates after emergency treatment) than people without psychological comorbidities [50–52].

The traditional organisation and delivery of services for patients reporting breathlessness does not facilitate a comprehensive assessment and a coordinated treatment of breathlessness and its underlying causes. Time-limited primary care consultations and distorted reimbursement systems can affect the assessment and diagnostic process. In primary care, there may be a tendency to attach a diagnosis to the symptom of breathlessness as soon as possible without allowing time to build a diagnosis. This has clear consequences on how breathlessness, the patient's reason for the encounter, is coded, but also affects the patient's adherence to a treatment plan [53, 54]. In addition, the approach to diagnosing, treating and managing breathlessness is not uniform across respiratory and cardiology specialist services. Moreover, the evidence suggests that patients who do not fall neatly into an organ-based specialty remit may become lost in the system or neglected [55–57]. Poor coordination of care between primary and secondary care, and between health and social care, can adversely affect a patient's outcome and increase waste [58, 59]. Lack of clinician confidence in behaviour change skills may also contribute to the problems of "hand-offs" to other services [41, 60].

When looking at management and treatment options for people with heart failure, COPD, asthma and, to some extent, obesity [61, 62], there is a substantial underuse of high-value interventions. It is likely that these interventions will be high-value interventions for breathlessness. They include: 1) flu vaccination and pneumococcal vaccination, which are cost-effective for COPD, heart failure and asthma and yet vaccination rates remain low [61, 63–67]; 2) smoking cessation [61, 68]: the prevalence of tobacco dependence in people with COPD, asthma, pulmonary fibrosis and heart failure is often higher than the average prevalence [69–74] and yet opportunities are not taken to help smokers quit in primary care or on admission [75–77]; 3) programmed rehabilitation programmes for people with COPD, heart failure or both, which have been shown to be cost-effective [78] and there are no safety reasons to exclude patients with heart failure except those with arrhythmias [79, 80], yet evidence suggests that there are insufficient pulmonary rehabilitation programmes for people with COPD, and that there is an even greater lack of cardiac rehabilitation programmes accessible to people with heart failure [81–84]; 4) physical activity [85], which reduces the risk of the underlying causes of breathlessness and yet lack of assessment of physical activity or active patient engagement remains a major challenge [31, 86]; 5) self-management and personal care planning [87, 88], which can be effective but are not widely used, and there is little evidence yet on the effectiveness in multimorbidity [89]; and

6) psychological and emotional support, for which there is a limited but growing evidence base of value in improving adherence to care plans, as well as reducing the impact that breathlessness has on the person's life, yet this is not routinely available as part of multidisciplinary teams to support the team and patients [90].

A second order of problems relates to the limited availability of evidence that can be meaningfully used in day-to-day clinical practice by health professionals faced with an ageing population and a growing prevalence of multimorbidity. Specifically, there seem to be three main interrelated issues: 1) the evidence that is generated by researchers; 2) what evidence-based guidelines are produced; and 3) how the evidence available informs clinical practice and service planning and delivery.

There are substantial blind spots in the literature with respect to both the epidemiology and the clinical management of breathlessness. Cost-effectiveness analyses are typically organised by diagnosis, and hence none is available for breathlessness. There is also a substantial deficit of research delivered by allied health professionals, such as physiotherapists, psychologists and dieticians, whose experience is underrepresented in the literature [41].

Evidence-based guidelines are usually organised around single diseases and conditions although people increasingly have more than one [91], are based on trials that exclude people with comorbidities [3], and ignore the fact that people present with symptoms that may have a number of root causes and that they often have both physical and mental health needs. By focusing on optimal treatments following diagnosis of a single disease, they may be of limited use for day-to-day clinical practice, especially in primary care. The fact that we observe wide variations in clinical practice confirms the struggle of practising evidence-based medicine [92].

Unsurprisingly, a by-product of disease-specific evidence-based guidelines has been the specialisation of medicine, with chronic disease management increasingly being provided within disease-specific clinics, to the detriment of generalist services in primary care or outpatient departments, which would be best placed to offer holistic, patient-centred and coordinated care [93].

The pitfalls of traditional evidence-based medicine in the current demographic context have been recognised, and an agenda for "real evidence-based medicine" [92] has already been put forward. In this framework, health professionals may use the best evidence available complemented by their intuition, experience, collective or tacit knowledge ("mindlines" [94]), which is probably more able to manage uncertainty and complexity. This framework also suggests that evidence about "know-what (works)" ought to be supplemented with "know-about" (*e.g.* comorbidity, psychological status, the local population), "know-why (*e.g.* the historical explanation of behaviours)", "know-how" (to translate and tailor the general evidence into patient-centred care personalised for the specific case) and "know-who" (to involve the correct people to implement it successfully) [95].

What are we aiming for?

As the previous section has described, traditional health and care systems are not equipped for dealing with the complexity of chronic breathlessness in adults. Care and services currently offered to patients with breathlessness are generating poor health outcomes and seem unaffordable, and therefore are providing low value.

An ideal service for adults with chronic breathlessness would aim to improve health outcomes and be cost-effective, financially viable and context specific. Such a service would encompass a triple aim: 1) to minimise the impact of the symptom and its underlying cause or causes on the person's life; 2) to use available resources in the optimal way, prioritising interventions with high value for the individual and for the population, reducing waste (*e.g.* avoiding repeat diagnostic tests or multiple appointments, and tackling avoidable hospitalisation and readmissions [96, 97]) and making every contact count [98]; and 3) to be sustainable over time and institutionalised within different settings with the necessary capacity provided by a trained and motivated workforce; the ultimate goal of a sustainable service is the continued achievement of desired population health outcomes [99], *e.g.* by reducing the incidence or severity of breathlessness and by reducing premature mortality associated with breathlessness. Thus, the overall aim would be to minimise the impact of adult chronic breathlessness within available resources and in a sustainable way.

The design and implementation of a breathlessness service needs to be highly context specific, depending on demography, local capacity (*e.g.* primary care, secondary care, palliative care) and leadership (*e.g.* a primary care physician with an overarching view or special interest, or a respiratory–cardiology team, or an integrated care physician), the role of the payer and available resources, and how the service sits in the broader care system.

In order to take account of these contextual factors, a gradual and incremental approach to designing, planning and implementing services or interventions for breathlessness is recommended.

In the short run, a decision support tool for the assessment of breathlessness, such as the one developed by IMPRESS, could be used by any health professional dealing with a patient presenting with breathlessness. A further or additional development in the medium term might be the development of a breathlessness assessment and treatment service for people with difficult-to-manage breathlessness, which could lead to the creation, in the long run, of a breathlessness system.

How can we get there in the short term? A decision support tool

In 2013, IMPRESS, a joint initiative of the British Thoracic Society and the Primary Care Respiratory Society UK, two leading professional societies for respiratory care in the UK, developed a decision support tool for the assessment of breathlessness (figure 1).

IMPRESS has an impressive record of achievement in working with general practice, community and hospital care, and across professions, culminating in a comprehensive assessment of the value of interventions for COPD [62, 101–103]. Building on these previous experiences and a strong base of trust among colleagues, IMPRESS invited experts with an interest in breathlessness drawn from different settings (general practice, hospital and community), specialties (respiratory, cardiology, obesity and mental health) and disciplines (medicine, nursing, physiotherapy, psychology, management, academia) across England to develop the decision support tool. A comprehensive review of the literature and other publicly available policy documents was complemented by expert case-based consensus when the evidence was not available or weak.

The tool recommends an assessment process to be followed with a chronically breathless adult in primary care, or at first contact elsewhere in the system (figure 1). It acknowledges

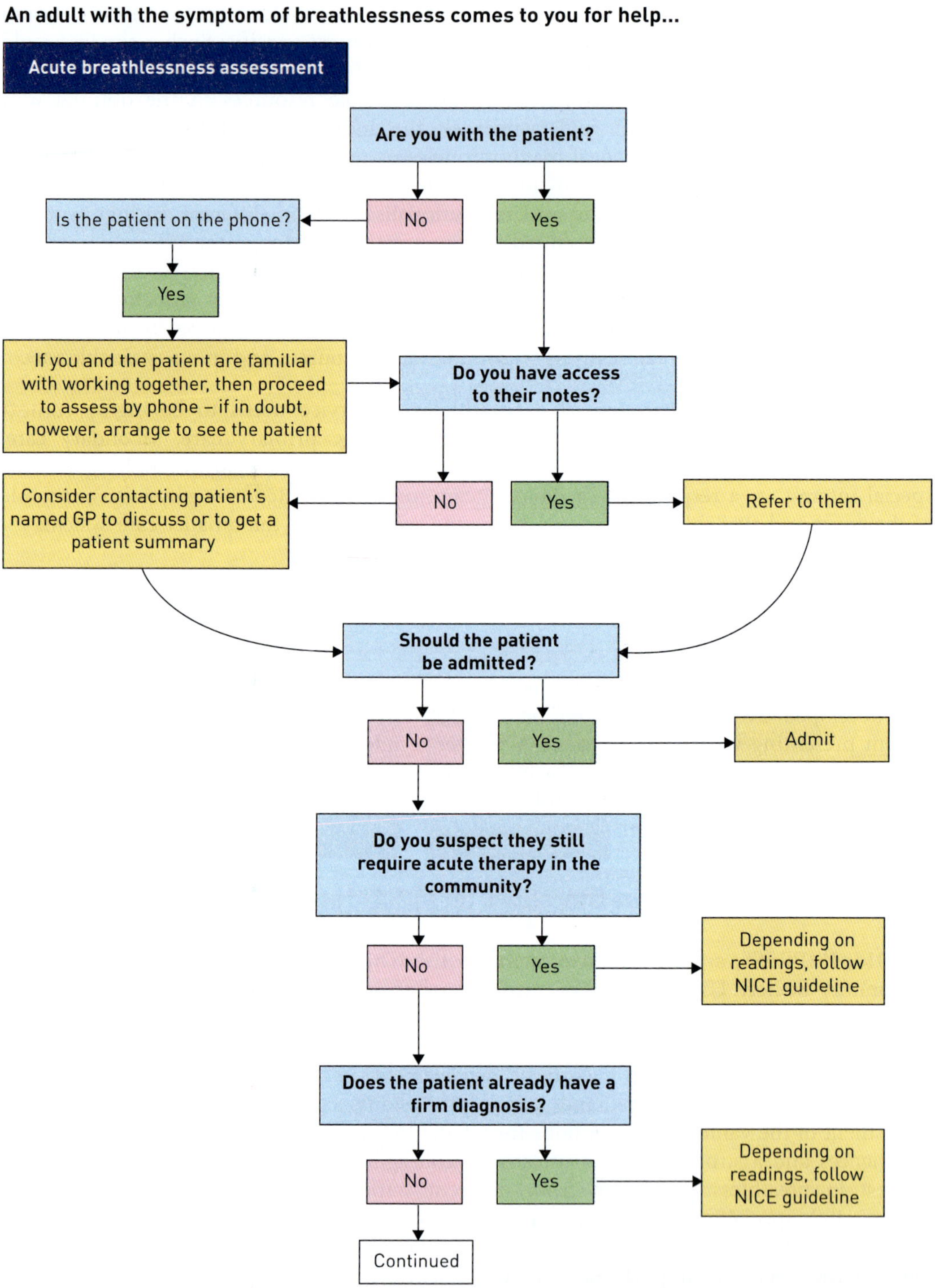

Figure 1. IMProving and Integrating RESpiratory Services in the NHS (IMPRESS) breathlessness algorithm. NICE: National Institute for Health and Care Excellence; MRC: Medical Research Council; NYHA: New York Heart Association. Reproduced and modified from [100] with permission.

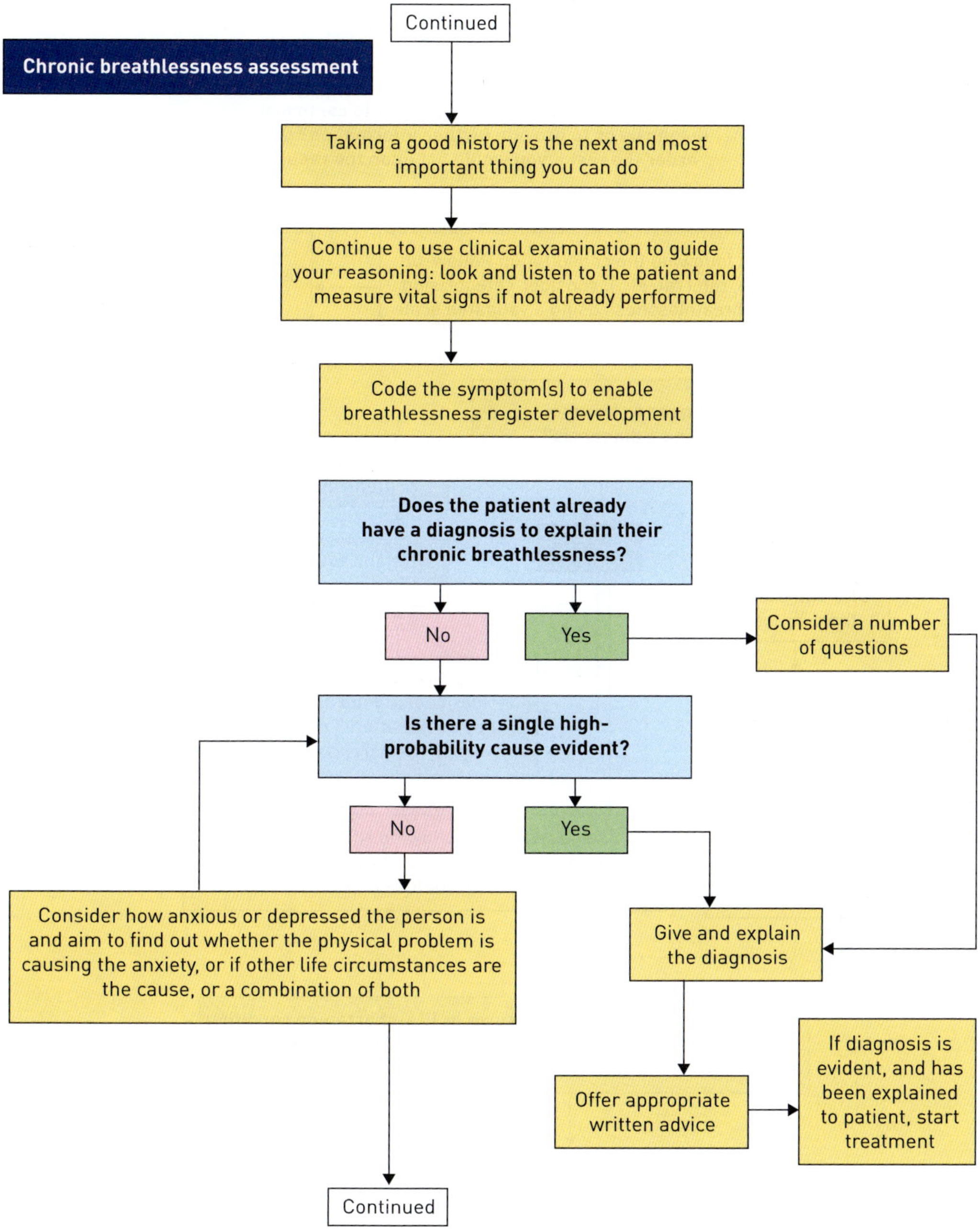

Figure 1. Continued.

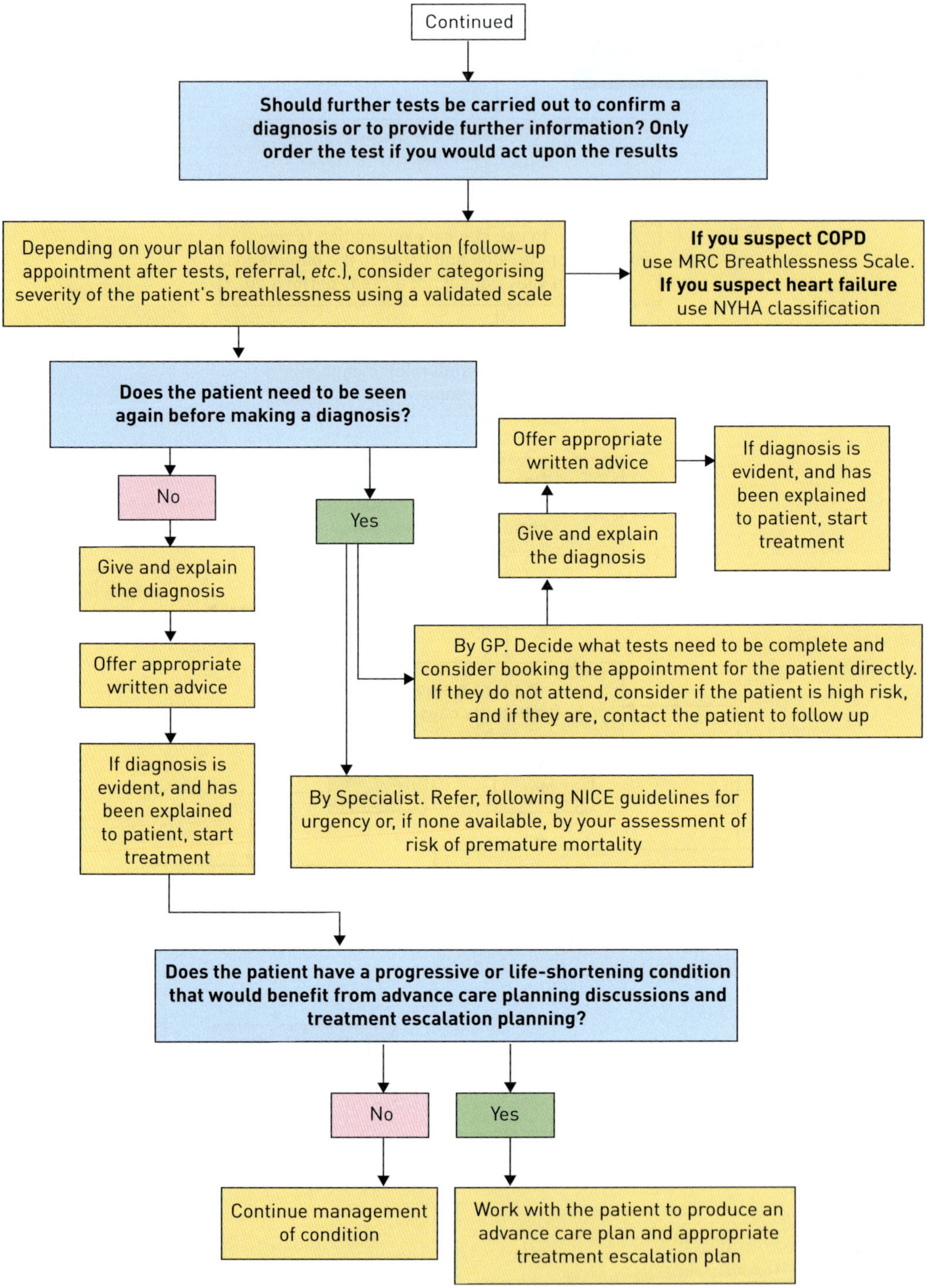

Figure 1. Continued.

the strengths of a family physician approach, given family physicians' training in holistic approaches, continuity and relationships of trust built over serial encounters [104]. It shows how the diagnostic process for breathlessness ought to be circular and iterative, rather than linear, in order to improve the certainty of diagnosis and treatment decisions. For experienced clinicians, it acts as a reminder of best practice, while it acts as a guide for less confident colleagues.

The guidance acknowledges that breathlessness is highly subjective and that, accordingly, the process of diagnosis ought to be individualised for each patient. The clinical decision support tool highlights the importance of good clinical judgement and acknowledges both the art and science of medical practice. The art relates to the tacit knowledge and soft skills of health professionals: their empathy in listening to patients' histories and in examining them, and, whenever a diagnosis is made, in explaining it clearly and compassionately. The science is application of the evidence by using validated questions and questionnaires and counselling, as well as near-patient testing and prescribing.

The decision support tool recommends 15 points that the family physician or other health professional with a chronically breathless adult patient should consider. This decision support tool could be embedded into an electronic record system in general practices:

1. Manage the acute component to the patient's condition, even where there is a pre-existing diagnosis of a chronic condition. Identify who needs admission, to be managed by the appropriate specialist team because this will improve outcomes [105, 106]. Pulse oximetry is a simple and discriminating test for respiratory failure (irrespective of the cause, which may be cardiac) and should be done first, because patients with new or worsening respiratory failure always need admission. A high respiratory rate, high pulse rate and worrying blood pressure, noting the presence of pulmonary oedema or extensive peripheral oedema, are also important and may suggest that admission is necessary. There are further reasons for admission, which may depend on knowing what is normal for that particular patient.

2. While assessment, diagnosis and treatment are normally sequential, in reality, if the patient's breathlessness is acute, diagnosis and treatment will merge (*e.g.* appropriate oxygen for hypoxia), and sometimes a trial of treatment is the most appropriate next diagnostic process.

3. For patients who do not need admission, take a full history, including smoking status, physical activity and psychological status; use the history to guide clinical examination in order to exclude diagnoses. There are three validated tools to assist:

3.1. Very Brief Advice: ask all chronically breathless patients about their current and past smoking history and calculate pack-years, where appropriate, to advise and act [107, 108]. The use of a carbon monoxide monitor to objectively check smoking status can also be a useful motivational tool to help a patient quit [74, 109].

3.2. The General Practice Physical Activity Questionnaire (GPPAQ) to ask about physical activity [85, 110].

3.3. Asking "What do you think causes your breathlessness?", which can sometimes directly bring out anxiety-inducing concerns. Where mental health problems may coexist, use validated screening tools, such as the Patient Health Questionnaire 4 (PHQ4) [111], the Generalized Anxiety Disorder 7 (GAD7) if anxiety seems likely [112] or the Patient Health Questionnaire 9 (PHQ9) if depression is likely [113].

Their value is in identifying the people who would benefit from a psychological assessment and intervention because their response to their breathlessness is creating a significant impact on their well-being and/or on health service use.

4. Ask about the impact of breathlessness on the person's life, using a mix of open and closed questions: "How does your breathing/breathlessness make you feel?", "Has your breathlessness been frightening to you or your family?", "What has your breathlessness stopped you doing that you want to do again, or would like to do for the first time?" Remember omissions (what is not said) can be equally important, and observe the length of sentences that are spoken and the ease of this [114].

5. Two-thirds of breathlessness is due to cardiac or pulmonary causes [115]. Start with diagnosing/excluding common causes using evidence-based tests for asthma, COPD, heart failure, obesity and anaemia. Recognise that anxiety may also be a cause or may coexist [26, 116]. Use low-cost physical measurements, such as waist circumference, if this is manageable. The strength of the association between BMI and heart failure events declines with a person's age, but increased waist size is a predictor of heart failure, even when measurements of BMI may fall within the normal range [117, 118].

6. Remember that, while common things do occur commonly, there may be an alternative explanation or additional explanation for the breathlessness. Patients with pulmonary or cardiac disease may not tolerate some small additional problem well, and so problems such as anaemia or infection may cause worsening breathlessness. It is better to be uncertain than to make the wrong diagnosis and have to correct it later.

7. If electronic records are being used, consider using a breathlessness symptom code (*e.g.* Read parent code 173 or International Classification of Primary Care RO2) until a diagnosis is confirmed, and maintain the symptom code as "active" and "significant" to encourage future review of breathlessness status and revisiting of the cause, and as a baseline measurement of performance.

8. During the primary care consultation, make sure to establish the patient's understanding, ideas and expectations. When giving the diagnosis, address Leventhal's five components [53]: 1) What is it? 2) How long will the problem and the treatment last? What treatment options are there? 3) What caused it? 4) What will happen now and in the future? 5) Can it be cured or controlled? The way in which the diagnosis becomes conceptualised by the patient will affect their self-management and outcomes.

9. Provide the right information tailored for the needs of the patient and/or their carers. IMPRESS has produced information for patients with breathlessness that has been well received by patients [119].

10. Test to confirm diagnosis. For example, if heart failure is a possible explanation, measure a natriuretic peptide and refer to specialist assessment, such as a rapid-access one-stop diagnostic clinic if the level is above the value that excludes heart failure. If there is a history of previous myocardial infarction, refer without measuring the level of natriuretic peptide [120].

11. Beware of assuming that previous mental health problems are the cause: death rates from physical causes, often caused by tobacco dependence, are much higher than average in people with mental health problems [121, 122].

12. Once a diagnosis is reached, provide high-value evidence-based treatments, following national guidelines where they exist. These will include both pharmacological and non-pharmacological treatments: flu and pneumoccocal vaccination, treatment for tobacco dependence, self-management support, medication, programmed rehabilitation and physical activity [123–126].

13. Recognise the risks of iatrogenic hospital admission [127] or harm, and aim for appropriate polypharmacy [128]. Recruit effective medicine reconciliation strategies [129].

14. Be familiar with the community resources that exist to help people learn to breathe better, *e.g.* swimming, yoga, Pilates, tai-chi and singing in a choir [130], as well as pulmonary and cardiac rehabilitation, walks and exercise classes. Personal care plans should include these options. Practice teams can be taught and engaged in population diagnosis and intervention design to improve population health [131].

15. If the patient has a progressive or life-shortening condition that would benefit from advance care planning discussions, work with the patient to produce an advance care plan and an appropriate treatment escalation plan. Specialist breathlessness clinics for people with advanced disease may also prolong survival [132].

New services to improve care for people at risk of poor outcomes

Where there is prolonged uncertainty, or the patient would benefit from multidisciplinary support, there may be a need for a new breathlessness service. This would consist of a pathway connecting the first point of contact, typically the GP, with additional multidisciplinary and integrated assessment and treatment services, with a feedback loop to the referrer to enable continuity of care. In terms of priority, decisions will be needed about where to target services to achieve the aim of minimising the impact of adult chronic breathlessness within available resources and in a sustainable way. This process may need to reallocate existing resources of clinical and patient time, tests and space (including beds) to improve the equity of access to care and of outcomes. Options that may be considered include: shared decision making; integration, including virtual clinics, administration and estates; substitution of location, skills, technology, model or organisation; segmentation of the breathlessness population; and simplification of processes [133].

The process of developing a breathlessness assessment and treatment service should build on the services or interventions currently available locally and requires data on the population at risk of poor health outcomes and of unscheduled care, including ambulance use. This is likely to include people with severe mental illness who have significant premature mortality from respiratory and heart disease [121], as well as people with complex psychological problems who would benefit from multidisciplinary support.

There may be opportunities to integrate existing teams and services. A review of inclusion criteria might enable a harmonisation of approaches between diseases, or the rethinking of referral systems and incentives. For example, more integration between heart failure and COPD services may provide more value than separate specialist services.

Increasing integration of services may also benefit from reinforcement of the natural "care coordinator" role delivered by the GP [134, 135] or by new professional roles, such as integrated care consultant posts and registrar schemes that benefit from an integrated training across settings [136, 137]. In some circumstances, there may be options for extending frontline staff capacity to deliver behavioural interventions, to "make every contact count" [138] and to ease the access to relevant tests and results.

In community settings, case management or care management can improve the delivery of clinical and social services to patients with complex needs, *e.g.* patients suffering from progressive, life-threatening chronic diseases that can be improved with proper treatment such as CHF and COPD, people with multiple morbidity or people at high risk with poor access to care such as homeless people, for whom supportive care can enhance independence and quality of life. For these patients, healthcare resources generally are available but may be inaccessible or poorly coordinated [58, 139–141]. Case or care managers or care navigators can help deliver care that is more seamless than routine care, for example by helping patients improve their self-management skills, identifying services that could meet their needs and facilitating access to these services, improving communication across providers, reviewing the needs of the patient over time or acting as a patient advocate. Electronic patient-held records, such as those enabled by Patients Know Best (www.patientsknowbest.com) or VitruCare (www.vitrucare.com), can also support better self-coordination of care.

In hospital settings, multidisciplinary care planning conferences held with patients and their family are also a promising approach that can be used during a hospital admission to diagnose and treat contributing causes and coordinate inputs from a range of professionals, including physical and mental health and social care. Care planning conferences aim to support the coordinated delivery of high-value interventions (*e.g.* treatment of tobacco dependence) started in hospital and continuing in the community, complemented by plans for risk reduction, for treatment escalation and for EOL care [142].

It is unlikely that there will be sufficient provision of programmed rehabilitation. To this aim, current provision should be reviewed, also taking into account seasonality, as adults with long-term breathlessness are a population whose health and use of services varies across the year [143, 144]. Shortages of programmed rehabilitation could be addressed by increasing the places available in cardiac rehabilitation programmes, and/or inviting people with heart failure to pulmonary rehabilitation clinics. Any increase in capacity needs to be accompanied by support for GP referrers to build their confidence in promoting programmed rehabilitation to their breathless patients.

People with a disproportionate response to their chronic breathlessness may benefit from breathing re-education [145] and psychological support, including relaxation and cognitive behavioural therapy [146–151]. The evidence for the effectiveness and cost-effectiveness of psychological interventions is promising [90, 152]. Therefore, a breathlessness service should also provide access to allied health professionals, including physiotherapists and psychologists. A breathlessness service could also signpost to additional activities, such as swimming, yoga, Pilates, tai-chi, choirs [130], walks and exercise classes, which may be offered by local-authority or third-sector organisations.

For those patients at the EOL whose breathlessness is caused by COPD or heart failure, the breathlessness service should provide advance care planning. This offers the healthcare professional, carer and patient an opportunity to discuss sensitively the choice of place to die, without a bias in favour of one location, as sick, frightened and breathless people may choose hospital [153, 154]. A breathlessness service for patients at the EOL should also provide an active management of each symptom [153].

Looking to the longer term: creating a breathlessness system

In the longer term, a healthcare system for the population at risk of, or with, breathlessness, with a defined budget, should be the planning goal. Such a system should enable the achievement of the triple aim of minimising the impact of adult chronic breathlessness within available resources and in a sustainable way. This requires collaboration between patients and carers, stakeholders and clinical leaders from primary care, respiratory, cardiology, mental health services, psychological services and obesity services to describe their needs, to share local experience of living and dealing with breathlessness, and to review the data and evidence.

The following nine steps are recommended when developing a breathlessness system [155]:

1. Define the scope of the breathlessness system.

2. Define the population to be served, which may include subpopulations or segments at different levels of complexity and activation requiring different services [156, 157]; it may include people with complex needs, such as homeless people, who are known to many service providers, including GPs, ambulance services, EDs and respiratory departments, and who would benefit from better care coordination to improve their breathlessness [139].

3. Reach agreement on the aim and objectives of the services provided by the system, also considering options for disinvestment.

4. For each objective, agree one or more criteria by which the performance of the service would be assessed.

5. For each of the criteria, identify levels of performance that can be used as quality standards, based on the data locally available.

6. Identify all the resources used in the system, thus creating a breathlessness budget, including clinical staff, equipment, diagnostic tests, hospital beds, prescribing budgets, estates and administration.

7. Identify who needs to be engaged in a clinical network that will provide collective leadership for the system and be accountable for its performance.

8. Produce a breathlessness system specification that can be used for contractual arrangements between providers and payers.

9. Agree an evaluation framework to assess the impact of the breathlessness system

With the London Respiratory Network, the collective leadership of respiratory care in the NHS in London, UK, we tested objectives and criteria for a breathlessness system aligned to the United Nations Sustainable Development Goals [158] and to the aims of the Global Monitoring Framework on Non-communicable Diseases set by the World Health Organization [159]: 1) by 2030, reduce by one-third premature mortality from non-communicable diseases through prevention and treatment and promote mental health and well-being; 2) achieve universal health coverage, including financial risk protection, access to quality essential healthcare services and access to safe, effective, quality and affordable essential medicines and vaccines for all; and 3) strengthen the implementation of the World Health Organization Framework Convention on Tobacco Control in all countries, as appropriate [158].

We offer these as a starting point for local discussion. Standards should be agreed using local baseline data. The main objectives and criteria for a breathlessness system are outlined in table 1.

Conclusions and guiding principles

Assessing and treating chronic breathlessness in resource-constrained health systems is a complex problem at both an individual and population level. Solutions ultimately require a whole-system approach engaging patients, carers, multiple specialties and multiple providers. A decision support tool for assessing and diagnosis breathlessness and the development of a breathlessness service are intermediate steps to a breathlessness system. Some implementation experiments have started, including plans to evaluate their impact. For example, in the London Boroughs of Lambeth and Southwark, an electronic record based on the IMPRESS decision support tool is being implemented and monitored. Several cardiorespiratory clinics that aim to integrate outpatient care for people with heart disease and respiratory disease are being piloted at Imperial and Hammersmith and Fulham hospitals in London. The UK Department of Health is planning a follow-up breathlessness public awareness campaign to encourage earlier diagnosis, building on the first 2014 pilot campaign.

Whatever the local context, resources available, pace of improvements and reasons for improving care for patients with breathlessness, the following five guiding principles [160] should be agreed by all stakeholders and used to guide local decisions: 1) use data to decide if breathlessness represents a problem that needs to be solved and if so, commit to sharing responsibility for solving it [161]; it may be useful to segment different population needs, using risk factors and severity, as well as psychological health and level of activation, and to address these separately; 2) use a framework of value to decide where to focus discussion about investment and disinvestment decisions; best-value services offer the right care for the right need, diagnose accurately and fully, and treat both the symptom and the underlying causes; 3) commit to a patient-centred approach and involve patients from the beginning in the diagnosis, care planning and delivery at an individual and population level; 4) unify approaches to training, recruitment, assessment and treatment across specialties and disciplines, building on local strengths and opportunities: there is no one size fits all model; and 5) commit to making public examples of service models, both negative and positive findings, including allied health professionals.

Continuing professional development: questions for reflection and review of local data

1. How is breathlessness coded in your primary care practice/office? Is there an agreed code? Is it used for every patient presenting with chronic disabling breathlessness? Do you ask about it prospectively for older people and those at risk?

2. If you have the data, how big a problem is breathlessness for your patients?

3. If you don't, how might you start to collect it?

4. Can you stratify/segment your breathless population and quantify how many patients might be in each level? This might be, for example, in terms of clinical segmentation (with and without respiratory failure; current, ex- and non-smokers; severity of mental illness; morbid obesity or not) or in terms of activation level: high patient activation measure (PAM) (levels 3 and 4) and low PAM (levels 1 and 2) [151, 152].

TABLE 1. Objectives and criteria for a breathlessness system

Proposed objectives	Suggested criteria
Improve accuracy and timeliness of the diagnosis to enable earlier treatment	At least one putative diagnosis of the cause of breathlessness made at first assessment in primary care/alternative setting Proportion of breathless people who have had a comprehensive assessment, including: smoking status measured with exhaled carbon monoxide monitor where necessary; peak flow; spirometry; chest radiograph; oximetry; height; weight; waist circumference; ECG; and BNP where appropriate Reduction in hospital admissions with undiagnosed COPD later confirmed by spirometry Reduction in hospital admissions with undiagnosed CHF Reduction in admissions or ED attendances for people with undiagnosed adult asthma Proportion of breathless people who have been assessed for morbidities in addition to main diagnosis
Achieve a 25% relative reduction in premature mortality for patients with COPD and heart failure aged 30–70 years by 2025, and a relative reduction in asthma deaths [159]	Mean age at death with COPD Mean age at death with heart failure Number of deaths at age <75 years in people with severe mental illness
Increase access to high-value interventions	Flu vaccination rate Prevalence of current tobacco use in people aged ≥15 years [159] Prevalence of overweight (BMI ≥25 $kg \cdot m^{-2}$) and obesity (BMI ≥30 $kg \cdot m^{-2}$) in people aged ≥18 years [159] Physical activity (*i.e.* 150 min of moderate-intensity activity per week or equivalent) in people aged ≥18 years [159] Proportion of breathless patients referred to rehabilitation services Completion rate of rehabilitation programme Availability of palliative care services for people with heart failure and COPD Availability of appropriate drug treatment for tobacco dependence, COPD and heart failure Proportion of people accessing weight reduction interventions for morbid obesity, including bariatric surgery as treatment for respiratory failure due to obesity
Improve the quality of life for people who have chronic disabling breathlessness	Increase in proportion of breathless people with written information that they can recall Increase in proportion of breathless people with an agreed care plan that is adjusted for their level of activation Increase in proportion of breathless people screened as having anxiety who are referred for psychological assessment Increase in proportion of breathless people without an underlying disease who are referred to a physiotherapist and/or psychologist for breathing technique training, relaxation and coping strategies

Continued

TABLE 1. Continued

Proposed objectives	Suggested criteria
Improve the experience of dying for people who have disabling and progressive breathlessness	Increase in proportion of patients with chronic breathlessness grade 5 (or MRC 4) and those with emergency hospital admission with breathlessness and/or respiratory failure, and their families and carers, who are offered advanced care planning conversations as part of routine care by staff skilled in these conversations, including discussions about the role of ICU, NIV, safe oxygen prescribing for respiratory failure, treatments for breathlessness and EOL preferences Increase in proportion of people with COPD, heart failure or ILD admitted as an emergency with breathlessness with a documented advanced care plan before admission
Reduce waste of resources	Reduction in proportion of hospital admissions for breathless people who do not have respiratory failure Reduction in total annual bed days for people with COPD and heart failure Reduction in number of people on triple therapy who have not been referred to pulmonary rehabilitation Reduction in resource use in the year prior to diagnosis Reduction in smoking-attributable bed days and admissions Reduction in proportion of current smokers with new lung cancer diagnosis Reduction in single outpatient appointments for patients with multiple conditions in a year Increase in patients admitted with breathlessness who have had a medicine reconciliation
Sustain the service through robust workforce development and support, stakeholder engagement, and slowing disease progression	Increase in proportion of staff trained in Very Brief Advice Increase in proportion of staff trained to use and act upon a psychological screening tool, such as PHQ4 Increase in proportion of staff trained to use a validated measure of physical activity and act upon the results Availability of multidisciplinary training Reduction in variation in the first six objectives Reduction in year-on-year vacancy levels in the service Reduction in smoking rates of the staff in the service Increase in flu vaccination rates of staff in the service
Code consultations for chronic breathlessness consistently and accurately to enable the collection of real data on the size of the problem, the outcomes and the cost	Consultations coded, *e.g.* by using the MRC breathlessness score or appropriate national coding systems, *e.g.* Read parent code 173 in UK general practice
Report annually on improvements	Annual report published
Promote and support interdisciplinary research on chronic breathlessness	Increase in published research on the management of breathlessness involving more than one discipline or specialty

BNP: brain natriuretic peptide; MRC: Medical Research Council; PHQ4: Patient Health Questionnaire 4.

5. Who would you bring together to discuss multispecialty provision of care?

6. Where is the best training and education for shared decision making in your system? How can your team share this?

7. Where is the best training and education for behaviour change, and specifically smoking cessation, in your system? How can your team share this?

8. What assessment tools do you use routinely to assess and treat your patients' psychological and mental health? Have you tried PHQ4? How is this recorded? Who has access to psychological support and how do they get it?

9. How do you assess and treat patients who have chronic disabling breathlessness who are tobacco dependent? Do you code this? What proportion of your breathless population/patient register are current smokers?

10. How do you assess the physical activity of patients with chronic disabling breathlessness and what options do they have to increase their activity?

11. What proportion of people discharged from hospital with heart failure/COPD should be offered rehabilitation?

12. Who has access to rehabilitation programmes? Are they available? Are they equally available to people with heart failure and CRD?

13. How are people without an underlying diagnosis who have problems breathing assessed and treated?

14. How can the evidence of best-value advance care planning be integrated into your practice for people with chronic disabling breathlessness and who would benefit at an earlier stage?

15. What equipment do you need to make it easy for you and your team to deliver a high-value breathlessness service?

16. Are you and your team confident to use this equipment?

17. What training needs do you and your team have to each deliver an agreed standardised breathlessness assessment?

References

1. Glouberman S, Zimmerman B. Complicated and complex systems: What would successful reform of Medicare look like? Discussion paper No. 8. Privy Council, Commission on the Future of Health Care in Canada, 2002.
2. Vanfleteren LEGW, Spruit MA, Groenen M, *et al.* Clusters of comorbidities based on validated objective measurements and systemic inflammation in patients with chronic obstructive pulmonary disease. *Am J Respir Crit Care Med* 2013; 187: 728–735.
3. Barnett K, Mercer SW, Norbury M, *et al.* Epidemiology of multimorbidity and implications for health care, research, and medical education: a cross-sectional study. *Lancet* 2012; 380: 37–43.
4. Bausewein C, Booth S, Gysels M, *et al.* Understanding breathlessness: cross-sectional comparison of symptom burden and palliative care needs in chronic obstructive pulmonary disease and cancer. *J Palliat Med* 2010; 13: 1109–1118.
5. Liaropoulos L, Goranitis I. Health care financing and the health system. *Int J Equity Health* 2015; 14: 80–84.
6. Thomson S, Figueras J, Evetovits T, *et al.* Economic Crisis, Health Systems and Health in Europe: Impact and Implications for Policy. Policy Summary. Copenhagen, World Health Organization Regional Office for Europe, 2014.

Available from: www.euro.who.int/__data/assets/pdf_file/0008/257579/Economic-crisis-health-systems-Europe-impact-implications-policy.pdf
7. Expert Panel on Effective Ways of Investing in Health. Access to Health Services in the European Union – Preliminary Opinion. Brussels, European Union, 2015. http://ec.europa.eu/health/expert_panel/opinions/docs/010_access_healthcare_en.pdf
8. Bowden J, To THM, Abernethy AP, *et al.* Predictors of chronic breathlessness: a large population study. *BMC Public Health* 2011; 11: 33.
9. Currow DC, Plummer JL, Crockett A, *et al.* A community population survey of prevalence and severity of dyspnea in adults. *J Pain Symptom Manage* 2009; 38: 533–545.
10. van Mourik Y, Rutten FH, Moons KGM, *et al.* Prevalence and underlying causes of dyspnoea in older people: a systematic review. *Age Ageing* 2014; 43: 319–326.
11. Parshall M, Schwartzstein R, Adams L, *et al.* An Official American Thoracic Society statement: update on the mechanisms, assessment, and management of dyspnea. *Am J Respir Crit Care Med* 2012; 185: 435–452.
12. Frostad A, Søyseth V, Andersen A, *et al.* Respiratory symptoms as predictors of all-cause mortality in an urban community: a 30-year follow-up. *J Intern Med* 2006; 259: 520–529.
13. Solano JP, Gomes B, Higginson IJ. A comparison of symptom prevalence in far advanced cancer, AIDS, heart disease, chronic obstructive pulmonary disease and renal disease. *J Pain Symptom Manage* 2006; 31: 58–69.
14. Sarkar S, Amelung PJ. Evaluation of the dyspneic patient in the office. *Prim Care* 2006; 33: 643–657.
15. Ambrosino N, Serradori M. Chronic respiratory disease determining the cause of dyspnoea: linguistic and biological descriptors. *Chron Respir Dis* 2006; 3: 117–122.
16. Elliott M, Adams L, Cockcroft A, *et al.* The language of breathlessness. Use of verbal descriptors by patients with cardiopulmonary disease. *Am Rev Respir Dis* 1991; 144: 826–832.
17. Mahler D, Harver A, Lentine T, *et al.* Descriptors of breathlessness in cardiorespiratory diseases. *Am J Respir Crit Care Med* 1996; 1154: 1357–1363.
18. Simon ST, Higginson IJ, Benalia H, *et al.* Episodic and continuous breathlessness: a new categorization of breathlessness. *J Pain Symptom Manage* 2012; 45: 1019–1029.
19. Banzett RB, Mossavi S. Dyspnea and pain: similarities and contrasts between two very unpleasant sensations. *APS Bulletin* 2001; 11: 1–8.
20. Wilson RC, Jones PW. Differentiation between the intensity of breathlessness and the distress it evokes in normal subjects during exercise. *Clin Sci* 1991; 80: 65–70.
21. Banzett RB, Pedersen SH, Schwartzstein RM, *et al.* The affective dimension of laboratory dyspnea: air hunger is more unpleasant than work/effort. *Am J Respir Crit Care Med* 2008; 177: 1384–1390.
22. Bausewein C, Farquhar M, Booth S, *et al.* Measurement of breathlessness in advanced disease: a systematic review. *Respir Med* 2007; 101: 399–410.
23. Edmonds PM, Rogers A, Addington-Hall JM, *et al.* Patient descriptions of breathlessness in heart failure. *Int J Cardiol* 2005; 98: 61–66.
24. Ekman I, Granger B, Swedberg K, *et al.* Measuring shortness of breath in heart failure (SOB-HF): development and validation of a new dyspnoea assessment tool. *Eur J Heart Fail* 2011; 13: 838–845.
25. Gysels MH, Higginson IJ. The lived experience of breathlessness and its implications for care: a qualitative comparison in cancer, COPD, heart failure and MND. *BMC Palliat Care* 2011; 10: 15.
26. Pratter MR, Abouzgheib W, Akers S, *et al.* An algorithmic approach to chronic dyspnea. *Respir Med* 2011; 105: 1014–1021.
27. Pedersen F, Mehlsen J, Raymond I, *et al.* Evaluation of dyspnoea in a sample of elderly subjects recruited from general practice. *Int J Clin Pract* 2007; 61: 1481–1491.
28. Nielsen LS, Svanegaard J, Wiggers P, *et al.* The yield of a diagnostic hospital dyspnoea clinic for the primary health care section. *J Intern Med* 2001; 250: 422–428.
29. Bailey PH. The dyspnea-anxiety-dyspnea cycle – COPD patients' stories of breathlessness: "It's scary when you can't breathe". *Qual Health Res* 2004; 14: 760–778.
30. Hopkinson NS, Polkey MI. Does physical inactivity cause chronic obstructive pulmonary disease? *Clin Sci* 2010; 118: 565–572.
31. Byberg L, Melhus H, Gedeborg R, *et al.* Total mortality after changes in leisure time physical activity in 50 year old men: 35 year follow-up of population based cohort. *BMJ* 2009; 338: b688.
32. Johnson MJ, Bland JM, Gahbauer EA, *et al.* Breathlessness in elderly adults during the last year of life sufficient to restrict activity: prevalence, pattern, and associated factors. *J Am Geriatr Soc* 2016; 64: 73–80.
33. Currow DC, Abernethy AP, Ko DN. The active identification and management of chronic refractory breathlessness is a human right. *Thorax* 2014; 69: 393–394.
34. Morgan R, Pendleton N, Clague JE, *et al.* Older people's perceptions about symptoms. *Br J Gen Pract* 1997; 47: 427–430.
35. Johnson MJ, Bowden JA, Abernethy AP, *et al.* To what causes do people attribute their chronic breathlessness? A population survey. *J Palliat Med* 2012; 15: 744–750.

36. DePaso WJ, Winterbauer RH, Lusk JA, *et al.* Chronic dyspnea unexplained by history, physical examination, chest roentgenogram, and spirometry. Analysis of a seven-year experience. *Chest* 1991; 100: 1293–1299.
37. Aspinall PJ. Scoping Research of Models of Care to Support Earlier Diagnosis of Diseases Related to Breathlessness as a Symptom. Leeds, NHS Improving Quality (NHS England), 2014. www.nhsiq.nhs.uk/media/2582027/breathlessness-scoping-research-full-report.pdf
38. Dept of Health, Medical Directorate, Respiratory Team. An Outcomes Strategy for Chronic Obstructive Pulmonary Disease (COPD) and Asthma in England. London, Dept of Health, 2011. www.gov.uk/government/uploads/system/uploads/attachment_data/file/216139/dh_128428.pdf
39. Tylee A, Walters P. Underrecognition of anxiety and mood disorders in primary care: why does the problem exist and what can be done? *J Clin Psychiatr* 2007; 68: Suppl. 2, 27–30.
40. Dept of Health Cardiovascular Team. Cardiovascular Disease Outcomes Strategy. Improving Outcomes for People With or At Risk of Cardiovascular Disease. London, Dept of Health, 2013. www.gov.uk/government/uploads/system/uploads/attachment_data/file/217118/9387-2900853-CVD-Outcomes_web1.pdf
41. Blane DN, Macdonald S, Morrison D, *et al.* Interventions targeted at primary care practitioners to improve the identification and referral of patients with co-morbid obesity: a realist review protocol. *Syst Rev* 2015; 4: 61.
42. Bastin AJ, Starling L, Ahmed R, *et al.* High prevalence of undiagnosed and severe chronic obstructive pulmonary disease at first hospital admission with acute exacerbation. *Chron Respir Dis* 2010; 7: 91–97.
43. Charles J, Ng A, Britt H. Presentations of shortness of breath in Australian general practice. *Aust Fam Physician* 2005; 34: 520–521.
44. Jolly DT. Dyspnea in primary care. *Can Fam Physician* 1978; 24: 983–988.
45. Frese T, Sobeck C, Herrmann K, *et al.* Dyspnea as the reason for encounter in general practice. *J Clin Med Res* 2011; 3: 239–246.
46. Currow DC, Clark K, Mitchell GK, *et al.* Prospectively collected characteristics of adult patients, their consultations and outcomes as they report breathlessness when presenting to general practice in Australia. *PLoS One* 2013; 8: e74814.
47. Prekker ME, Feemster LC, Hough CL, *et al.* The epidemiology and outcome of prehospital respiratory distress. *Acad Emerg Med* 2014; 21: 543–550.
48. Parshall MB. Adult emergency visits for chronic cardiorespiratory disease: does dyspnea matter? *Nurs Res* 48: 62–70.
49. Saracino A, Weiland TJ, Jolly B, *et al.* Verbal dyspnoea score predicts emergency department departure status in patients with shortness of breath. *Emerg Med Australas* 2010; 22: 21–29.
50. Dahlén I, Janson C. Anxiety and depression are related to the outcome of emergency treatment in patients with obstructive pulmonary disease. *Chest* 2002; 122: 1633–1637.
51. Turan O, Yemez B, Itil O. The effects of anxiety and depression symptoms on treatment adherence in COPD patients. *Prim Health Care Res Dev* 2014; 15: 244–251.
52. Yohannes AM, Willgoss TG, Baldwin RC, *et al.* Depression and anxiety in chronic heart failure and chronic obstructive pulmonary disease: prevalence, relevance, clinical implications and management principles. *Int J Geriatr Psychiatry* 2010; 25: 1209–1221.
53. Leventhal II, Meyer D, Nerenz D. The common sense representations of illness danger. *In*: Rachman S, ed. Contributions to Medical Psychology. New York, Pergamon, 1980.
54. Tate P. Ideas, concerns and expectations. *Medicine* 2005; 33: 26–27.
55. Patterson L. Wrong Bed, Wrong Ward. London, The King's Fund, 2012. www.kingsfund.org.uk/sites/files/kf/linda-patterson-wrong-bed-wrong-ward-poor-transitional-care-patient-outcomes-kingsfund-dec12.pdf
56. Future Hospital Commission. Future Hospital: Caring for Medical Patients. A Report from the Future Hospital Commission to the Royal College of Physicians. London, Royal College of Physicians, 2013. Available from: www.rcplondon.ac.uk/projects/outputs/future-hospital-commission
57. Evans T. Future Hospital Commission: the time for action. *Br J Gen Pract* 2013; 63: 571–572.
58. Øvretveit J. Does Clinical Coordination Improve Quality and Save Money? London, The Health Foundation, 2011. Available from: www.health.org.uk/publication/does-clinical-coordination-improve-quality-and-save-money
59. Schoen C, Osborn R, Squires D, *et al.* New 2011 survey of patients with complex care needs in eleven countries finds that care is often poorly coordinated. *Health Aff* 2011; 30: 2437–2448.
60. Howie JG, Porter AM, Forbes JF. Quality and the use of time in general practice: widening the discussion. *BMJ* 1989; 298: 1008–1010.
61. Dept of Health. Achieving World Class Productivity in the NHS 2009/10–2013/14: Detailing the Size of the Opportunity. London, Dept of Health, 2009. http://webarchive.nationalarchives.gov.uk/20130107105354/http://www.dh.gov.uk/prod_consum_dh/groups/dh_digitalassets/documents/digitalasset/dh_116521.pdf
62. IMProving and Integrating RESpiratory Services in the NHS (IMPRESS). IMPRESS Guide to the Relative Value of COPD Interventions. London, British Thoracic Society and Primary Care Respiratory Society UK, 2012. www.impressresp.com/index.php?option=com_docman&task=doc_view&gid=51&Itemid=82

63. Santaularia J, Hou W, Perveen G, *et al.* Prevalence of influenza vaccination and its association with health conditions and risk factors among Kansas adults in 2013: a cross-sectional study. *BMC Public Health* 2016; 16: 185.
64. Centers for Disease Control and Prevention. People at High Risk of Developing Flu-Related Complications. www.cdc.gov/flu/about/disease/high_risk.htm Date last updated: May 25, 2016. Date last accessed: July, 2016.
65. Nyweide DJ, Anthony DL, Bynum JPW, *et al.* Continuity of care and the risk of preventable hospitalization in older adults. *JAMA Intern Med* 2013; 173: 1879–1885.
66. Hak E, van Essen GA, Buskens E, *et al.* Is immunising all patients with chronic lung disease in the community against influenza cost effective? Evidence from a general practice based clinical prospective cohort study in Utrecht, The Netherlands. *J Epidemiol Community Health* 1998; 52: 120–125.
67. Mowls DS, Cheruvu VK, Zullo MD. Influenza vaccination in adults with chronic obstructive pulmonary disease: the impact of a diagnostic breathing test on vaccination rates. *PLoS One* 2013; 8: e67600.
68. Hoogendoorn M, Feenstra TL, Hoogenveen RT, *et al.* Long-term effectiveness and cost-effectiveness of smoking cessation interventions in patients with COPD. *Thorax* 2010; 65: 711–718.
69. Restrick L, Stern M, Baxter N. Tiotropium *versus* salmeterol in COPD. *N Engl J Med* 2011; 364: 2552–2554.
70. Dempsey OJ, Miller D. Idiopathic pulmonary fibrosis. *BMJ* 2013; 347: f6579.
71. To T, Stanojevic S, Moores G, *et al.* Global asthma prevalence in adults: findings from the cross-sectional World Health Survey. *BMC Public Health* 2012; 12: 204.
72. Suskin N, Sheth T, Negassa A, *et al.* Relationship of current and past smoking to mortality and morbidity in patients with left ventricular dysfunction. *J Am Coll Cardiol* 2001; 37: 1677–1682.
73. Mullen K-A, Coyle D, Manuel D, *et al.* Economic evaluation of a hospital-initiated intervention for smokers with chronic disease, in Ontario, Canada. *Tob Control* 2015; 24: 489–496.
74. Shahab L, West R, McNeill A. A randomized, controlled trial of adding expired carbon monoxide feedback to brief stop smoking advice: evaluation of cognitive and behavioral effects. *Health Psychol* 2011; 30: 49–57.
75. van Schayck OCP, Pinnock H, Ostrem A, *et al.* IPCRG Consensus statement: tackling the smoking epidemic – practical guidance for primary care. *Prim Care Respir J* 2008; 17: 185–193.
76. Siddiqi K, Dodgar OF, Siddiqi N. Smoking cessation in long-term conditions: is there "an opportunity in every difficulty"? *Int J Popul Res* 2013; 2013: 251048.
77. Papadakis S, Pipe A, Kelly S, *et al.* Strategies to improve the delivery of tobacco use treatment in primary care practice (Protocol). *Cochrane Database Syst Rev* 2015; 3: CD011556.
78. Griffiths TL. Cost effectiveness of an outpatient multidisciplinary pulmonary rehabilitation programme. *Thorax* 2001; 56: 779–784.
79. Evans RA, Singh SJ, Collier R, *et al.* Generic, symptom based, exercise rehabilitation; integrating patients with COPD and heart failure. *Respir Med* 2010; 104: 1473–1481.
80. Evans RA. Developing the model of pulmonary rehabilitation for chronic heart failure. *Chron Respir Dis* 2011; 8: 259–269.
81. NHS Medical Directorate. COPD Commissioning Toolkit. A Resource for Commissioners. London, Dept of Health, 2012. Available from: www.gov.uk/government/publications/commissioning-toolkit-for-respiratory-services
82. Dalal HM, Wingham J, Palmer J, *et al.* Why do so few patients with heart failure participate in cardiac rehabilitation? A cross-sectional survey from England, Wales and Northern Ireland. *BMJ Open* 2012; 2: e000787.
83. Jaarsma T, Lesman I, van Veldhuisen DJ. Psychology and cardiology: do not forget the heart failure patient. *Eur Heart J* 2008; 29: 1208.
84. British Heart Foundation. National Audit of Cardiac Rehabilitation. 2010. Available from: www.cardiacrehabilitation.org.uk/docs/2010.pdf Date last accessed: March 22, 2016.
85. National Institute for Health and Care Excellence (NICE). Physical Activity: Brief Advice for Adults in Primary Care. NICE Guidelines PH44. London, NICE, 2013. Available from: www.nice.org.uk/guidance/ph44
86. British Heart Foundation National Centre (BHFNC) for Physical Activity and Health. Economic Costs of Physical Inactivity. Loughborough, BHFNC for Physical Activity and Health, Loughborough University, 2013. www.bhfactive.org.uk/userfiles/Documents/eonomiccosts.pdf
87. Tsai AC, Morton SC, Mangione CM, *et al.* A meta-analysis of interventions to improve care for chronic illnesses. *Am J Manag Care* 2005; 11: 478–488.
88. Taylor SJ, Pinnock H, Epiphaniou E, *et al.* A rapid synthesis of the evidence on interventions supporting self-management for people with long-term conditions: PRISMS – Practical systematic Review of Self-Management Support for long-term conditions. *Heal Serv Deliv Res* 2014; 2.53.
89. Royal College of General Practitioners, NHS Improvement Lung. Managing Multi-morbidity in Practice… What Lessons can be Learnt from the Care of People with COPD and Co-morbidities? Leicester, NHS Improvement, 2013. www.rcgp.org.uk/clinical-and-research/clinical-resources/~/media/Files/CIRC/RCGP-COPD-Multi-Morbidities-April-2013.ashx
90. Mental Health Network – NHS Confederation. Investing in Emotional and Psychological Wellbeing for Patients with Long-term Conditions. London, The NHS Confederation, 2012.

91. Fabbri LM, Boyd C, Boschetto P, *et al.* How to integrate multiple comorbidities in guideline development: article 10 in Integrating and coordinating efforts in COPD guideline development. An official ATS/ERS workshop report. *Proc Am Thorac Soc* 2012; 9: 274–281.
92. Greenhalgh T, Howick J, Maskrey N, *et al.* Evidence based medicine: a movement in crisis? *BMJ* 2014; 348: g3725.
93. Salisbury C. Multimorbidity: redesigning health care for people who use it. *Lancet* 2012; 380: 7–9.
94. Wieringa S, Greenhalgh T. 10 years of mindlines: a systematic review and commentary. *Implement Sci* 2015; 10: 45.
95. Davies H, Nutley S, Walter I. Why 'knowledge transfer' is misconceived for applied social research. *J Health Serv Res Policy* 2008; 13: 188–190.
96. Porter M. What is value in health care? *N Engl J Med* 2010; 363: 2477–2481.
97. Gray M. Evidence-Based Healthcare and Public Health: How to Make Decisions about Health Services and Public Health. 3rd Edn. Elsevier Limited, 2009.
98. National Institute for Health and Care Excellence (NICE). Behaviour Change: Individual Approaches. NICE Guidelines PH49. London, NICE, 2014. Available from: www.nice.org.uk/guidance/ph49
99. Chambers D, Glasgow R, Stange K. The dynamic sustainability framework: addressing the paradox of sustainment amid ongoing change. *Implement Sci* 2013; 8: 117.
100. British Thoracic Society, Primary Care Respiratory Society UK. IMPRESS Breathlessness Algorithm. www.respiratoryfutures.org.uk/knowledge-portal/impress-documents/impress-breathlessness-algorithm/ Date last updated: October 2014. Date last accessed: April 2016.
101. IMProving and Integrating RESpiratory Services in the NHS (IMPRESS). More for Less. London, IMPRESS, 2010. www.respiratoryfutures.org.uk/knowledge-portal/impress-documents/impress-more-for-less/
102. IMProving and Integrating RESpiratory Services in the NHS (IMPRESS). IMPRESS Guide to Pulmonary Rehabilitation. London, British Thoracic Society and Primary Care Respiratory Society UK, 2011. www.respiratoryfutures.org.uk/media/1107/impress-pulmrehab-191211-lres.pdf
103. Gray M, El Turabi A. Optimising the value of interventions for populations. *BMJ* 2012; 345: e6192.
104. Starfield B, Shi L, Macinko J. Contribution of primary care to health systems and health. *Milbank Q* 2005; 83: 457–502.
105. National Institute for Cardiovascular Outcomes Research (NICOR). National Heart Failure Audit: April 2012–March 2013. London, NICOR, 2013. www.ucl.ac.uk/nicor/audits/heartfailure/documents/annualreports/hfannual12-13.pdf
106. Royal College of Physicians of London, British Thoracic Society, British Lung Foundation. Report of The National Chronic Obstructive Pulmonary Disease Audit 2008: Clinical Audit of COPD Exacerbations Admitted to Acute NHS Units Across the UK. London, Royal College of Physicians, 2008. Available from: www.rcplondon.ac.uk/projects/outputs/national-copd-audit-2008
107. West R. Smoking cessation guidelines for health professionals: an update. *Thorax* 2000; 55: 987–999.
108. Stead LF, Buitrago D, Preciado N, *et al.* Physician advice for smoking cessation. *Cochrane Database Syst Rev* 2013; 5: CD000165.
109. London Clinical Senate. Helping Smokers Quit: Adding Value to Every Clinical Contact by Treating Tobacco Dependence. www.londonsenate.nhs.uk/helping-smokers-quit/ Date last updated May 2016. Date last accessed July 2016.
110. Dept of Health. General Practice Physical Activity Questionnaire (GPPAQ). London, Dept of Health, 2013. Available from: www.gov.uk/government/publications/general-practice-physical-activity-questionnaire-gppaq
111. Löwe B, Wahl I, Rose M, *et al.* A 4-item measure of depression and anxiety: validation and standardization of the Patient Health Questionnaire-4 (PHQ-4) in the general population. *J Affect Disord* 2010; 122: 86–95.
112. Spitzer RL, Kroenke K, Williams JB, *et al.* A brief measure for assessing generalized anxiety disorder: the GAD-7. *Arch Intern Med* 2006; 166: 1092–1097.
113. Kroenke K, Spitzer RL, Williams JB. The PHQ-9: validity of a brief depression severity measure. *J Gen Intern Med* 2001; 16: 606–613.
114. Neighbour RH. The Inner Consultation: How to Develop an Effective and Intuitive Consulting Style. Lancaster, Kluwer Academic Press, 1987.
115. Gillespie DJ, Staats BA. Unexplained dyspnea. *Mayo Clin Proc* 1994; 69: 657–663.
116. Karnani NG, Reisfield GM, Wilson GR. Evaluation of chronic dyspnea. *Am Fam Physician* 2005; 71: 1529–1537.
117. Levitan EB, Yang AZ, Wolk A, *et al.* Adiposity and incidence of heart failure hospitalization and mortality: a population-based prospective study. *Circ Heart Fail* 2009; 2: 202–208.
118. World Health Organization. Waist Circumference and Waist–Hip Ratio. Report of a WHO Expert Consultation. Geneva, 8–11 December 2008. Geneva, World Health Organization, 2011. Available from: www.who.int/nutrition/publications/obesity/WHO_report_waistcircumference_and_waisthip_ratio/en/
119. IMProving and Integrating RESpiratory Services in the NHS (IMPRESS). IMPRESS breathlessness resources. www.networks.nhs.uk/nhs-networks/impress-improving-and-integrating-respiratory/news/impress-breathlessness-resources Date last updated: October 2014. Date last accessed: July 2016.

120. National Institute for Health and Care Excellence (NICE). Chronic Heart Failure. Shared Learning: Use of the Scenarios Simulation in the Introduction of Serum Natriuretic Peptide Testing. Implementing NICE Guidance. London, NICE, 2011. www.nice.org.uk/guidance/cg108/resources/use-of-scenario-simulation-in-the-introduction-of-serum-natriuretic-peptide-136055341
121. McManus S, Meltzer H, Brugha T, *et al.* Adult Psychiatric Morbidity in England, 2007. Results of a Household Survey. Leeds, The NHS Information Centre for Health and Social Care, 2009. www.hscic.gov.uk/catalogue/PUB02931/adul-psyc-morb-res-hou-sur-eng-2007-rep.pdf
122. Hoang U, Stewart R, Goldacre MJ. Mortality after hospital discharge for people with schizophrenia or bipolar disorder: retrospective study of linked English hospital episode statistics, 1999–2006. *BMJ* 2011; 343: d5422.
123. National Institute for Health and Care Excellence (NICE). Chronic Heart Failure: National Clinical Guideline for Diagnosis and Management in Primary and Secondary Care. Full version of NICE Clinical Guideline No. 108. London, National Clinical Guideline Centre, 2010. www.nice.org.uk/guidance/cg108/evidence/full-guideline-136060525
124. National Institute for Health and Care Excellence (NICE). Chronic Obstructive Pulmonary Disease in Over 16s: Diagnosis and Management. NICE Guidelines CG101. London, NICE, 2010. Available from: www.nice.org.uk/guidance/CG101
125. National Institute for Health and Care Excellence (NICE). Chronic Obstructive Pulmonary disease in Adults. NICE Quality Standard QS10. London, NICE, 2011. Available from: www.nice.org.uk/guidance/qs10
126. National Institute for Health and Care Excellence (NICE). Chronic Heart Failure in Adults. NICE Quality Standard QS9. London, NICE, 2011. Available from: www.nice.org.uk/guidance/qs9
127. Gallego Munoz C, Dominguez Cantero M, Rodriguez Mateos M, *et al.* PS-097 Admissions caused by iatrogenic disease in a reference hospital. *Eur J Hosp Pharm Sci Pract* 2015; 22: Suppl. 1, A174–A175.
128. World Health Organization. The World Health Report 2003. Shaping the Future. Geneva, World Health Organization, 2003. Available from: www.who.int/whr/2003/en/
129. National Institute for Health and Care Excellence (NICE). Medicines Optimisation: The Safe and Effective Use of Medicines to Enable the Best Possible Outcomes. NICE Guidelines NG5. London, NICE, 2015. Available from: www.nice.org.uk/guidance/ng5
130. Lord VM, Hume VJ, Kelly JL, *et al.* Singing classes for chronic obstructive pulmonary disease: a randomized controlled trial. *BMC Pulm Med* 2012; 12: 69.
131. Gillam S, Schamroth A. The community-oriented primary care experience in the United Kingdom. *Am J Public Health* 2002; 92: 1721–1725.
132. Higginson IJ, Bausewein C, Reilly CC, *et al.* An integrated palliative and respiratory care service for patients with advanced disease and refractory breathlessness: a randomised controlled trial. *Lancet Respir Med* 2014; 2: 979–987.
133. Curry N, Ham C. Clinical and Service Integration: The Route to Improved Outcomes. London, The King's Fund, 2010. www.kingsfund.org.uk/sites/files/kf/Clinical-and-service-integration-Natasha-Curry-Chris-Ham-22-November-2010.pdf
134. Bodenheimer T. Coordinating care – a perilous journey through the health care system. *N Engl J Med* 2008; 358: 1064–1071.
135. Bodenheimer T. Primary care physicians should be coordinators, not gatekeepers. *JAMA* 1999; 281: 2045.
136. British Thoracic Society. The Role of the Respiratory Specialist in the Integrated Care Team. A Report from the British Thoracic Society. London, British Thoracic Society, 2014. www.brit-thoracic.org.uk/document-library/delivery-of-respiratory-care/integrated-care/role-of-the-respiratory-specialist-in-the-integrated-care-team-june-2014/
137. British Thoracic Society. Integrated Care. www.brit-thoracic.org.uk/delivery-of-respiratory-care/integrated-care/working-in-integrated-care/ Date last updated: May 2016. Date last accessed: July 2016.
138. NHS Yorkshire and the Humber. Making Every Contact Count. www.makingeverycontactcount.co.uk/ Date last updated: 2012. Date last accessed: March 29, 2016.
139. Hickam DH, Weiss JW, Guise JM, *et al.* Outpatient Case Management for Adults With Medical Illness and Complex Care Needs. Comparative Effectiveness Review No. 99. Rockville, Agency for Healthcare Research and Quality, 2013. www.effectivehealthcare.ahrq.gov/ehc/products/240/733/CER99_OutpatientCaseManagement_FinalReport_20130102.pdf
140. Low L-F, Yap M, Brodaty H. A systematic review of different models of home and community care services for older persons. *BMC Health Serv Res* 2011; 11: 93.
141. Martínez-González NA, Berchtold P, Ullman K, *et al.* Integrated care programmes for adults with chronic conditions: a meta-review. *Int J Qual Heal Care* 2014; 26: 561–570.
142. The King's Fund. Whittington Respiratory Service. Specialists in Out-of-Hospital Settings. London, The King's Fund, 2014. www.kingsfund.org.uk/sites/files/kf/media/whittington-respiratory-service-kingsfund-oct14.pdf
143. Donaldson GC, Goldring JJ, Wedzicha JA. Influence of season on exacerbation characteristics in patients with COPD. *Chest* 2012; 141: 94–100.
144. Gallerani M, Boari B, Manfredini F, *et al.* Seasonal variation in heart failure hospitalization. *Clin Cardiol* 2011; 34: 389–394.

145. Hough A. Physiotherapy in Respiratory Care: a Problem-solving Approach to Respiratory and Cardiac Management. 2nd Edn. Cheltenham, Nelson Thornes, 1996.
146. Smith SMS, Sonego S, Ketcheson L, *et al.* A review of the effectiveness of psychological interventions used for anxiety and depression in chronic obstructive pulmonary disease. *BMJ Open Respir Res* 2014; 1: e000042.
147. Livermore N, Sharpe L, McKenzie D. Prevention of panic attacks and panic disorder in COPD. *Eur Respir J* 2010; 35: 557–563.
148. Lamers F, Jonkers CCM, Bosma H, *et al.* Improving quality of life in depressed COPD patients: effectiveness of a minimal psychological intervention. *COPD* 2010; 7: 315–322.
149. Jiang X, He G. Effects of an uncertainty management intervention on uncertainty, anxiety, depression, and quality of life of chronic obstructive pulmonary disease outpatients. *Res Nurs Health* 2012; 35: 409–418.
150. Alexopoulos GS, Kiosses DN, Sirey JA, *et al.* Personalised intervention for people with depression and severe COPD. *Br J Psychiatry* 2013; 202: 235–236.
151. British Psychological Society. Health Psychology and Long-term Conditions. www.bps.org.uk/news/health-psychology-and-long-term-conditions Date last updated: June 15, 2012. Date last accessed: April 2016.
152. Howard C, Dupont S, Haselden B, *et al.* The effectiveness of a group cognitive-behavioural breathlessness intervention on health status, mood and hospital admissions in elderly patients with chronic obstructive pulmonary disease. *Psychol Health Med* 2010; 15: 371–385.
153. Lynn J, Goldstein NE. Advance care planning for fatal chronic illness: avoiding commonplace errors and unwarranted suffering. *Ann Intern Med* 2003; 138: 812–818.
154. IMProving and Integrating RESpiratory Services in the NHS (IMPRESS). IMPRESS Guide for Commissioners on Supportive and End of Life Care for People with COPD. London, IMPRESS, 2012.
155. Healthcare Public Health. Design and Development of a System for People at Risk of Stroke and Vascular Dementia from Atrial Fibrillation – A New Model. www.healthcarepublichealth.net/people-with-atrial-fibrillation.php Date last updated: December 2014. Date last accessed: April 2016.
156. Hibbard J, Greene J, Sacks R, *et al.* adding a measure of patient self-management capability to risk assessment can improve prediction of high costs. *Health Aff* 2016; 35: 489–494.
157. Hibbard JH, Greene J, Overton V. Patients with lower activation associated with higher costs; delivery systems should know their patient "scores". *Health Aff* 2013; 32: 216–222.
158. United Nations Department of Economic and Social Affairs. Sustainable Development Goals Knowledge Platform. https://sustainabledevelopment.un.org/sdgs Date last updated: October 2015. Date last accessed: April 2016.
159. World Health Organization. Noncommunicable Diseases – Global Monitoring Framework. Comprehensive Global Monitoring Framework and Targets for the Prevention and Control of Noncommunicable Diseases. Geneva, World Health Organization, 2013. www.who.int/nmh/global_monitoring_framework/en/
160. Plsek PE. Working Paper: Some Emerging Principles for Managers of Complex Adaptive Systems (CAS). www.directedcreativity.com/pages/ComplexityWP.html Date last updated: September 23, 1997. Date last accessed: March 2016.
161. Heineman M, Froemke S, Berwick D, *et al.* Escape Fire: the Fight to Rescue American Healthcare. Santa Monica, Lionsgate, 2013.

Acknowledgements: Thanks to Mara Airoldi (Departmental Lecturer in Economics and Public Policy, Blavatnik School of Government, University of Oxford, Oxford, UK), who encouraged us to publish and who facilitated the original IMPRESS work. We have enjoyed challenging and helpful discussions with members of the London Respiratory Network about the aims, objectives and criteria for a system of care for people with chronic disabling breathlessness. In particular, we would like to thank Louise Restrick (Integrated Consultant Respiratory Physician, Whittington Health and Islington Clinical Commissioning Group, London Respiratory Network Co-lead, London, UK); Noel Baxter (GP, Southwark and Southwark Clinical Commissioning Group, London Respiratory Network Co-lead, London, UK); Nicholas Hopkinson (Reader in Respiratory Medicine and Honorary Consultant Chest Physician, National Heart and Lung Institute Royal Brompton Hospital, London, UK); Vince Mak (Consultant Physician in Respiratory Integrated Care at Imperial College Healthcare and Central London Community Healthcare Trusts, London, UK); Irem Patel (Consultant Respiratory Physician, Integrated Care, Kings Health Partners, Honorary Senior Lecturer, King College London School of Medicine, London, UK); Sarah Elkin (Lead in Respiratory Medicine at Imperial College NHS Trust and Honorary Senior Lecturer at Imperial College London, London, UK); Maria Buxton (Consultant Respiratory Physiotherapist, North West London Hospitals Trust and Ealing Hospital Trust, Brent, London, UK); Daniel O'Toole (Principal Clinical Psychologist, Hammersmith and Fulham Specialist Respiratory Service, Central London Community Healthcare NHS Trust, London, UK); Jane Hutton (Consultant Clinical Psychologist in Psychological Medicine at King's College Hospital, London, UK); Samantha Prigmore (Respiratory Nurse Consultant, St George's Healthcare NHS Trust, London, UK); Debbie Roots (Lead Respiratory Nurse, Bromley Healthcare, London, UK); and Grainne D'Ancona (Principal Pharmacist, Guys and St Thomas' NHS Trust, London, UK). As ever, we benefited from carer insights from Sasha Wilson (Carer and Clinical Nurse Specialist, Transfusion, University College Hospital, University College Hospitals NHS Trust, London, UK) and welcomed the patient's perspective from Chris Warburton (London, UK). It was useful to compare primary care coding systems with Jaime Correia de Sousa (Community Health, School of Health Sciences, University of Minho, Braga, Portugal) and Miguel Roman-Rodriguez (GP, Centro de Salud Son Pisa, Palma de Mallorca, Spain). We also acknowledge and thank the experts involved in the original work on the decision support tool and Tips for Clinicians, Commissioners, Patients and Researchers (affiliations listed refer to those held at the time of the original work): Noel Baxter (GP, Southwark, London, UK); Angel Chater (Registered Health Psychologist and Sport and Exercise Psychologist, Lecturer in Behavioural Medicine, UCL School of Pharmacy Centre for Behavioural Medicine, London, UK); Mark Dancy (Consultant Cardiologist, North West London Hospitals Trust, London, UK); Sarah Elkin (Lead in Respiratory Medicine at Imperial College NHS Trust and Honorary Senior Lecturer at Imperial College London, London, UK); Ahmet Fuat (Professor of Primary Care Cardiology, Durham University, Durham, UK; GP, GP Tutor and GPSI Cardiology, Darlington, UK); Steve Holmes (GP, Shepton Mallet, Somerset, UK; Co-chair of IMPRESS); Mike Kirby (Visiting Professor, University of Hertfordshire, Hatfield, UK; UK Editor of *Primary Care Cardiovascular Journal*); Basil Penney (GP, Darlington, UK; GPSI Respiratory Medicine and GP Respiratory Lead, Darlington Clinical Commissioning Group, Darlington, UK); Louise Restrick (Integrated Consultant Respiratory Physician, Whittington Health and Islington CCG, London Respiratory Network Lead, London, UK); Sam Roberts (Director of Community Academic Partnerships, UCL Partners, London, UK); Jane Scullion (Respiratory Nurse Consultant, University Hospitals of Leicester NHS Trust, Respiratory Clinical Lead Midlands and East, Leicester, UK); and Shahrad Taheri (Bariatric physician and lead for Weight Management Services and Senior Lecturer in Medicine, University of Birmingham, Birmingham Heartlands Hospital and Royal College of Physicians Action on Obesity nominee, Birmingham, UK). David Kingdon (Professor of Mental Health Care Delivery, University of Southampton, Southampton, UK), nominated by Geraldine Strathdee (NHS England National Clinical Director for Mental Health, London, UK), commented on mental health issues. Matt Kearney (GP and Advisor to the National Clinical Directors for Respiratory Disease at the time the decision tool was produced, Runcorn, UK) also provided learning from the original breathlessness campaign pilot run by the UK Department of Health.

Support statement: We are indebted to the British Thoracic Society and the Health Foundation for the generous financial support they gave in the development of the decision support tool.

Disclosures: S. Williams was paid by IMPRESS as a part-time contracted project manager on the original decision support tool, and received payment as a part-time contractor for Programme Management of the London Respiratory Network. C. De Poli received a grant from the Health Foundation while contributing to the development of the original IMPRESS decision support tool for the assessment of breathlessness.

Chapter 12

Palliative care in respiratory disease in low-resource settings

Talant M. Sooronbaev

Palliative care for respiratory diseases is a separate and serious problem for low-income countries. Many patients with advanced COPD and other chronic lung diseases who have reached the terminal stage often have disabling symptoms, such as breathlessness, cough, anxiety, depression, pain and fatigue. These patients need to be able to access health professionals with skills in palliative care in order to ensure optimal symptom control. In turn, these patients depend on the adoption of palliative care policies at local and national levels to ensure such access. These networks are, generally, far better developed in high-income countries than in low- and middle-income countries. That is why it is important to develop palliative care in low- and middle-income countries for patients with advanced, progressive respiratory diseases.

There are significant social and healthcare differences between high-, middle- and low-income countries. Many of the underlying causes of these differences are rooted in the long history of development of such nations, and include social, cultural and economic variables, historical and political elements, international relations, and geographic factors. According to the United Nations, a developing country is one with a relatively low standard of living, an undeveloped industrial base and a moderate-to-low Human Development Index. This index is a comparative measure of poverty, literacy, education, life expectancy and other factors that has been reported for countries worldwide [1].

CRDs are currently ranked fifth as a cause of disability [2]. CRDs are the third most frequent cause of mortality globally and are becoming more important in planning health services [3]. Most deaths among patients with CRD occur in patients with COPD. Thus, it has a high prevalence in low-resource settings [4]. According to the *European Lung White Book* [4], it should also be noted that the mortality rate of all respiratory diseases in low-resource settings occupies a leading position among the European countries and amounts to 143.9 deaths per 100 000 people in Kyrgyzstan. Unfortunately, to date, there are no data for the prevalence or mortality from CRDs in low- and middle-income countries.

According to World Health Organization (WHO) estimates, every year, about 20 million people around the world need palliative care at the EOL [5]. 80% of these people currently

Respiratory Medicine, Intensive Care and Sleep Medicine Department of NCCIM, Bishkek, Kyrgyzstan.

Correspondence: Talant M. Sooronbaev, Respiratory Medicine, Intensive Care and Sleep Medicine Department of NCCIM, 3 Togolok Moldo str, 720040, Bishkek, Kyrgyzstan. E-mail: sooronbaev@yahoo.com

 Print ISBN: 978-1-84984-071-2. Online ISBN: 978-1-84984-072-9. Print ISSN: 2312-508X. Online ISSN: 2312-5098.

live in low- and middle-income countries, about two-thirds are over the age of 60 years and it is estimated that about 6% are children. Most adult patients in need of palliative care die from cardiovascular disease (38.5%), cancer (34%), CRD (10.3%), HIV/AIDS (5.7%) and diabetes (4.6%) [5, 6].

Many patients with advanced COPD and other chronic lung diseases who have reached the terminal stage often have disabling symptoms: breathlessness, cough, anxiety, depression, pain and fatigue. Such patients need to be able to access health professionals with skills in palliative care in order to ensure optimal symptom control. In turn, these people depend on the adoption of palliative care policies at local and national levels to ensure such access. These networks are, generally, far better developed in high-income countries than in low- and middle-income countries. That is why it is important to develop palliative care in low- and middle-income countries for people with advanced, progressive respiratory diseases.

Key definitions and concepts

Definitions of terms used in the field of palliative care are discussed in more detail in the first chapter of this *Monograph*, but are summarised here to provide context for this discussion [7]. Palliative care is an approach that seeks to optimise the quality of life of patients and their families who face the problem of life-limiting illnesses, to optimise a person's continued independence for as long as possible, and to reduce suffering by early identification and accurate assessment of the whole person including their clinical care [8]. Palliative care is an important part of public healthcare. It also has goals related to preserving and improving human dignity, and actively identifying the unmet needs of patients and their families throughout the course of the life-limiting illness and, for families and friends, during bereavement [8].

Chronic, progressive diseases are accompanied by various symptoms and various levels of functional impairment. Chronic diseases often occur in combination with other chronic conditions, especially as people age, all of which may impact on a person's quality of life. Despite the different clinical causes of advanced, life-limiting illnesses, many people experience a similar pattern of symptoms late in life. The intensity of these symptoms and the functional impairment that they cause can vary from person to person and from life-limiting illness to life-limiting illness.

Palliative care should be delivered when a patient needs such care and before the symptoms become uncontrolled. It should not be delivered exclusively by specialised medical teams, palliative care services or hospices [9]. Such care needs to be available from a range of health and clinical services, with specialist services being involved when symptom management becomes more difficult. Specialist palliative care is intensive support for patients or their families with the most complex needs.

Low-income countries

Palliative care is a separate and serious problem for low-income countries. The lack of widespread access to palliative care in low-resource settings is generated by a number of factors, the main one of which is the overall lack of access to adequate health services. There is also sometimes a traditional cultural taboo in sharing patients' diagnosis and prognosis with them in the setting of a life-limiting illness.

For the successful development of palliative care in low-resource settings, it is necessary to create policies and strategies to create and expand the scope of services, train health personnel, and redistribute financial resources so as to meet the increasing demand as the health of whole populations improves. Initially, this will require a careful analysis of existing policies that can facilitate palliative care, and evaluate the gaps between ideal policies and those currently in place. This gap can then be addressed through policy development.

Since 1987, palliative care has been recognised as branch of medicine in its own right. In 1990, for the first time, the WHO defined palliative care with an emphasis on how this approach can be introduced in low-, medium- and high-resource countries. Two concepts of palliative care developed by WHO are presented in figure 1 [10].

Palliative care: 1) respects human life and accepts human mortality; 2) respects the dignity of the patient and their independence, and prioritises their needs; 3) is delivered to all patients suffering from an advanced, progressive disease, regardless of their age; 4) is focused on optimal control and reduction of symptoms, including pain, breathlessness and fatigue; and 5) includes diagnostic measures necessary for the most accurate assessment of the nature of clinical complications causing the patient's symptoms, adequate treatment of underlying causes when this is appropriate, and optimising the patient's quality of life.

Palliative care offers: 1) a system of care that supports the sick person, helping them to ensure the best possible quality of life until the death; and 2) support for the patient's family and friends who provide the majority of care, both during the patient's life and after their death in bereavement.

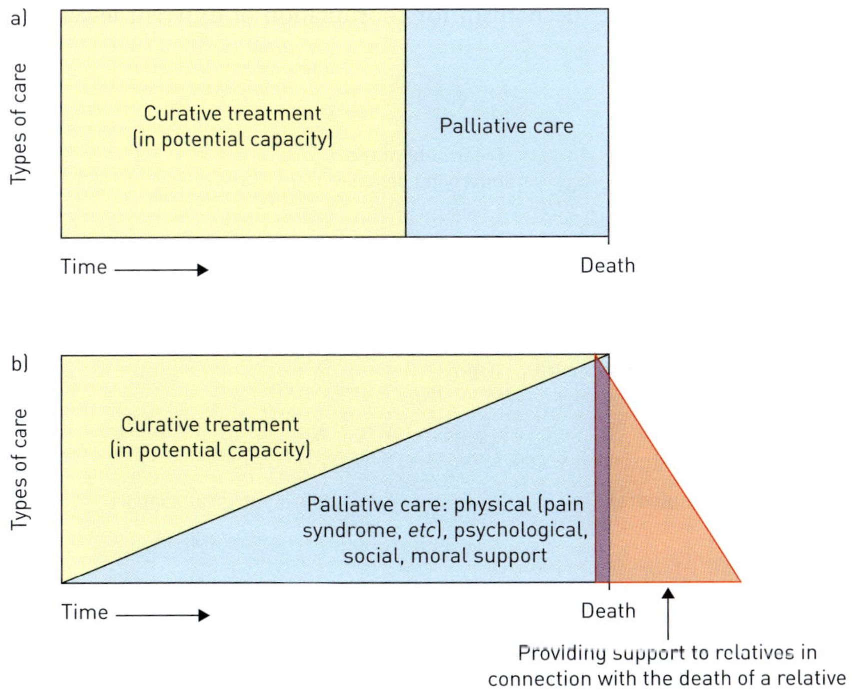

Figure 1. a) A traditional concept of palliative care. b) A new concept of palliative care. Reproduced and modified from [10] with permission.

In low-resource settings, there is a lack of accurate information about where and how people are dying. At a more detailed level, there is almost no information on the symptom burden of people with life-limiting illnesses. A life-limiting illness causes more than physical symptoms: it can cause emotional, spiritual and social problems for patients and their families. The terminal stages of chronic, progressive diseases (cardiovascular diseases, COPD, diabetes, cancer, HIV/AIDS, tuberculosis and malaria) cause patients' suffering, accompanied by a range of symptoms. In this regard, it is important to understand and implement the basic principles of palliative care, based on simple, available evidence-based approaches (figure 2). In this construct of a framework for quality palliative care, none of the spheres will be effective without interaction with the other two. This requires close and effective interdisciplinary cooperation.

The development of national standards and models for palliative care, especially in low- and medium-resource settings, will pave the way for improving the quality of palliative care in each country that adopts this approach. The WHO recommends that in resource-limited settings, it is important to ensure that minimum standards have been adopted for palliative care at all levels of healthcare, with particular emphasis on providing home-based services [12].

The analysis of the current situation of palliative care in low-resource settings

Despite palliative care being an essential component of healthcare in low-resource settings, it is currently insufficient and fragmented due to the lack of the following [5, 6]. 1) Public policy and national programmes providing guidance for and priority to palliative care. In some countries there are also legislative and regulatory barriers to providing adequate palliative care. 2) Appropriate interagency and interdisciplinary collaboration both at the central and local levels. 3) The mechanism for coordination of different levels of healthcare

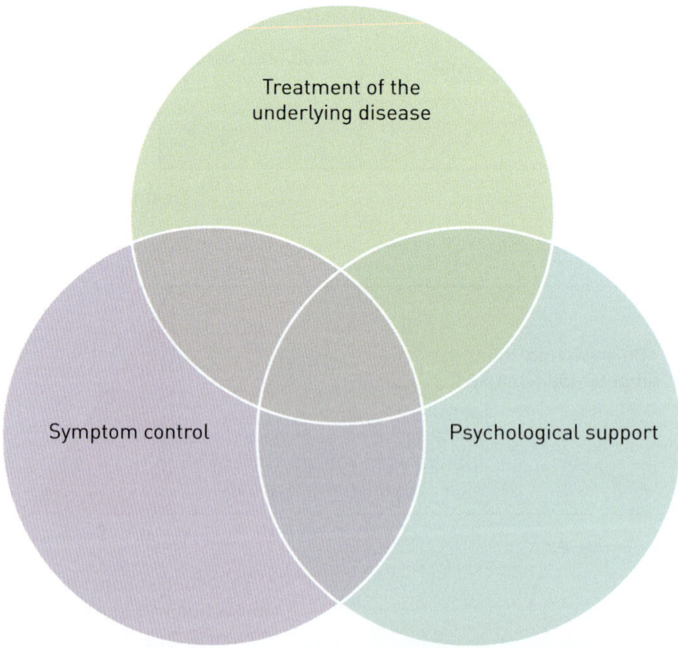

Figure 2. The principles of palliative care adopted in the Kyrgyz Republic [11].

delivery systems. 4) Institutional and human resources to create a network of palliative care organisations and services, with standard protocols for key components of care. 5) A system of training and skills development for healthcare workers including social workers and pharmacists on palliative care provision. 6) One of the main problems is the lack of financial resources allocated to the health sector as a whole but this is exacerbated greatly when there is no infrastructure for palliative care on which to build.

Palliative care services have also failed to agree on criteria for referral to specialist palliative care at national, regional or international levels. This makes it difficult to educate primary and secondary care services about how best to use palliative care services. This situation is worsened when there are no local assessment or treatment protocols for palliative care providers (whether they are from primary care or specialised services).

In addition, in low-resource settings, many patients who have a life-limiting illness have complex needs that will ideally be met through support from a combination of resources from health and from social services. Often, there is very poor cooperation between the social welfare and healthcare systems. The system of educating the community more broadly requires the active involvement of public health services, the media, civil society, patients and family members.

The basic principles of palliative care in respiratory pathology

Minimum standards for developing countries

Currently, there are no unified standards or specific recommendations for palliative care in people with respiratory diseases for developing countries, and developing such recommendations is complicated and resource intensive. In this context, the experience of certain countries in development of national palliative care guidelines is of great interest [13, 14].

Difficulties in providing palliative care in low-resource settings

Throughout the world, providing palliative care encounters serious obstacles: in many countries, public health policy is formed without due regard to the needs of palliative care; often, corresponding scientific work or professional training is not conducted at all or is insufficient; and there is poor access to opioid analgesics. According to recent study of the state of palliative care in 234 countries, regions and administrative–territorial entities, in only in 20 was this type of care properly integrated into the health system; in 42% of cases, palliative care services do not exist, and in 32% of cases, access to these services is provided only for small part of the population [15].

Among obstacles, one can include a lack of awareness of the extent of the need for palliative care; insufficient or improperly implemented public policies to improve the delivery of palliative care system; lack of knowledge of palliative care among healthcare workers; limitations in availability and affordability of opioids (especially oral) and other essential medicines needed for palliative care, in many counties; the existence of misconceptions about palliative care; and financial, organisational and structural constraints faced by public health system. Social and cultural barriers (for example, beliefs and perceptions of dying and death) and difficulties in providing an ethical approach to decision-making related to patients with life-threatening diseases have a significant impact on the availability of palliative care.

Activities to strengthen palliative care at the country level

Many of the measures needed to provide good palliative care for respiratory patients can be already realised today at the national level in low- and middle-income countries. Measures that can contribute to expanding and strengthening the system of palliative care at the country level include (but are not limited to) [8, 16] the following. 1) Development and implementation of national policies aimed at inclusion of evidence-based palliative care into the process of continuous delivery of health services to patients with life-threatening diseases, including respiratory disease, at all levels of health care with a particular emphasis on primary health care and organisation of palliative care for community care at home. 2) Advocacy for the provision of palliative care aimed at achieving universal coverage by healthcare services. 3) The adoption of policy measures to ensure affordable and consistent access to essential medicines for symptom control. This must include ensuring adequate access to controlled drugs such as opioids while having measures to limit the likelihood of illicit diversion. Such local or national frameworks must reflect the WHO guidelines for controlled substances. 4) Use needs assessment tools in palliative care to direct it to the patients and their families who most need care. 5) Focus on measures to continuously improve the quality and safety of palliative care. 6) Work towards fully implementing, and monitoring progress on implementation of, the recommendations proposed in WHO Global Action Plan for the Prevention and Control of Noncommunicable Diseases 2013–2020 and inclusion of provisions of this document into action plans of national health programmes to ensure universal coverage by healthcare services. 7) Inclusion in curricula of medicine, nursing and allied health of content to develop the skills, beliefs and competencies, and ethical understanding required for quality palliative care. There also needs to be appropriate postgraduate training for generalist and specialists in palliative care. 8) Ensuring provision of all components of palliative care (primary healthcare, and psychological and spiritual support for patients and their families) are under the supervision of trained health professionals. 9) Development of guidelines dedicated to ethical aspects of palliative care, such as ensuring equitable access to this type of care, providing services with due respect to a patient, and involvement of local communities in the development and implementation of these policies and subsequent programmes. 10) Actively create partnerships with other sectors in order to develop research activities in refining the evidence base for the practice of palliative care, including developing local cost-effective models of these services. All these measures, combined with committed political leadership, are deemed as necessary for effective and efficient development of palliative care services.

There are many models of palliative care service delivery and many ways in which they have been introduced into local and national policies and service delivery systems. The keys to success are interdisciplinary and intersectoral approaches, adjusting to specific cultural, social and economic conditions. Such a process requires that palliative care is incorporated into existing healthcare structures, with a particular emphasis on primary healthcare and organisation of patient-centred community care. In countries with limited resources, where the number of patients in need of care is high and there is currently inadequate nursing and medical staff to provide this care, an effective approach can be to augment the health professionals with volunteers from local communities who can work under the supervision of health professionals.

Palliative care is an integral part of healthcare services. It is the best approach to care for patients in severe stages of disease and it should be included into the national health systems of all countries around the world.

References

1. O'Sullivan A, Sheffrin SM. Economics: Principles in Action. Upper Saddle River, Pearson Prentice Hall, 2003.
2. Vos T, Flaxman AD, Naghavi M, *et al.* Years lived with disability (YLDs) for 1160 sequelae of 289 diseases and injuries 1990–2010: a systematic analysis for the Global Burden of Disease Study 2010. *Lancet* 2012; 380: 2163–2196.
3. Lozano R, Naghavi M, Foreman K, *et al.* Global and regional mortality from 235 causes of death for 20 age groups in 1990 and 2010: a systematic. *Lancet* 2013; 380: 2095–2128.
4. Strachan D. The burden of lung disease. *In:* Gibson JB, Loddenkemper R, Sibille Y, *et al.*, eds. European Lung White Book. 2nd Edn. Sheffield, European Respiratory Society, 2013; pp. 2–15.
5. How many people are in need of palliative care worldwide? *In:* Connor R, Sepulveda Bermedo MC, eds. Global Atlas of Palliative Care at the End of Life. Geneva, World Health Organization and Worldwide Palliative Care Alliance, 2014; pp. 10–26.
6. Burney P, Patel J, Newson R, *et al.* Global and regional trends in COPD mortality, 1990–2010. *Eur Respir J* 2015; 45: 1239–1247.
7. Kayser JB, Mooney-Doyle K, Lanken PN. Definitions and policy. *In*: Bausewein C, Currow DC, Johnson MJ, eds. Palliative Care in Respiratory Disease (ERS Monograph). Sheffield, European Respiratory Society, 2016, pp. 1–20.
8. National Cancer Control Programmes: Policies and Managerial Guidelines. 2nd Edn. Geneva, World Health Organization, 2002.
9. World Health Organization. Palliative care. Convincing facts. Geneva, World Health Organization, 2005.
10. World Health Organization. Cancer Pain Relief and Palliative Care: Report of a WHO Expert Committee. Technical Report Series 804. Geneva, World Health Organization, 1990. http://apps.who.int/iris/bitstream/10665/39524/1/WHO_TRS_804.pdf.
11. Palliative care strategy of Ministry of Health of the Kyrgyz Republic for 2012–2016. Order of the Ministry of Health. Bishkek. 2011; p. 14.
12. Rajagopal M, Joad AK, Muckaden M, *et al.* Creation of minimum standard tool for palliative care in india and self-evaluation of palliative care programs using it. *Indian J Palliat Care* 2014; 20: 201–207.
13. Watson M, Lucas C, Hoy A, *et al.*, eds. Palliative Care Guidelines. http://book.pallcare.info Date last updated: July 28, 2016.
14. Sabyrbekova T, Zhumabaev A, Zhargalbekova RT. Palliative Care. Clinical guidelines for organizations, engaged in preventive health activities in the Kyrgyz Republic. Expert Council of the Ministry of Health of the KR. Bishkek. 2012; p. 99.
15. Lynch T, Connor S, Clark D. Mapping levels of palliative care development: a global update. *J Pain Symptom Manage* 2013; 45: 1094–1106.
16. World Health Organization. Cancer Control Knowledge Into Action. WHO Guide for Effective Programmes. Module 5: Palliative Care. Geneva, World Health Organization, 2007.

Disclosures: None declared.

Chapter 13

Recognising advanced disease, advance care planning and recognition of dying for people with COPD

Karen Margaret Detering[1], Elizabeth Anne Sutton[1] and Christine Faye McDonald[2]

COPD is a common, complex, progressive and incurable disease. Many patients with advanced disease experience debilitating physical, psychological and social impairments over relatively long periods of time. Currently, despite evidence showing that there is a wish and need for advance care planning (ACP), most patients with COPD do not have access to this. While prognosis for the COPD patient is difficult, mortality is high, and patient education regarding the implications of a COPD diagnosis is often lacking but wanted. Potential barriers to the discussion of prognosis include the uncertain illness trajectory in COPD and uncertainty among health professionals as to how to have these discussions. Health professionals need to be aware of the importance of holding these discussions in a timely fashion, and need to prioritise these discussions during routine care. In order to improve the quality of life and reduce the suffering of people with advanced COPD and their families, ACP and palliative care need to be incorporated as part of usual care and earlier into the trajectory of COPD.

COPD is one of the leading causes of morbidity and mortality worldwide, and is the only leading cause for which mortality is rising globally [1]. COPD is a complex, chronic, incurable and life-limiting illness. It is a systemic disease that is usually progressive, and people with the condition often experience debilitating physical, psychological and social impairments over relatively long periods of time. Despite this significant burden of disease, patients with COPD frequently have unmet needs, especially when their disease is advanced. These unmet needs include access to advance care planning (ACP) opportunities and quality palliative care. The typical disease trajectory in COPD is one of gradual decline in health status over years, punctuated by acute exacerbations that are associated with an increased risk of dying. ACP is often not considered until during a crisis situation, such as a severe exacerbation. This chapter examines the reasons why

[1]Advance Care Planning Dept, Austin Health, Heidelberg, Australia. [2]Dept of Respiratory and Sleep Medicine, Austin Health, Heidelberg, Australia.

Correspondence: Karen Margaret Detering, Advance Care Planning Dept, Austin Health, 145 Studley Road, Heidelberg, Victoria 3084, Australia. E-mail: karen.detering@austin.org.au

 Print ISBN: 978-1-84984-071-2. Online ISBN: 978-1-84984-072-9. Print ISSN: 2312-508X. Online ISSN: 2312-5098.

patients with COPD do not have access to ACP services and offers clinicians an opportunity to introduce ACP into their work as part of standard practice, and earlier in the disease trajectory than commonly occurs at present.

How do we know a patient with COPD has advanced disease?

Patients with advanced COPD experience significant morbidity, disability and increased healthcare resource utilisation. These patients commonly have severe, refractory breathlessness that may be profoundly distressing to them, and to their families and carers [2–4]. One study showed that <50% of COPD patients experience relief from dyspnoea during their last 6 months of life [5]. Patients with COPD also have a large burden of symptoms beyond breathlessness. These symptoms are complex and both interact with, and further impact on, functional capacity and social isolation. This may include being housebound, which may add to the social impact of the disease. Other common symptoms include fatigue, persistent cough, pain, weight loss and difficulty sleeping [4, 6, 7]. Furthermore, patients with COPD often also experience unrecognised and uncontrolled anxiety and depression [6, 8], both of which are associated with poor health outcomes, including increased frequency of hospital admission, decreased quality of life (QoL) and early death [8]. Studies comparing symptom burden and QoL among patients with COPD with patients with cancer and other diseases have shown similar or worse outcomes for the COPD patients [9–12].

Typical disease trajectories for people with progressive illness are illustrated in figure 1. The trajectory in COPD is one of a gradual decline in health status and physical capacities over many years, punctuated by episodic acute exacerbations that may require hospitalisation, and these episodes are associated with an increased risk of dying (figure 1b) [13, 14].

In-hospital mortality following an acute exacerbation of COPD may be as high as 25%, while of those who survive, 25–55% will be readmitted and 25–50% will die within 1 year [15]. Thus, patients may survive many acute episodes before death [15]. This episodic course of COPD makes the exact timing of death difficult to predict, and it often seems unexpected and abrupt for both families and clinicians, particularly given that the patient may have survived many seemingly similar episodes in the past [15]. By way of example, in a study of patients who were later found to be in their last week of life, 40% were estimated by their physicians to have an expected survival of at least 6 months [16]. Another study showed that 5 days before death, physicians estimated that their patients with COPD were more than 50% likely to be alive in 6 months [17]. Furthermore, while some patients with COPD die from progressive respiratory failure, other comorbidities, such as cardiovascular disease, stroke and cancer, can also affect survival [18, 19], further complicating prognosis in individual patients. This makes the need to introduce ACP earlier in the disease course essential.

Factors assisting prognosis in the patient with COPD

While the classic trajectory applies to the general population of COPD patients, the natural history of COPD varies greatly among individuals [15, 19–21], and therefore prognosis in an individual patient is difficult. Although an FEV_1 of <30% is associated with increased mortality [22–24], the degree of lung function impairment is often not correlated to the patient's symptom burden or disease course [20], and spirometric measures, such as FEV_1, are not good predictors in individual patients. Indices that capture the pulmonary and

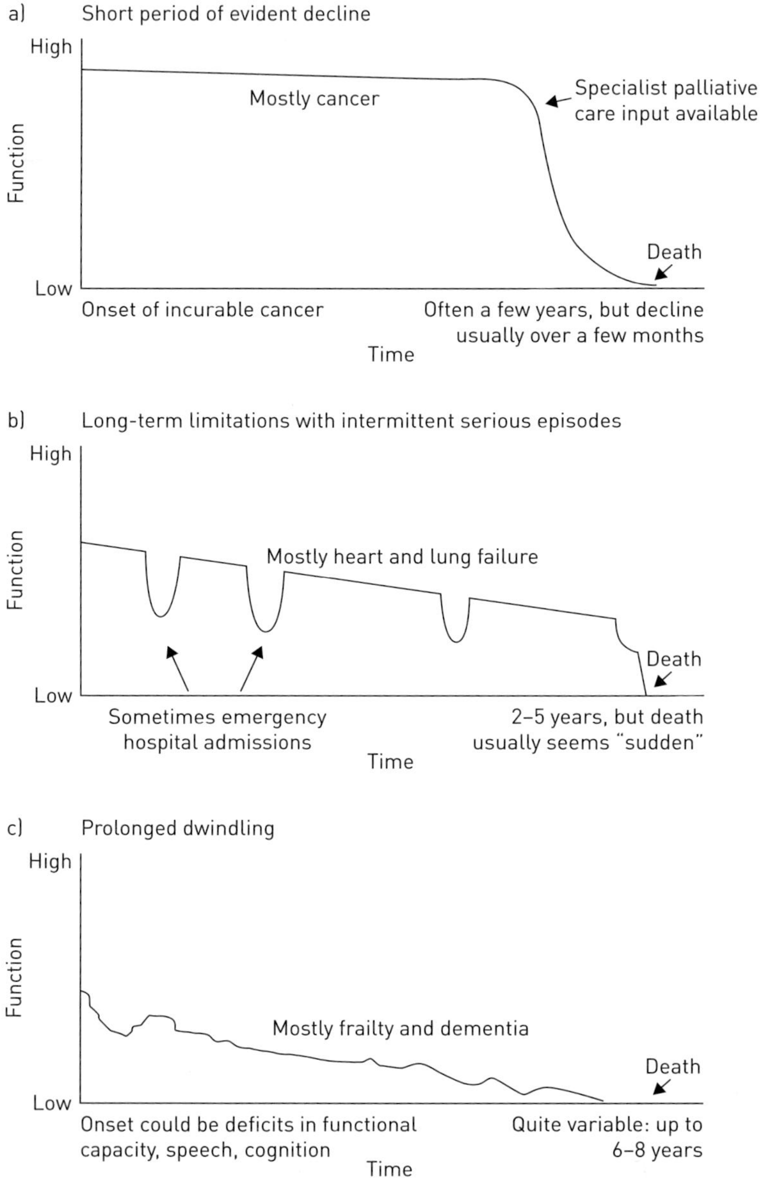

Figure 1. The three "typical" illness trajectories described for people with chronic progressive illnesses. a) Short period of evident decline. b) Long-term limitations with intermittent serious episodes. c) Prolonged dwindling. Reproduced from [13] with permission.

systematic manifestations of COPD perform better than FEV_1 alone as predictors of mortality. The BODE index (BMI, airflow obstruction, dyspnoea and exercise capacity) [25], and the ADO index (age, dyspnoea and obstruction) [26] perform better than FEV_1 alone and relatively well for populations of patients, but are less useful for individual patients.

Studies have also examined the predictors of mortality during and following acute exacerbations of COPD. Factors suggesting a poorer outcome include advanced age, prior admissions for COPD exacerbations, severity of underlying lung disease, presence of significant comorbidities, severity of dyspnoea, a low BMI, degree of functional impairment and health-related QoL [4, 15, 23, 27–29]. Although in-hospital mortality is related to the severity of underlying disease, the main influence on in-hospital mortality is the severity of the associated acute illness [15]. If the patient survives to discharge, however, the severity of the acute illness has less impact on subsequent mortality, with the severity of the underlying disease becoming the more important factor [15].

What is ACP and why is it important?

ACP is a coordinated communication process between a person, their family and healthcare providers that aims to clarify the person's values, treatment preferences and goals of medical treatment should the person lose capacity to make or communicate such decisions in the future [30]. Although completion of documents (advance directives), which set out the person's wishes, may be a desired outcome, the discussions that are central to the ACP process are valuable in their own right [31]. Completion of advance directives alone, without further discussion, may not influence future medical care [32, 33]. Rather, ACP discussions, a central element of person-centred care, enables the person to explore their specific goals for care and to determine their own healthcare priorities, and also to assist them and their clinicians to align their healthcare preferences with the care they receive.

Palliative care is an approach that improves the QoL of patients and their families facing the problems associated with life-threatening illness through the prevention and relief of suffering by means of early identification and impeccable assessment [34]. Palliative care is not limited to EOL care and has important roles throughout the COPD disease trajectory.

ACP is not a single event but an ongoing process, which should be revisited regularly during the course of a person's life and illness. This is especially important as a person's medical situation changes. The traditional objectives of ACP have been to assist patients to make treatment decisions in advance and to plan for possible future incapacity. However, ACP can also facilitate and clarify current decision making in a patient who retains capacity [35], and can ensure that care aligns with the person's goals.

Due to the inherent challenges of prognosis in many diseases, coupled with the difficulty of predicting the course of a person's illness, it is suggested that the main focus of ACP should be on preparing patients and surrogate decision makers to participate with clinicians in making the best possible "in-the-moment" decisions [36]. Preparation for "in-the-moment" decision making shifts the focus away from premature treatment decisions based on incomplete or hypothetical information. Rather, the aim is to ensure that complex health decisions are based on a more complete set of considerations, such as the current clinical context, shifting and evolving goals, the patient's wishes and, finally, the decision makers' needs [36]. This may be especially relevant when caring for patients with COPD, where prognosis is difficult. Importantly, ACP also provides an opportunity to introduce the concept of palliative care earlier in the disease process for people with COPD [37].

In both prospective studies and randomised trials, ACP has been shown to significantly improve outcomes for patients and their families. ACP improves the quality of care, including EOL care [35, 38], and increases the likelihood that a person will die in their preferred place [35, 39]. It is associated with an increase in utilisation of hospice services, a reduction in hospitalisation and a reduction in the use of unwanted intensive treatments at the EOL [31, 35, 40]. Furthermore, ACP decreases the burden experienced by surrogate decision makers [41, 42] and improves psychological outcomes in both surviving relatives [35, 38] and treating healthcare providers [43]. More recently, ACP has been shown to be feasible and acceptable in people from culturally and linguistically diverse backgrounds in Australia [44]. Finally, there are data showing that ACP reduces the cost of EOL care [40, 45], without increasing mortality [31]. A 2014 review on the efficacy of ACP concluded that "considering the positive effects of ACP on multiple outcomes, implementation into regular clinical care is recommended" [31].

ACP in COPD: perspectives of patients, family and physicians

ACP is likely to be of particular importance and relevance for patients with COPD, especially when one considers the unique and uncertain disease trajectory, the high burden of debilitating symptoms, the frequent coexistence of other potentially fatal conditions and the risk of sudden death. Patients with COPD report wanting information about their diagnosis and expected disease process, treatment, prognosis, what dying might be like and ACP [46].

Despite this desire for information, many patients report that they lack information about their disease and its implications [9, 16]. They may be unaware that COPD is progressive, incurable and, for many, ultimately a fatal disease [47–49]. For example, one study showed that only 63% of patients with advanced COPD who were housebound, had extensive symptoms and had had recent admissions knew that they were likely to die from COPD [50]. COPD patients also report deficits in their clinicians with respect to them discussing what the dying process might be like [48]. This is despite the patients' desire to have emotional support and to discuss their EOL care [46], and despite patients identifying communication as one of the most important skills required by their clinicians [51]. Interestingly, it has been shown that, although COPD patients rated their clinicians' general communication skills highly, they concurrently rated their clinicians' skills at discussing EOL topics, such as prognosis or what dying might be like, as poor [48]. Other studies have shown that healthcare professionals' communication about ACP, palliative care and EOL care is lacking or of poor quality [6, 12, 48, 52].

Family and caregivers also have needs. Studies have shown that family/caregivers also desire information regarding the expected course of the disease, the process of death and dying, care requirements and specifically how to deal with an emergency [53, 54]. However, this need for information is often not met. In a study of bereaved relatives of patients with COPD, almost half reported that they were not aware that their loved one might die from COPD, and yet most of these stated that they would have preferred to know [5]. There is also variation in the family experiences, depending on the disease their family member has. A qualitative study exploring the experiences of bereaved family caregivers and decision making regarding LSTs found differences between patients with COPD and those with cancer [55]. For the cancer group, caregivers reported that patients reached a point in their illness when it was accepted that there were no longer any treatment options available to prolong life. In contrast, the caregivers of patients with COPD experienced the need to make specific treatment decisions about LSTs at the EOL [55]. For example, studies have found that, despite similar preferences for intensity of care as patients with cancer, COPD patients are more likely than patients with cancer to die in the ICU or on a ventilator [56, 57] and not to be treated with symptom-relieving medications [56].

Healthcare professionals themselves also report a deficiency in discussing EOL care with patients who have COPD [49]. Apart from issues relating to prognosis, other cited reasons for not having these conversations include feeling ill-prepared to deliver bad news, viewing ACP as conceding to the disease, anticipating conflict with the patient or family, and a lack of time or training [58, 59]. While clinicians acknowledge that the appropriate timing for ACP is when a patient's disease is stable, they note that these discussions are often initiated during a crisis and when patients are too ill to make their own decisions about their care [49].

Clinicians also voice concerns that discussing COPD prognosis and offering ACP and palliative care will remove hope [60] and cause anxiety and depression in their patients, thus potentially having a detrimental effect on their patients' QoL and mortality [61]. This is not borne out by the evidence. A central aspect of ACP discussions is the emphasis on the importance of maintaining hope [62]. ACP has not been shown to be associated with negative psychological outcomes for patients [35, 63], and discussions regarding prognosis in patients with COPD show decreased anxiety and improved satisfaction with care [61]. Similarly, data from cancer patients show that patient–physician communication about EOL care is not associated with an increase in anxiety or depression [64], and studies in ESRD requiring dialysis, another progressive chronic disease, have shown that ACP has beneficial outcomes in relation to a person's hope [65]. Thus, the available evidence shows that ACP does not result in harm but rather is associated with improved psychological outcomes for patients.

What is the current status of ACP in patients with COPD?

Despite the information and ACP needs of COPD patients and their family, as outlined in the previous section, this need is largely unmet. Of COPD patients entering a pulmonary rehabilitation programme, only one-fifth had discussed advance directives with their clinician, with even lower numbers believing that their clinician understood their wishes for EOL care [66]. Another study showed that only one-quarter of patients with COPD had discussed their wishes regarding cardiopulmonary resuscitation before they were hospitalised [67], while another study reported that only one-third of oxygen-dependent patients with COPD had discussed their EOL wishes with their clinicians [61]. All of these results are of great importance, given that it is very likely that the majority of these patients had advanced COPD.

Despite the perceived need for ACP discussions to occur during periods of stability, ACP discussions are more likely to occur during periods of crisis [49, 68] or in the ICU [69], when patients are too ill to make decisions and caregivers may feel ill equipped to make such decisions. Additionally, physicians may not be aware that patients are interested in discussing prognosis [58].

Incorporating ACP into routine COPD management

Although it is often recommended that ACP should be initiated early and during relatively stable phases of the disease, and not in the midst of a crisis such as a hospital or ICU admission, formal studies comparing the optimal timing of ACP for patients with COPD are lacking. Most patients do not initiate these discussions but will wait for clinicians to do so, and may perceive an absence of such discussions as evidence that they are not yet needed [37, 70, 71]. Given that the typical disease trajectory in COPD is characterised by episodic deteriorations and partial recoveries, clinicians, patients and caregivers may be lulled into a false belief that ACP can wait until a future time. What then can occur is that patients deteriorate and treatment decisions need to be made, but ACP has not yet taken place. Difficulties with prognosis for individual patients with COPD may further complicate this situation. It is worth noting that ACP can be opportunistic, and specific events or circumstances may act as prompts for initiating or revisiting ACP [72]. These may include the following [6, 36, 37, 70, 73]: 1) the patient or family indicate that they wish to discuss ACP; 2) FEV_1 of <30–40%; 3) severe refractory dyspnoea; 4) oxygen dependence or commencement; 5) use of NIV; 6) a recent hospitalisation, or one or more admissions in last year; 7) Functional decline; 8) increasing dependence on others; 9) weight loss; 10) a new or worsening comorbid condition; and 11) pulmonary rehabilitation (referral/attendance).

Therefore, ACP needs to be incorporated into routine management and offered in a nonthreatening and systematic way. This may be assisted by considering the dual agendas of "hoping for the best and planning for the worst" [74]. ACP has many potential benefits for patients and their family/caregivers and helps align the person's specific healthcare goals with the care they receive.

As COPD progresses, patients usually have increasingly frequent interactions with healthcare services, as depicted in figure 2. These contacts offer important opportunities to proactively initiate or review ACP, as well as incorporating other important aspects of care, such as palliative care. Clinicians need skills to discuss topics such as ACP and EOL care [61]. These skills do not reliably improve with experience alone [75] but are teachable [76–79]. Nonphysician facilitators have been shown to be effective in conducting ACP and EOL conversations with patients

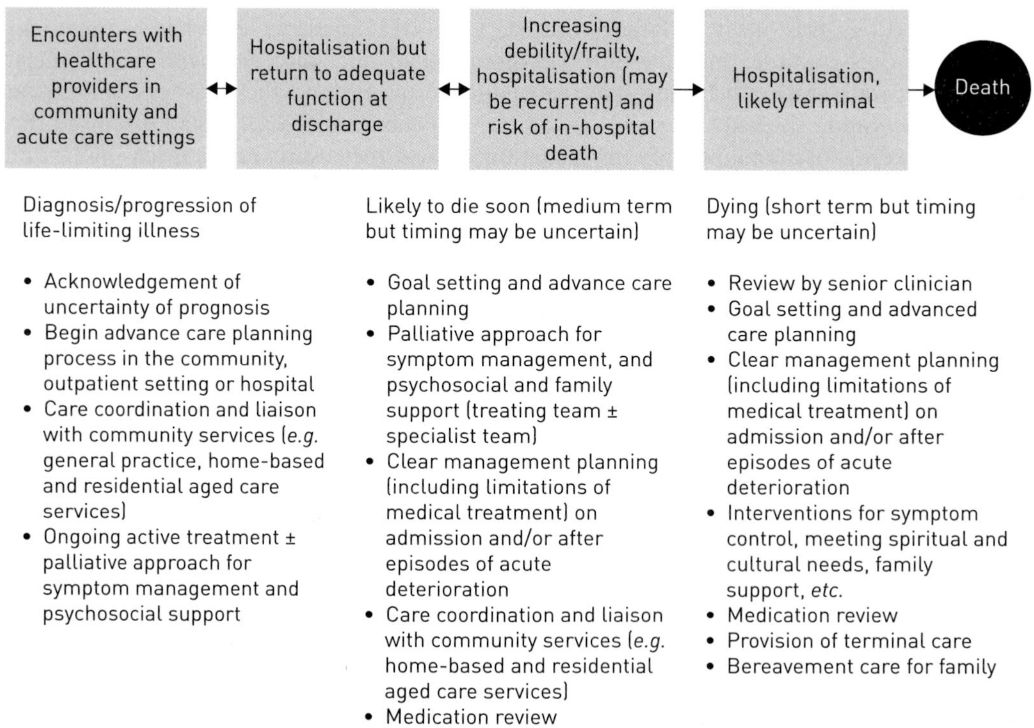

Figure 2. Interaction between deterioration in the patient, health service usage and timing for medical planning. Reproduced from [30] with permission.

[38, 61, 80], and this is a feasible option, with the potential to increase opportunities for patient access to ACP. It is particularly relevant to consider important ACP opportunities, such as pulmonary rehabilitation, or chronic disease case management where nonphysician healthcare professionals may routinely interact with people with COPD.

Internationally, in support of the growing recognition of the needs of patients with COPD, ACP and palliative care recommendations are being included in guidelines. For example, in the Australian COPD X guidelines, there is a specific section pertaining to palliative care and ACP [81]. The EOL care strategy for England [82] advocates that all patients with advanced, progressive chronic illness have access to ACP. Furthermore, the 2008 American Thoracic Society clinical policy statement on palliative care for patients with respiratory diseases and critical illnesses has also recommended that communication and ACP should be one of the core competencies for pulmonary clinicians [83]. Such initiatives are important in supporting healthcare professionals and healthcare services to provide ACP opportunities to patients with advanced COPD.

The ACP process in COPD patients

An ACP conversation is essentially a structured discussion, which follows a broad outline. The order the ACP discussion follows will vary depending on the patient and clinician, the current clinical situation and how the discussion progresses [84]. Patients and family need time to think and reflect, so it is expected that the ACP process will extend over time.

Patients may not wish to have an ACP discussion, and patients with COPD differ in the extent to which they want to receive information regarding their prognosis [16]. Thus, prior to an ACP discussion, it is important to seek permission to have the discussion and to ascertain how much information they would like to know.

The key components of an ACP discussion are outlined in the following sections [36, 84, 85]. Table 1 outlines some suggested questions and comments relevant to these key steps.

Ensure the relevant people are present during discussions

Having others, including surrogates, involved in discussions provides support for the patient and provides the opportunity to receive information first hand regarding COPD, possible treatments and the likely disease course. Furthermore, when surrogates are present during discussions, the completion of advance directives is more likely [38], and the surrogate is more able to follow a person's wishes [86]. Surrogates find decision making more difficult if they do not have a sense of what the patient may have wanted [36]. Thus, having them present helps to better prepare them for their possible future surrogate decision-making role.

Establish how decisions are to be made if the person does not wish to or is unable to make their own decisions

This often involves appointment of a surrogate decision-maker(s), and establishing how that person will make treatment decisions. This step includes the preparation for making in-the-moment decisions [36], and discussing how much scope or leeway the patient would like the decision-maker to have. Patients and surrogates may not realise the importance of preparing for future decision making. Most patients want their loved ones to have leeway in

Table 1. Advance care planning (ACP) discussion tips

Step	Purpose	Question/comment
Obtain permission and wish for prognostic information	Invites the patient to discuss their current condition and desires regarding future medical care. This helps to ascertain how much information the patient (and family/carers if present) wish regarding their likely prognosis. It is important to note that not everyone wishes to participate in ACP (not now or possibly not ever).	Would you like to talk about what to expect or what to prepare for as your illness worsens? Often people with COPD have lots of questions about what might happen to them in the future. "Is this something that we could talk about?" Some people like to know everything that is going on with them and what may happen in the future; others prefer not to know too many details. What do you prefer?
Surrogate decision-making	To identify how and who will make decisions if the person is unable to or does not wish to do this for themselves.	If you cannot, or choose not to, participate in healthcare decisions, how would you want decisions regarding your medical treatment to be made? Is there a specific person(s) that you would like your doctors to speak to regarding your medical care?
Education regarding the role of the surrogate	To facilitate understanding relating to how the surrogate decision-maker would make decisions in the future.	Does this person know you have chosen them for the role? Would they know what your wishes are? What if, based on the situation with your health, your doctor recommends something different to what you have told your loved one? What would you want to happen in this circumstance? Are there certain decisions about your healthcare that you would not want your loved one to change under any circumstances?
Explore values and beliefs, and what it means to live well	To help the patient define what it means to "live well". It is important to note that, for many people, they may not ever have thought about life as an abstract concept and may not have a ready answer. Many people have concerns besides simply prolonging life. Other priorities may include avoiding suffering, being with family, being mentally aware and not being a burden to others.	What types of things do you like to do? How can we help you to live well? What things are important for you to be able to enjoy your life? When you look at the future, what do you hope for? What concerns you? Do you have any thoughts about how you would like to be cared for if you became much sicker? Is there anything that you worry about happening if you were very ill? Do you have spiritual or cultural beliefs that you would like the healthcare team to know about?

Continued

Table 1. Cont nued

Step	Purpose	Question/comment
Current and future goals for treatment	To ascertain what the patient would want both now and in the future, being mindful of the nature of the disease.	If you were to become more unwell, what would be most important to you? Is there anything that you worry about happening if you were very ill? What goals do you have, now and in the future? What would you like to achieve in the next year? How do you think your current and future health will affect your chance of achieving your goals?
Understanding of the illness and possible treatments	To determine what the patient's understanding is regarding their medical situation at the present time.	Do you feel you have a good understanding of your illness and what can be done? What further information do you need? What do you understand about where things stand right now with your illness? What have you been told about your illness? At what point (if any) during your illness would you consider stopping treatments and changing the focus of care to supportive care? With who and how would these decisions be made?
Provide information	To provide clear information about the choices that may be faced in the future, individualised to the patient's own current medical situation.	Your illness is getting worse, and it is likely you will have more admissions to hospital. Your lung tests are much worse and show...
Hoping for the best, preparing for the worst	Facilitating a dual agenda, which may be especially relevant in COPD where exact prognosis is uncertain.	Hoping for the best and preparing for the worst does not mean giving up. It means arranging the best medical care for you, no matter what happens. It's a good plan to hope for the best but at the same time to make some decisions in case things don't go as well as we hope.
Treatments not wanted	To determine whether there are any specific treatments that a patient would not want, regardless of outcome.	Are there medical treatments you have experienced or seen others experience that have caused you concern? Are there any specific treatments you would definitely not want to receive? Encourage the patient to be specific. For the patient who is interested in trials of life support, ask them to specify how long a trial should be, and what criteria should be used to decide to stop the treatment.

Continued

Table 1. Continued

Step	Purpose	Question/comment
Documentation	Encourages the patient to complete advance directives if they wish to.	It is great we have had this discussion. The decisions you have made are really important. It would be great to write these down. Is that OK with you? Encourage distribution among the family to ensure that ACP decisions of the patient are known to their loved ones and to surrogate decision makers. It is important to let family members know of your wishes and desires for the future. This includes letting everyone know who you have chosen as your surrogate decision-maker.
Encourage distribution among family	To ensure that ACP decisions of the patient are known to their loved ones and surrogate decision makers.	It is important to let family members know of your wishes and desires for the future. This includes letting them know who you have chosen as your surrogate decision-maker.
Review	A review of these plans on a regular basis ensures that the ACP discussions accurately reflect the decisions of the patient.	These are discussions we may need to revisit from time to time, especially if there are any changes in your health.

decision making [33, 87], and surrogates' consideration of additional factors beyond patients' advance treatment preferences may lead to better decisions and improved patient care [88]. Patients and surrogates may also need to re-evaluate pre-specified wishes in light of unforeseen clinical contexts [71, 89].

Explore the person's values and beliefs and what it means to live well

This step involves discussion of the patient's values, beliefs and what it means to them to "live well". It includes discussion of current and future goals and what they would consider to be a "reasonable outcome" from treatment. The central focus here is on the person themselves, to help align the person's goals for care with the healthcare that they receive. Many people may not have thought about these concepts in detail and may require time to understand what is important to them.

Understanding illness, treatment and prognosis (where desired)

This step involves assessing the current understanding of the illness, the likely trajectory and prognosis. Specific information related to COPD can be provided, but also acknowledging the uncertainty related to prognosis in individuals with COPD is important. This helps correct any misconceptions that patients and family may have and assists them in a better understanding of the disease and potential future treatment decisions, which may be required. There may be specific treatments not wanted under any circumstance, and trials of treatment may be also considered and discussed.

Studies have shown that accurate information is preferred as long as it is not delivered bluntly, or with too much hard factual or detailed information [90, 91]. Therefore, it is best to balance sensitivity and honesty when discussing prognosis or delivering bad news [53, 92]. Patients also vary in how they like to receive prognostic information. Some COPD patients desire direct and explicit information, while others require a more general approach, such as describing what may happen to other people with COPD [9, 60].

When discussing COPD it is important to acknowledge that the diagnosis of COPD does mean a degree of uncertainty. Clinicians should also be mindful that there is an important interaction between preferences for hope and desire for prognostic information [60]. One way to address this is to consider the dual agendas of "hoping for the best and planning for the worst" [74].

During the ACP discussion, fostering realistic hope is important. This may be facilitated by emphasising what can be done (particularly when disease-specific treatments are no longer working). Patients may hope for many things, not just a cure. Exploring this with patients may help to facilitate setting realistic goals. Be honest without being blunt [53].

Patients and caregivers want health professionals to provide empathy, consistency and a sense that they will stay the course, and that they will not be abandoned as the illness progresses [53, 93].

Documentation and dissemination

While documentation in an advance directive is not essential to the process of ACP, it is ideal and increases the likelihood of a person's wishes being known and respected. Even when a surrogate has been appointed, completing an advance directive documenting values and future treatment wishes is useful. This is because it functions to remind the surrogate of the wishes, and to support them in decision making, particularly if there is disagreement between surrogates and healthcare providers. It is also available if the surrogate is not contactable in an emergency.

Once completed, advance directives need to be available when treatment decisions are required. Conversion of a person's wishes as outlined in advance directives into clear and actionable medical orders may be especially important for patients with advanced COPD. For example, the POLST (Physician Orders for LST) programme has specifically addressed these issues and has been shown to improve outcomes and care for people with advanced chronic disease and frailty [94]. A key element of the POLST programme is the use of a standardised form containing actionable medical orders that transfer between healthcare settings.

Review and update as appropriate

ACP is an ongoing process that requires regular reviews and updating as appropriate, because the patient's needs and wishes may change over time and as their condition changes. For those patients who initially refuse an ACP discussion, reintroduction of the concept is part of good care to ensure that they are given the opportunity to complete ACP if they are now ready to do so. Furthermore, review of an ACP means that patients can change their wishes and appointments of surrogate decision-makers should they wish to do so. It is important to ensure patients understand that they can change their minds and update plans at any time.

Conclusion

In order to improve the QoL and reduce the suffering of people with advanced COPD and their families, ACP and palliative care need to be incorporated earlier into the trajectory of the illness. Currently, both clinicians and patients/family are waiting until identification of the terminal phase of illness. This creates major difficulties, given that the terminal phase is often indistinguishable from the slow, chronic decline punctuated by repeated acute exacerbations that are typically seen in advanced COPD. Rather, ACP and palliative care need to be timely in order to facilitate a better QoL for people with COPD, regardless of where they are on the disease trajectory.

Frontline healthcare providers should focus on symptom management, ACP and support for patients as part of usual, comprehensive and patient-centred care. Patients with COPD have a serious life-limiting illness that is not curable and that often causes a significant burden of symptoms and a dramatic reduction in QoL. The current underprovision of ACP and palliative care may reflect a combination of difficulty in predicting when a patient with COPD is near or at the EOL, failure to recognise poor symptom control and reduced QoL, and a greater emphasis on providing palliative care for patients with malignant rather than non-malignant disease.

ACP must become an important part of routine care for patients with advanced COPD. Information needs in COPD are often unmet, and patients with COPD and their families seldom have a complete understanding of the condition and its prognosis. While prognosis in COPD is difficult, mortality is ultimately high, and patient education regarding the implications of a COPD diagnosis is often lacking. Potential barriers to the discussion of prognosis may include the uncertain illness trajectory in COPD, and uncertainty among health professionals as to how to have these discussions. An awareness of the importance to patients of holding these discussions in a timely fashion, as well as tips to help initiate the ACP conversation, may assist in ensuring that clinicians prioritise these discussion during routine care.

References

1. Lopez AD, Shibuya K, Rao C, *et al.* Chronic obstructive pulmonary disease: current burden and future projections. *Eur Respir J* 2006; 27: 397–412.
2. Currow DC, Abernethy AP, Ko DN. The active identification and management of chronic refractory breathlessness is a human right. *Thorax* 2014; 69: 393–394.
3. Bausewein C, Booth S, Gysels M, *et al.* Understanding breathlessness: cross-sectional comparison of symptom burden and palliative care needs in chronic obstructive pulmonary disease and cancer. *J Palliat Med* 2010; 13: 1109–1118.
4. Hardin KA, Meyers F, Louie S. Integrating palliative care in severe chronic obstructive lung disease. *COPD* 2008; 5: 207–220.
5. Elkington H, White P, Addington-Hall J, *et al.* The healthcare needs of chronic obstructive pulmonary disease patients in the last year of life. *Palliat Med* 2005; 19: 485–491.
6. Vermylen JH, Szmuilowicz E, Kalhan R. Palliative care in COPD: an unmet area for quality improvement. *Int J Chron Obstruct Pulmon Dis* 2015; 10: 1543–1551.
7. Blinderman CD, Homel P, Billings JA, *et al.* Symptom distress and quality of life in patients with advanced chronic obstructive pulmonary disease. *J Pain Symptom Manage* 2009; 38: 115–123.
8. Maurer J, Rebbapragada V, Borson S, *et al.* Anxiety and depression in COPD: current understanding, unanswered questions, and research needs. *Chest* 2008; 134: Suppl. 4, 43S–56S.
9. Gore JM, Brophy CJ, Greenstone MA. How well do we care for patients with end stage chronic obstructive pulmonary disease (COPD)? A comparison of palliative care and quality of life in COPD and lung cancer. *Thorax* 2000; 55: 1000–1006.
10. Walke LM, Byers AL, Tinetti ME, *et al.* Range and severity of symptoms over time among older adults with chronic obstructive pulmonary disease and heart failure. *Arch Intern Med* 2007; 167: 2503–2508.
11. Solano JP, Gomes B, Higginson IJ. A comparison of symptom prevalence in far advanced cancer, AIDS, heart disease, chronic obstructive pulmonary disease and renal disease. *J Pain Symptom Manage* 2006; 31: 58–69.
12. Janssen DJ, Spruit MA, Uszko-Lencer NH, *et al.* Symptoms, comorbidities, and health care in advanced chronic obstructive pulmonary disease or chronic heart failure. *J Palliat Med* 2011; 14: 735–743.
13. Murray SA, Kendall M, Boyd K, *et al.* Illness trajectories and palliative care. *BMJ* 2005; 330: 1007–1011.
14. Lynn J, Adamson DM. Living Well at the End of Life. Santa Monica, RAND Coorporation, 2003.
15. Steer J, Gibson GJ, Bourke SC. Predicting outcomes following hospitalization for acute exacerbations of COPD. *QJM* 2010; 103: 817–829.
16. Gardiner C, Gott M, Small N, *et al.* Living with advanced chronic obstructive pulmonary disease: patients concerns regarding death and dying. *Palliat Med* 2009; 23: 691–697.
17. The SUPPORT Principal Investigators. A controlled trial to improve care for seriously ill hospitalized patients. The study to understand prognoses and preferences for outcomes and risks of treatments (SUPPORT). *JAMA* 1995; 274: 1591–1598.
18. Sin DD, Anthonisen NR, Soriano JB, *et al.* Mortality in COPD: role of comorbidities. *Eur Respir J* 2006; 28: 1245–1257.
19. Seamark DA, Seamark CJ, Halpin DM. Palliative care in chronic obstructive pulmonary disease: a review for clinicians. *J R Soc Med* 2007; 100: 225–233.
20. Casanova C, de Torres JP, Aguirre-Jaíme A, *et al.* The progression of chronic obstructive pulmonary disease is heterogeneous: the experience of the BODE cohort. *Am J Respir Crit Care Med* 2011; 184: 1015–1021.
21. Han MK, Agusti A, Calverley PM, *et al.* Chronic obstructive pulmonary disease phenotypes: the future of COPD. *Am J Respir Crit Care Med* 2010; 182: 598–604.
22. Gudmundsson G, Gislason T, Lindberg E, *et al.* Mortality in COPD patients discharged from hospital: the role of treatment and co-morbidity. *Respir Res* 2006; 7: 109.
23. Groenewegen KH, Schols AM, Wouters EF. Mortality and mortality-related factors after hospitalization for acute exacerbation of COPD. *Chest* 2003; 124: 459–467.
24. Curtis JR. Palliative and end-of-life care for patients with severe COPD. *Eur Respir J* 2008; 32: 796–803.
25. Celli BR, Cote CG, Marin JM, *et al.* The body-mass index, airflow obstruction, dyspnea, and exercise capacity index in chronic obstructive pulmonary disease. *N Engl J Med* 2004; 350: 1005–1012.

26. Puhan MA, Garcia-Aymerich J, Frey M, *et al.* Expansion of the prognostic assessment of patients with chronic obstructive pulmonary disease: the updated BODE index and the ADO index. *Lancet* 2009; 374: 704–711.
27. Almagro P, Calbo E, Ochoa de Echagüen A, *et al.* Mortality after hospitalization for COPD. *Chest* 2002; 121: 1441–1448.
28. Connors AF Jr, Dawson NV, Thomas C, *et al.* Outcomes following acute exacerbation of severe chronic obstructive lung disease. The SUPPORT investigators (Study to Understand Prognoses and Preferences for Outcomes and Risks of Treatments). *Am J Respir Crit Care Med* 1996; 154: 959–967.
29. McGhan R, Radcliff T, Fish R, *et al.* Predictors of rehospitalization and death after a severe exacerbation of COPD. *Chest* 2007; 132: 1748–1755.
30. Australian Commission on Safety and Quality in Health Care. National Consensus Statement: Essential Elements for Safe and High-quality End-of-life Care. Available from: www.safetyandquality.gov.au/publications/national-consensus-statement-essential-elements-for-safe-high-quality-end-of-life-care/ Date last accessed: March 1, 2016. Date last updated: 2015.
31. Houben CH, Spruit MA, Groenen MT, *et al.* Efficacy of advance care planning: a systematic review and meta-analysis. *J Am Med Dir Assoc* 2014; 15: 477–489.
32. Tulsky JA. Beyond advance directives: importance of communication skills at the end of life. *JAMA* 2005; 294: 359–365.
33. Prendergast TJ. Advance care planning: pitfalls, progress, promise. *Crit Care Med* 2001; 29: Suppl. 2, 34–N39.
34. World Health Organisation. WHO Definition of Palliative Care. www.who.int/cancer/palliative/definition/en/ Date last accessed: April 30, 2016.
35. Brinkman-Stoppelenburg A, Rietjens JA, van der Heide A. The effects of advance care planning on end-of-life care: a systematic review. *Palliat Med* 2014; 28: 1000–1025.
36. Sudore RL, Fried TR. Redefining the "planning" in advance care planning: preparing for end-of-life decision making. *Ann Intern Med* 2010; 153: 256–261.
37. Heffner JE. Advance care planning in chronic obstructive pulmonary disease: barriers and opportunities. *Curr Opin Pulm Med* 2011; 17: 103–109.
38. Detering KM, Hancock AD, Reade MC, *et al.* The impact of advance care planning on end of life care in elderly patients: randomised controlled trial. *BMJ* 2010; 340: c1345.
39. Molloy DW, Russo R, Pedlar D, *et al.* Implementation of advance directives among community-dwelling veterans. *Gerontologist* 2000; 40: 213–217.
40. Teno JM, Gruneir A, Schwartz Z, *et al.* Association between advance directives and quality of end-of-life care: a national study. *J Am Geriatr Soc* 2007; 55: 189–194.
41. Handy CM, Sulmasy DP, Merkel CK, *et al.* The surrogate's experience in authorizing a do not resuscitate order. *Palliat Support Care* 2008; 6: 13–19.
42. Vig EK, Starks H, Taylor JS, *et al.* Surviving surrogate decision-making: what helps and hampers the experience of making medical decisions for others. *J Gen Intern Med* 2007; 22: 1274–1279.
43. Elpern EH, Covert B, Kleinpell R. Moral distress of staff nurses in a medical intensive care unit. *Am J Crit Care* 2005; 14: 523–530.
44. Detering K, Sutton E, Fraser S, *et al.* Feasibility and acceptability of advance care planning in elderly Italian and Greek speaking patients as compared to English-speaking patients: an Australian cross-sectional study. *BMJ Open* 2015; 5: e008800.
45. Zhang B, Wright AA, Huskamp HA, *et al.* Health care costs in the last week of life: associations with end-of-life conversations. *Arch Intern Med* 2009; 169: 480–488.
46. Curtis JR, Wenrich MD, Carline JD, *et al.* Patients' perspectives on physician skill in end-of-life care: differences between patients with COPD, cancer, and AIDS. *Chest* 2002; 122: 356–362.
47. Gardiner C, Gott M, Payne S, *et al.* Exploring the care needs of patients with advanced COPD: an overview of the literature. *Respir Med* 2010; 104: 159–165.
48. Curtis JR, Engelberg RA, Nielsen EL, *et al.* Patient-physician communication about end-of-life care for patients with severe COPD. *Eur Respir J* 2004; 24: 200–205.
49. Gott M, Gardiner C, Small N, *et al.* Barriers to advance care planning in chronic obstructive pulmonary disease. *Palliat Med* 2009; 23: 642–648.
50. Elkington H, White P, Addington-Hall J, *et al.* The last year of life of COPD: a qualitative study of symptoms and services. *Respir Med* 2004; 98: 439–445.
51. Curtis JR, Wenrich MD, Carline JD, *et al.* Understanding physicians' skills at providing end-of-life care perspectives of patients, families, and health care workers. *J Gen Intern Med* 2001; 16: 41–49.
52. Houben CH, Spruit MA, Schols JM, *et al.* Patient-clinician communication about end-of-life care in patients with advanced chronic organ failure during one year. *J Pain Symptom Manage* 2015; 49: 1109–1115.
53. Parker SM, Clayton JM, Hancock K, *et al.* A systematic review of prognostic/end-of-life communication with adults in the advanced stages of a life-limiting illness: patient/caregiver preferences for the content, style, and timing of information. *J Pain Symptom Manage* 2007; 34: 81–93.

54. Currow DC, Ward A, Clark K, *et al.* Caregivers for people with end-stage lung disease: characteristics and unmet needs in the whole population. *Int J Chron Obstruct Pulmon Dis* 2008; 3: 753–762.
55. Fried TR, O'Leary JR. Using the experiences of bereaved caregivers to inform patient- and caregiver-centered advance care planning. *J Gen Intern Med* 2008; 23: 1602–1607.
56. Au DH, Udris EM, Fihn SD, *et al.* Differences in health care utilization at the end of life among patients with chronic obstructive pulmonary disease and patients with lung cancer. *Arch Intern Med* 2006; 166: 326–331.
57. Claessens MT, Lynn J, Zhong Z, *et al.* Dying with lung cancer or chronic obstructive pulmonary disease: insights from SUPPORT. *J Am Geriatr Soc* 2000; 48: Suppl. 5, S146–S153.
58. Morrison RS, Morrison EW, Glickman DF. Physician reluctance to discuss advance directives. An empiric investigation of potential barriers. *Arch Intern Med* 1994; 154: 2311–2318.
59. Patel K, Janssen DJ, Curtis JR. Advance care planning in COPD. *Respirology* 2012; 17: 72–78.
60. Curtis JR, Engelberg R, Young JP, *et al.* An approach to understanding the interaction of hope and desire for explicit prognostic information among individuals with severe chronic obstructive pulmonary disease or advanced cancer. *J Palliat Med* 2008; 11: 610–620.
61. Knauft E, Nielsen EL, Engelberg RA, *et al.* Barriers and facilitators to end-of-life care communication for patients with COPD. *Chest* 2005; 127: 2188–2196.
62. Philip J, Gold M, Brand C, *et al.* Negotiating hope with chronic obstructive pulmonary disease patients: a qualitative study of patients and healthcare professionals. *Intern Med J* 2012; 42: 816–822.
63. Wong JS, Gottwald M. Advance care planning discussions in chronic obstructive pulmonary disease: a critical review. *J Palliat Care* 2015; 31: 258–264.
64. Wright AA, Zhang B, Ray A, *et al.* Associations between end-of-life discussions, patient mental health, medical care near death, and caregiver bereavement adjustment. *JAMA* 2008; 300: 1665–1673.
65. Davison SN, Simpson C. Hope and advance care planning in patients with end stage renal disease: qualitative interview study. *BMJ* 2006; 333: 886.
66. Heffner JE, Fahy B, Hilling L, *et al.* Attitudes regarding advance directives among patients in pulmonary rehabilitation. *Am J Respir Crit Care Med* 1996; 154: 1735–1740.
67. Hofmann JC, Wenger NS, Davis RB, *et al.* Patient preferences for communication with physicians about end-of-life decisions. *Ann Intern Med* 1997; 127: 1–12.
68. Gelberg J, McIvor RA. Overcoming gaps in the management of chronic obstructive pulmonary disease in older patients: new insights. *Drugs Aging* 2010; 27: 367–375.
69. McNeely PD, Hébert PC, Dales RE, *et al.* Deciding about mechanical ventilation in end-stage chronic obstructive pulmonary disease: how respirologists perceive their role. *CMAJ* 1997; 156: 177–183.
70. McCormick JR. Pulmonary rehabilitation and palliative care. *Semin Respir Crit Care Med* 2009; 30: 684–699.
71. Perkins HS. Controlling death: the false promise of advance directives. *Ann Intern Med* 2007; 147: 51–57.
72. Reinke LF, Shannon SE, Engelberg RA, *et al.* Supporting hope and prognostic information: nurses' perspectives on their role when patients have life-limiting prognoses. *J Pain Symptom Manage* 2010; 39: 982–992.
73. Reinke LF, Engelberg RA, Shannon SE, *et al.* Transitions regarding palliative and end-of-life care in severe chronic obstructive pulmonary disease or advanced cancer: themes identified by patients, families, and clinicians. *J Palliat Med* 2008; 11: 601–609.
74. Back AL, Arnold RM, Quill TE. Hope for the best, and prepare for the worst. *Ann Intern Med* 2003; 138: 439–443.
75. Wilson IB, Green ML, Goldman L, *et al.* Is experience a good teacher? How interns and attending physicians understand patients' choices for end-of-life care. *Med Decis Making* 1997; 17: 217–227.
76. Detering K, Silvester W, Corke C, *et al.* Teaching general practitioners and doctors-in-training to discuss advance care planning: evaluation of a brief multimodality education programme. *BMJ Support Palliat Care* 2014: 4: 313–321.
77. Clayton JM, Adler JL, O'Callaghan A, *et al.* Intensive communication skills teaching for specialist training in palliative medicine: development and evaluation of an experiential workshop. *J Palliat Med* 2012; 15: 585–591.
78. Clayton JM, Butow PN, Waters A, *et al.* Evaluation of a novel individualised communication-skills training intervention to improve doctors' confidence and skills in end-of-life communication. *Palliat Med* 2013; 27: 236–243.
79. Back AL, Arnold RM, Tulsky JA, *et al.* Teaching communication skills to medical oncology fellows. *J Clin Oncol* 2003; 21: 2433–2436.
80. Kirchhoff KT, Hammes BJ, Kehl KA, *et al.* Effect of a disease-specific planning intervention on surrogate understanding of patient goals for future medical treatment. *J Am Geriatr Soc* 2010; 58: 1233–1240.
81. Lung Foundation Australia. COPD Guidelines: The COPD-X plan. Version 2.45. http://copdx.org.au/copd-xplan/ Date last accessed: March 1, 2016. Date last updated: March 2016.
82. Dept of Health. End of Life Care Strategy: Promoting High Quality Care for All Adults at the End of Life. London, Dept of Health, 2008. www.gov.uk/government/uploads/system/uploads/attachment_data/file/136431/End_of_life strategy.pdf
83. Lanken PN, Terry PB, Delisser HM, *et al.* An official American Thoracic Society clinical policy statement: palliative care for patients with respiratory diseases and critical illnesses. *Am J Respir Crit Care Med* 2008; 177: 912–927.

84. Advance Care Planning Australia. What is Advance Care Planning? http://advancecareplanning.org.au/advance-care-planning Date last accessed: March 1, 2016. Date last updated: February 2016.
85. Clayton JM, Hancock KM, Butow PN, *et al.* Clinical practice guidelines for communicating prognosis and end-of-life issues with adults in the advanced stages of a life-limiting illness, and their caregivers. *Med J Aust* 2007; 186: Suppl., S77–S108.
86. Silveira MJ, Kim SY, Langa KM. Advance directives and outcomes of surrogate decision making before death. *N Engl J Med* 2010; 362: 1211–1218.
87. Winzelberg GS, Hanson LC, Tulsky JA. Beyond autonomy: diversifying end-of-life decision-making approaches to serve patients and families. *J Am Geriatr Soc* 2005; 53: 1046–1050.
88. High DM. Families' roles in advance directives. *Hastings Cent Rep* 1994; 24: S16–S18.
89. Gillick MR. Advance care planning. *N Engl J Med* 2004; 350: 7–8.
90. Jones I, Kirby A, Ormiston P, *et al.* The needs of patients dying of chronic obstructive pulmonary disease in the community. *Fam Pract* 2004; 21: 310–313.
91. Clayton JM, Butow PN, Arnold RM, *et al.* Discussing life expectancy with terminally ill cancer patients and their carers: a qualitative study. *Support Care Cancer* 2005; 13: 733–742.
92. Wenrich MD, Curtis JR, Shannon SE, *et al.* Communicating with dying patients within the spectrum of medical care from terminal diagnosis to death. *Arch Intern Med* 2001; 161: 868–874.
93. Quill TE, Arnold R, Back AL. Discussing treatment preferences with patients who want "everything". *Ann Intern Med* 2009; 151: 345–349.
94. Hickman SE, Keevern E, Hammes BJ. Use of the physician orders for life-sustaining treatment program in the clinical setting: a systematic review of the literature. *J Am Geriatr Soc* 2015; 63: 341–350.

Disclosures: None declared.

Chapter 14

Symptom management at the end of life

Jane L. Phillips and Meera R. Agar

Optimal EOL care addresses the physical, practical, psychosocial and spiritual needs of dying patients and their families. Effective EOL care can readily be provided by the patients' usual care team and delivered in the community, as an inpatient or in a nursing home setting. Initiating EOL care is dependent on clinicians' timely recognition that the patient is dying, and sensitively communicating this reality to the patient, their family and other members of the interdisciplinary care team. Recognition of dying focuses the goals of care on comfort and dignity in accordance with the patients and their families' wishes. It acknowledges the importance of assessing and managing the patient's symptoms, as well as their psychological, social and spiritual care needs.

Adults with advanced respiratory disease have significant symptom burden at the EOL, which is comparable to, if not greater than, the symptoms experienced by people dying from cancer. These patients also experience poorer quality of life and significant social isolation as a result of their symptom burden, yet are less likely to be referred to specialist palliative care services than patients with cancer [1, 2]. Drawing from the palliative care guidance statement from the American Thoracic Society [3], this chapter focuses on the EOL care that can readily be provided by the patients' usual care team, and outlines when referral to specialist palliative care is indicated. It details the importance of clinicians responding to the unpredictable respiratory disease trajectory and the changing needs of the patient and family as death approaches. An overview of the best evidence-based pharmacological and non-pharmacological symptom management strategies for adults dying of advanced respiratory disease, whose prognosis is measured in days to hours, is also provided. This chapter also touches briefly on the care needs of those whose death is sudden (*i.e.* sudden cardiac death, massive haemoptysis or acute pulmonary obstruction) and the bereavement requirements of their families.

Defining EOL care

While chronic respiratory disease increases the risk of sudden cardiac death [4], the majority of patients will die an anticipated death. Globally, the term "EOL care" has been used variously to describe the final stages of a person's life. The time period that "EOL"

Centre for Cardiovascular and Chronic Care, Faculty of Health, University of Technology Sydney, Sydney, Australia.

Correspondence: Jane L. Phillips, Centre for Cardiovascular and Chronic Care, Faculty of Health, University of Technology Sydney, P.O. Box 123, Ultimo, Sydney, NSW 2007, Australia. E-mail: jane.phillips@uts.edu.au

 Print ISBN: 978-1-84984-071-2. Online ISBN: 978-1-84984-072-9. Print ISSN: 2312-508X. Online ISSN: 2312-5098.

encompasses has been variably defined, ranging from the last 12 months of life to the final hours or days of life [3]. For the purposes of this chapter, EOL care refers to the care and support that dying patients and their families require in the last days and hours of life. As described in another chapter of this *Monograph* [5], all clinicians have a responsibility to provide primary palliative care, *i.e.* to provide the necessary physical, psychological, social and spiritual care that advanced respiratory disease patients require at the EOL to optimise their comfort and that their families require to have better bereavement outcomes. If the patient has complex EOL care or their care exceeds the expertise of the interdisciplinary respiratory teams, then referral to the local specialist palliative care team is indicated [6].

Recognising dying and managing the terminal care transition

People living with advanced respiratory disease face the usual challenges of daily living but in a context of increasing exacerbations and deepening dependency as activities and mobility decrease, and their life becomes increasingly confined [7]. Reduced FEV_1, increased breathlessness, reduced physical activity and an increased number of hospital admissions in the past 2 years are all hallmarks of a terminal respiratory disease (table 1). Any one of these acute exacerbations may be a terminal event. The risk of sudden death within 5 years of a COPD diagnosis increases in patients with frequent exacerbations [4]. Faced with a sudden death, the focus of care during these final hours or minutes of life is on minimising the distress and suffering of the patients and their families.

Although acute or chronic respiratory failure is the final common pathway for many patients with advanced respiratory disease [8], too few will have been provided with an opportunity to discuss their EOL care preferences prospectively and to plan accordingly. In high-income countries, the majority of patients now die in hospital, and many receive medically futile, unnecessary and potentially distressing care [9]. A survey of patients with advanced COPD found that less than one-third (32%) had discussed the care they would want in the event that they were unable to communicate their wishes to their treating physician [9]. Clinicians' reluctance to discuss prognosis contributes to the limited understanding of patients and families about their illness trajectory [3]. Failure to plan also leads to patients receiving care that they may otherwise have declined, especially as a proportion may spend their final days ventilated in the ICU or requiring NIV [7].

In clinical situations where the patient has not responded to maximum treatment, and a decision has been made to withdrawal mechanical ventilation or NIV with the expectation that death will follow, clinicians need to communicate to the family the expected symptoms, the time course for deterioration and the expected time to death after withdrawal [10]. Consideration should be given to the likely symptoms that may occur after extubation based on the clinical situation of the individual, in particular the occurrence of breathlessness, and it may be necessary to commence opioids and sedative medication prior to and/or during the withdrawal process, titrating to effect [11].

For most clinicians, dying is viewed as a nonreversible physiological process or a series of negative physiological events from which the patient cannot recover [12]. Recognising when patients have only days or hours to live continues to be challenging for many clinicians, especially given the somewhat unpredictable course of advanced respiratory disease. The dying patient is typically profoundly weak and essentially bed-bound. For much of the day, they can be drowsy and disorientated to time, with a severely limited attention span. They are

Table 1. Criteria for identifying terminal respiratory disease

American Thoracic Society criteria for identifying terminal respiratory disease [3]	**Gold Standards Prognostic Indicator Framework – COPD [8]**
Patients with pulmonary disease will be considered to be requiring terminal care (life expectancy <6 months) if they: 1. Have severe chronic lung disease characterised by both: a) disabling dyspnoea at rest, poor or no response to bronchodilators resulting in decreased functional capacity (*e.g.* bed-to-chair existence), fatigue and cough; and b) progression of end-stage pulmonary disease, as evidenced by increased ED visits or hospitalisations for pulmonary infections and/or respiratory failure or increasing physician home visits (serial decrease of FEV_1 >40 $mL \cdot year^{-1}$ is objective evidence for disease progression). 2. Hypoxia at rest on ambient air (P_{aO_2} $\leqslant$55 mmHg); or oxygen saturation $\leqslant$88% on supplemental oxygen determined by either arterial blood gases or oxygen saturation; or hypercapnia, as evidenced by P_{CO_2} $\geqslant$50 mmHg. These values may be obtained from recent hospital records. 3. Right heart failure secondary to pulmonary disease (cor pulmonale) (*e.g.* not secondary to left heart disease or valvulopathy). 4. Unintended progressive weight loss of >10% of body weight over the preceding 6 months. 5. Resting tachycardia >100 $beats \cdot min^{-1}$.	At least two of the indicators below: Disease assessed to be severe (*e.g.* FEV_1 <30% predicted). Recurrent hospital admissions (at least three in last 12 months due to COPD). Fulfils long-term oxygen therapy criteria. Medical Research Council grade 4/5, *i.e.* shortness of breath after 100 m on the level or confined to house. Signs and symptoms of right heart failure. Combination of other factors (*i.e.* anorexia, previous intensive therapy unit/NIV-resistant organisms). >6 weeks of systemic steroids for COPD in preceding 6 months.

P_{aO_2}: arterial oxygen tension; P_{CO_2}: carbon dioxide tension.

increasingly disinterested in food and water, and find it difficult to swallow medication [13]. There may also be periods of apnoea and/or Cheyne–Stokes respirations, audible respirations, and/or mottling or cyanosed extremities. Considering these changes within the context of each individual patient helps identify when they are dying.

While much attention has been placed on prognostic tools and clinical markers, these measures cannot be reliably applied in everyday clinical practice [3]. The variable effectiveness of new therapeutic interventions adds to the challenges associated with prognosis.

Ruling out all reversible causes needs to be individualised and requires balancing the burden and risks associated with additional diagnostic tests or treatments. Understanding that some palliative treatments aimed at symptom control may also result in an improvement in the patient's condition requires a preparedness to tailor the goals of care to the patient's condition and their values/wishes, and to respond accordingly. Communicating with patients and families about these uncertainties is central to optimising EOL care outcomes [12]. The familiarity, understanding and trust that many long-term doctor–patient relationships have established provides a solid foundation for the respiratory physician to take the lead in sensitively initiating and facilitating EOL discussions with their patients and families. The patient's deteriorating status signals the need to reappraise both the patient's and their family's care and support needs, to avoid medically futile treatments and to be prepared for the remote possibility that, if the patient's condition improves, they will be afforded the opportunity to recover [14]. Managing these uncertainties in conjunction with providing optimal EOL care requires the treating physician to commit to continuously assessing their patient's symptoms, optimising symptom management, minimising distress, and facilitate appropriate and timely communication with the patient, their family and the interdisciplinary team [4].

Confirming the preferred place of death is required, as this location may differ from the patient's and/or family's preferred place of care [15]. If an advance care plan has not been completed previously, then seeking agreement and documenting the goals of care in accordance with the patients' wishes and preferences is a priority, making sure that their cardiopulmonary resuscitation orders are clearly documented and conveyed to the interdisciplinary team.

Families also need clear and regular explanations about the symptoms and signs to expect during the dying process, particularly as, for many, this will be the first death that they have witnessed. They also need to be aware that cardiopulmonary resuscitation offers little benefit for dying patients and may cause more harm and discomfort. Preparing for these conversations makes it easier for clinicians to confirm or elicit the patient's and family's preferences, provide the necessary information, acknowledge concerns, and provide realistic hope and reassurance that the patient's comfort will be maximised [16]. Reassuring families and friends about the teams' commitment to providing comfort is crucial for minimising distress and suffering.

Management of common symptoms

A palliative approach to care is recommended and needs to have been initiated long before the patient is dying [3]. The range of symptoms that patients living with advanced respiratory disease experience during the last days and hours of life can largely be managed by their interdisciplinary respiratory team. A number of international guidelines detail the palliative management of patients with advanced respiratory disease; however, few provide guidance for managing the last days or hours of life [15]. In addition to attending to the patient's physical needs, providing psychosocial and spiritual support to both the patient and family becomes increasingly important as death nears. Not being burdened by symptoms is one the major EOL care concerns of patients and their families.

Polypharmacy is common in patients at the EOL. Rational deprescribing of nonessential medication(s) (*i.e.* statins, hypoglycaemics, antihypertensives and anticoagulants) is also indicated at this time [17]. If maintenance of specific medications is indicated, changing the route of administration or drug may be required once the patient has difficulty swallowing.

Optimising the management of EOL symptoms is a key element of effective EOL care. A brief overview of the current evidence for the management of EOL symptoms experienced by patients dying from advanced respiratory disease is detailed below.

Breathlessness

Breathlessness (dyspnoea) is a complex, subjective symptom that is almost universally experienced by people dying of advanced respiratory disease. Nearly all (95%) patients with COPD experience breathlessness, and it is also common in patients with lung fibrosis, heart failure and terminal cancer. Breathlessness increases as death approaches [18]. Regular screening is needed to detect the presence of breathlessness, using the 11-point NRS to determine intensity, unpleasantness and/or distress. The presence of breathlessness on screening should prompt further assessment. Clinical judgement needs to be used to select the best assessment tool, as there is no one tool that has been validated in a dying COPD population, and patients will vary in their capacity to self-report, in particular if their level of consciousness or ability to talk in sentences is impaired [19]. It is important to note that observed signs (*e.g.* tachypnoea) do not necessarily correlate with the perceived breathlessness, so self-reporting, wherever possible, assists in optimising symptom management. When the person is no longer able to self-report, understanding how observed signs had correlated previously to their symptom experience can also be helpful information.

In terms of pharmacological management, oral or parental opioids are the only medications that impact positively on breathlessness [20]. There is good evidence that opioids, if carefully titrated, are safe to use in this population [21]. Many patients will already have been prescribed opioids, so once they are unable to swallow, their usual opioid dose needs to be converted to an equivalent subcutaneous dose (*e.g.* using the eviQ online Opioid Conversion Calculator at www.eviq.org.au). For the opioid-naïve patient, small doses of parenteral (subcutaneous) morphine of 1–2.5 mg can be given regularly (frequency of 4 hourly) for breathlessness (and/or pain), with access to as-required doses for breakthrough and titrated for effect. A subcutaneous continuous infusion of morphine over 24 h may be considered once the dose requirements are stable, which can minimise the need for frequent dose administration, in particular if the person is being cared for at home by family.

However, there is no evidence that nebulised opioids are any better than nebulised saline [20]. It is also important to consider the possibility of acute changes in renal function, and to alter opioid dosing or the agent accordingly to avoid acute accumulation. Although they are widely used, there is no evidence that benzodiazepines relieve breathlessness in patients with advanced respiratory disease. Given their adverse side-effects, benzodiazepines should only be considered if opioids and all other non-pharmacological interventions have failed to relieve the patient's breathlessness [22].

There is also limited evidence for the feasibility and usefulness of NIV at the EOL for comfort and to minimise adverse effects [23]. Oxygen therapy is helpful for reducing breathlessness in advanced respiratory disease patients with hypoxaemia [3]. If oxygen is indicated, the use of nasal prongs at the EOL may be more appropriate than a mask. Regular mouth care is required to minimise the drying effects of oxygen. If the patient is still conscious, giving them small chips of ice also helps keep their mouth moist. Teaching and supporting families to attend to the patient's mouth care in between routine care ensures that their mouth remains moist and clean. Other non-pharmacological approaches that are comforting include raising the head of the bed so that the patient's head and torso are elevated or positioning the patient with the affected lung downwards. Positioning the patient near an open window or placing a fan in the room may also provide some comfort.

Pain

After breathlessness, pain is the most commonly experienced EOL symptom. Unrelieved pain is the symptom that most patients fear and is the one symptom that bereaved families perceive to have been managed ineffectively [24]. Routinely assessing dying patients using a validated screening tool, such as the NRS [25], and undertaking a comprehensive pain assessment using a validated tool, such as the Brief Pain Inventory, is required to prevent the patient's pain from being undetected and unrelieved [26]. If the pain is new, differentiating between nociceptive and neuropathic pain enables the most appropriate pain management plan to be initiated. Most pain(s) can readily be controlled with an appropriate individually tailored analgesic regimen, which may include simple analgesics, opioids and/or non-pharmacological interventions, while more complex pain will require the input of the specialist palliative care or pain management team.

Respiratory secretions

Respiratory tract secretions are common and are predictive of imminent death within hours to days. The prevalence rates for respiratory tract secretions vary, with most available estimates generated for cancer patient populations [27]. Impairment of effective swallowing and coughing reflexes causes secretions to accumulate in the pharynx and/or airways [27]. It is thought that respiratory tract secretions are more common when pulmonary pathology exists, such as infection or lung cancer [28, 29]. It is unclear whether patients perceive the presence of respiratory secretions as distressing [27, 29]. Experiences from families who have witnessed the patient's respiratory secretions at the EOL also vary, but at least half found this symptom to be distressing [30, 31]. Health professionals providing care, as well as other patients, may also find the sound distressing [27]. Interpretation is influenced by the patient's appearance, and whether families believed it indicated that the person was drowning or choking [31]. Some families understood it as a useful warning sign that death was imminent [31]. It is important for families to be prepared for the possibility of respiratory secretions, and also for clinicians to spend time dispelling unfounded fears [27].

There is currently no evidence that pharmacological intervention with antimuscarinic medication is superior to placebo in the management of respiratory secretions [27, 32]. Studies that have been conducted have been limited to cancer, have lacked placebo controls, are unable to establish if the reduction in noise intensity is associated with a change in the patient's experience, and vary in the degree of objectivity of the measurement efficacy measure [32]. If a choice to use anticholinergics is made, it is critical that they are regularly re-evaluated for therapeutic benefit and adverse effects. They should be discontinued if there is no benefit and/or there are side-effects that are likely to be associated with greater patient distress [32]. Anticholinergic medications are commonly associated with side-effects such as dry mouth, urinary retention and delirium [27]; however, these effects are frequently under-recognised, as patients at the EOL are usually semi- or unconscious.

Avoidance of the use of parenteral hydration to prevent or reduce secretions is also an unestablished practice. Therapies to treat increased sputum production, purulence, and lower respiratory tract infections refractory to antibiotics and other treatments are yet to be evaluated for COPD patients in the EOL phase. It is unclear whether antibiotics offer symptom relief in this situation [33].

Non-pharmacological interventions, such as repositioning or removal of secretions by oropharyngeal suction, have also had minimal evaluation but can be considered in individual circumstances [32]. Most interventions are unable to eliminate existing secretions completely [27]. Indiscriminate use of anticholinergics is not supported, but current evidence, and careful and ongoing explanations to relatives covering the cause and implications and also addressing their fears about the secretions, should be the focus of care.

Delirium

Delirium is a recognised medical complication of serious and advanced illness. Delirium prevalence has been reported to be as high as 88% in people in the days to hours before death [34]. The clinical features of delirium develop acutely and fluctuate over time; they include disturbed consciousness, attention and awareness, disorientation, perceptual disturbance, sleep–wake cycle abnormalities and psychomotor disturbance (agitation or hypoactivity) [35]. Delirium in this setting is often a result of irreversible factors such as multiorgan failure, refractory infection or metabolic abnormalities [36]. However, even in the setting of irreversible delirium, it is important to review possible contributing factors (*e.g.* psychoactive medication, urinary retention, constipation or uncontrolled pain), which may make delirium symptoms worse, in particular if the issue is still amenable to simple noninvasive treatments. It is important to avoid nonspecific descriptive terms as diagnoses (*e.g.* terminal restlessness, terminal agitation), and instead to consider the specific differential diagnoses as much as is practicable, although it is acknowledged that this can be challenging. Differential diagnoses may include other uncontrolled symptoms (such as pain), urinary retention or constipation, seizures and metabolic causes of myoclonus, all which have specific approaches to management.

There is no current evidence that parenteral hydration improves delirium symptom control, and a change in opioid or a reduction in dose is only recommended where there are clear indications of opioid neurotoxicity. Current evidence does not support the use of antipsychotics to treat delirium symptoms [37, 38]. Families vary in their level of distress in witnessing delirium symptoms and need support during this time [35, 36]. It is important to ensure that discussions about prognosis are had, as delirium is often a predictor of death. Families also need an explanation about what delirium is (a medical condition due to multiple causes altering brain function, rather than a psychiatric condition), and acknowledgement that it causes distress to the patient and their family. Clinicians also need to recognise that being mentally aware is highly valued at the EOL, and should not assume that sedation is the treatment choice that would be chosen by all patients or their surrogate decision makers [35, 36]. Non-pharmacological approaches such as having familiar family in attendance, familiar objects in the room, maximising hearing and vision by ensuring the use of glasses and hearing aids, and minimising changes in the environment, such as room changes, can also minimise symptoms and distress for the dying patient and their family.

Anxiety

Anxiety is commonly experienced by two-thirds of patients with advanced respiratory disease [39]. It can be related to the disease itself or can emerge as a result of an underlying anxiety disorder, premorbid drug and alcohol issues, unrelieved pain, breathlessness or other symptoms [39]. Lower ego integrity, more physical problems and more psychological problems are predictive of higher levels of death anxiety in elderly people [40].

Although a range of pharmacological agents is routinely used to manage anxiety, there is little evidence for their effectiveness in patients during their last days and hours [41]. While addressing the underlying drivers of anxiety offers the best course of action, a low-dose anxiolytic may be required to manage escalating anxiety; however, its introduction needs to be balanced against its potential harm (*i.e.* increased drowsiness, reduced ability to communicate with family). Although benzodiazepines are commonly prescribed at the EOL, they can impair the patient's memory and cause dizziness, drowsiness, increased falls and anterograde amnesia [42].

If the patient is alert enough, social work or pastoral care input may help alleviate anxiety related to psychological or spiritual distress. Providing the patient with an opportunity to have their questions answered and supporting the family to stand by the patient can also do much to minimise anxiety at the EOL.

Cough

Cough is a prevalent and distressing symptom that can persist up to the time of death. Advanced disease, an accumulation of secretions, asthenia, muscle weakness and/or the inability to coordinate swallowing all contribute to ineffective, persistent involuntary coughing at the EOL. A moist cough in a patient dying of COPD is best managed with anticholinergic medications [43]. Although there is no convincing evidence that any of the commonly used drugs (*i.e.* opioids or over-the-counter cough syrups) are effective for cough in COPD patients [44, 45], there is some evidence that dextromethorphan may be helpful [45]. While there is some evidence for the use of mucolytic agents for the management of cough for patients with COPD, the effectiveness of these drugs at the EOL has not been investigated [43]. There is also no evidence to support the use of nebulised lignocaine or other local anaesthetics, and even less evidence for non-pharmacological intervention that minimises the burden of cough at the EOL.

Management of refractory symptoms

There are occasions when a dying patient's breathlessness, pain or delirium is not relieved by the optimal use of recommended palliative treatment regimes and the patient is experiencing significant distress as a result of this persistent symptom(s). In the context of refractory symptoms, palliative sedation may be indicated, but only after the patient has been thoroughly assessed by an interdisciplinary team (*i.e.* palliative physician, pain expert, psychosocial counsellor and pastoral care) and with the prior informed consent of the patient themselves. The interdisciplinary team needs to determine that all possible treatments have been optimised and that, based on their repeated and careful assessments,

Table 2. Essential domains of EOL care

Effective communication and shared decision making
- Communicate to the patient/family why no further investigation/treatment is indicated
- Ensure that there is an agreed plan of care and that a cardiopulmonary resuscitation order that reflects the wishes of the patient and their family is in place
- Actively involve the patient and family in the decision-making process
- Continue to orientate the patient to place, time and person

Respectful and compassionate care
- Maintain the patient's comfort and dignity
- Maintain mobility for as long as possible (*i.e.* support the patient to sit up, to sit out of bed for short periods and to use a bedside commode, if desired and safe to do so)
- Maintain hydration and diet for as long as possible (*i.e.* support the patient to sit up and assist them with eating or drinking as desired)
- Manage hygiene (*i.e.* personal hygiene, mouth care, eye care and continence – use incontinence aids but avoid catheterisation)
- Encourage families to continue to speak, touch and comfort the patient
- If comfortable and acceptable to the patient, allow the family to assist with the provision of personal care (*i.e.* mouth care, massage of hands and feet)

Expert care
- Regularly assess the patient's symptoms and adjust management accordingly
- Initiate rationale deprescribing of unnecessary oral medications
- Convert necessary medications to the subcutaneous or sublingual route
- Vital signs – limited to the parameters of interest where a response is required to ensure comfort
- Maintain skin integrity (*i.e.* pressure area care, repositioning, use of pressure-relieving mattresses, wound care and infusion site care, as required)

Trust and confidence in clinicians
- Identifying and communicate with the patient and family that the patient is dying
- Prepare the family for the physiological changes they are likely to observe during the dying process (*i.e.* explain the changes that are expected/occurring as death approaches)
- Provide ongoing emotional and practical support to the patient and family
- Refer the patient/family to the counsellor, social worker and pastoral care, as required
- Be prepared to offer but not impose spiritual care
- Provide volunteers' input/support as required for the patient and family, especially if the family are unable to stay and the patient does not wish to be alone
- After the death, provide the family with the opportunity to spend time with the deceased, as well as information about bereavement support services

Adequate environment for care and minimising burden (patient priority)
- Ensure privacy and space for the dying patient and their family
- Access to a single room may be preferred
- Provide the family with onsite access to a kitchenette and a place to rest

Financial affairs (family priority)
- Be mindful of the financial implications of EOL care for families (*i.e.* accommodation/travel, healthcare, homecare and childcare costs, and the need to take unpaid leave)
- Ensure that the patient's legal affairs are in order, and refer for social work support

no other methods are available for alleviation of the refractory symptoms within the life expectancy time frame. There needs to be consensus within the team that the benefits of palliative sedation outweigh the risks of what the patient can tolerate [46]. There are also cases where acute distressing events (*i.e.* massive bleeding, grand mal seizures or acute airway obstruction) require the use of palliative sedation. In these situations, the monitored use of nonopioid drugs (*i.e.* benzodiazepines, barbiturates and propofol) at a dose and in a manner that are ethically acceptable to the patient, family and healthcare team may be indicated to relieve the burden of otherwise intractable suffering. The patient and family need to be aware that administering palliative sedation will induce unconsciousness, which is likely to be irreversible and is in the context of death being expected [45].

Achieving a good death

Across the developed world, dying patients and families have identified maintaining control, good symptom management, an opportunity for closure, affirmation of the dying person, recognition of and preparation for impending death, and not being a burden as necessary for a "good death" [47–49]. A recent systematic review similarly confirmed that 1) effective communication and shared decision making, 2) expert care, 3) respectful and compassionate care, and 4) trust and confidence in clinicians are the most important EOL care elements for dying in both patients and their families [50]. The fifth next most important element differs, with financial affairs being important to families, while an adequate environment for care and minimising the burden are both important to patients [50]. In addition to effective symptom management, the type of care that dying patients and their families desire is person-centred, holistic interdisciplinary palliative care (table 2). Importantly, care for the family after the person's death is also critical, and health professionals have a role to provide support at the time of death, and also to refer them if necessary for ongoing bereavement support.

Conclusion

The provision of person-centred, holistic interdisciplinary EOL care is care that is grounded in best evidence-based symptom management and is focused on comfort and dignity; most importantly, it is care that is readily achievable within our current healthcare system. Regardless of the care setting, person-centred, holistic interdisciplinary EOL care offers the best chance of meeting the EOL care needs of patients dying of advanced respiratory disease and of minimising their family's distress. It is care that can readily be provided by the patient's usual care team or in partnership with the specialist palliative care team if the patient has complex EOL care needs. The greatest barrier to providing this type of EOL care is the failure of clinicians to recognise when the patient with advanced respiratory disease is dying and to initiate crucial and timely EOL conversations. Failure to initiate these conversations makes it difficult to put in place all of the necessary treatments and care that patients and their families require to minimise suffering and distress at the EOL.

References

1. Brown CE, Jecker NS, Curtis JR. Inadequate palliative care in chronic lung disease. An issue of health care inequality. *Ann Am Thorac Soc* 2016; 13: 311–316.
2. Ahmadi Z, Lundström S, Janson C, *et al.* End-of-life care in oxygen-dependent COPD and cancer: a national population-based study. *Eur Respir J* 2015; 46: 1190–1193.

3. Lanken PN, Terry PB, Delisser HM, *et al.* An official American Thoracic Society clinical policy statement: palliative care for patients with respiratory diseases and critical illnesses. *Am J Respir Crit Care Med* 2008; 177: 912–927.
4. Lahousse L, Niemeijer MN, van den Berg ME, *et al.* Chronic obstructive pulmonary disease and sudden cardiac death: the Rotterdam study. *Eur Heart J* 2015; 36: 1754–1761.
5. Kayser JB, Mooney-Doyle K, Lanken PN. Definitions and policy. *In*: Bausewein C, Currow DC, Johnson MJ, eds. Palliative Care in Respiratory Disease (ERS Monograph). Sheffield, European Respiratory Society, 2016; pp. 1–20.
6. Quill TE, Abernethy AP. Generalist plus specialist palliative care – creating a more sustainable model. *N Engl J Med* 2013; 368: 1173–1175.
7. Nava S, Sturani C, Hartl S, *et al.* End-of-life decision-making in respiratory intermediate care units: a European survey. *Eur Respir J* 2007; 30: 156–164.
8. Thomas K. The GSF Prognostic Indicator Guidance. London, The Gold Standards Framework Centre, 2011.
9. Stapleton RD, Randall Curtis J. End of life considerations in older patients with lung disease. *Clin Chest Med* 2007; 28: 801–811.
10. Long AC, Muni S, Treece PD, *et al.* Time to death after terminal withdrawal of mechanical ventilation: specific respiratory and physiologic parameters may inform physician predictions. *J Palliat Med* 2015; 18: 1040–1047.
11. Epker JL, Bakker J, Lingsma HF, *et al.* an observational study on a protocol for withdrawal of life-sustaining measures on two non-academic intensive care units in the Netherlands: few signs of distress, no suffering? *J Pain Symptom Manage* 2015; 50: 676–684.
12. Taylor PM, Johnson M. Recognizing dying in terminal illness. *Br J Hosp Med* 2011; 72: 446–450.
13. Palliative Care Outcomes Collaboration. PCOC: Assessment Tool Definitions: Phase. Wollongong, Australia, University of Wollongong, 2008.
14. Kennedy C, Brooks-Young P, Brunton Gray C, *et al.* Diagnosing dying: an integrative literature review. *BMJ Support Palliat Care* 2014; 4: 263–270.
15. Siouta N, van Beek K, Preston N, *et al.* Towards integration of palliative care in patients with chronic heart failure and chronic obstructive pulmonary disease: a systematic literature review of European guidelines and pathways. *BMC Palliat Care* 2016; 15: 1–12.
16. Clayton JM, Hancock KM, Butow PN, *et al.* Clinical practice guidelines for communicating prognosis and end-of-life issues with adults in the advanced stages of a life-limiting illness, and their caregivers. *Med J Aust* 2007; 186: Suppl., S77–S108.
17. Therapeutic Guidelines Ltd. Therapeutic Guidelines: Palliative Care (version 3). Melbourne, Therapeutic Guidelines Ltd, 2010.
18. Currow DC, Smith J, Davidson PM, *et al.* Do the trajectories of dyspnea differ in prevalence and intensity by diagnosis at the end of life? A consecutive cohort study. *J Pain Symptom Manage* 2010; 39: 680–690.
19. Bausewein C, Farquhar M, Booth S, *et al.* Measurement of breathlessness in advanced disease: a systematic review. *Respir Med* 2007; 101: 399–410.
20. Jennings A-L, Davies AN, Higgins JPT, *et al.* A systematic review of the use of opioids in the management of dyspnoea. *Thorax* 2002; 57: 939–944.
21. Ekström MP, Bornefalk-Hermansson A, Abernethy AP, *et al.* Safety of benzodiazepines and opioids in very severe respiratory disease: national prospective study. *BMJ* 2014; 348: g445.
22. Simon ST, Higginson IJ, Booth S, *et al.* Benzodiazepines for the relief of breathlessness in advanced malignant and non-malignant diseases in adults. *Cochrane Database Syst Rev* 2010; 1: CD007354.
23. Curtis JR, Cook DJ, Sinuff T, *et al.* Noninvasive positive pressure ventilation in critical and palliative care settings: understanding the goals of therapy. *Crit Care Med* 2007; 35: 932–939.
24. Lynn J, Teno J, Phillips R, *et al.* Perceptions by family members of the dying experience of older and seriously ill patients. *Ann Intern Med* 1997; 126: 97–106.
25. Hjermstad MJ, Fayers PM, Haugen DF, *et al.* Studies comparing Numerical Rating Scales, Verbal Rating Scales, and Visual Analogue Scales for assessment of pain intensity in adults: a systematic literature review. *J Pain Symptom Manage* 2011; 41: 1073–1093.
26. Dudgeon DJ, Harlos M, Clinch JJ. The Edmonton Symptom Assessment Scale (ESAS) as an audit tool. *J Palliat Care* 1999; 15: 14–19.
27. Mercadamte S. Death rattle: critical review and research agenda. *Support Care Cancer* 2013; 22: 571–575.
28. Morita T, Hyodo I, Yoshimi T, *et al.* Incidence and underlying etiologies of bronchial secretion in terminally ill cancer patients: a multicenter, prospective, observational study. *J Pain Symptom Manage* 2004; 27: 533–539.
29. Lokker ME, van Zuylen L, van der Rijt CC, *et al.* Prevalence, impact, and treatment of death rattle: a systematic review. *J Pain Symptom Manage* 2014; 47: 105–122.
30. Wee BL, Coleman PG, Hillier R, *et al.* The sound of death rattle I: are relatives distressed by hearing this sound? *Palliat Med* 2006; 20: 171–175.
31. Wee BL, Coleman PG, Hillier R, *et al.* The sound of death rattle II: how do relatives interpret the sound? *Palliat Med* 2006; 20: 177–181.

32. Wee B, Hillier R. Interventions for noisy breathing in patients near to death. *Cochrane Database Syst Rev* 2008; 1: CD005177.
33. Juthani-Mehta M, Malani PN, Mitchell SL. Antimicrobials at the end of life: an opportunity to improve palliative care and infection management. *JAMA* 2015; 314: 2017–2018.
34. Hosie A, Davidson PM, Agar M, *et al.* Delirium prevalence, incidence, and implications for screening in specialist palliative care inpatient settings: a systematic review. *Palliat Med* 2013; 27: 486–498.
35. Breitbart W, Alici Y. Agitation and delirium at the end of life: "We couldn't manage him". *JAMA* 2008; 300: 2898–910. E1.
36. Bush SH, Bruera E, Lawlor PG, *et al.* Clinical practice guidelines for delirium management: potential application in palliative care. *J Pain Symptom Manage* 2014; 48: 249–258.
37. Agar M, Lawlor P, Quinn S, *et al.* Phase III randomized double-blind controlled trial of oral risperidone, haloperidol or placebo with rescue subcutaneous midazolam for delirium management in palliative care. *J Am Geriatr Soc* 2015; 63: S99–S99.
38. Neufeld KJ, Yue J, Robinson TN, *et al.* Antipsychotic medication for prevention and treatment of delirium in hospitalized adults: a systematic review and meta-analysis. *J Am Geriatr Soc* 2016; 64: 705–714.
39. Solano JP, Gomes B, Higginson IJ. A comparison of symptom prevalence in far advanced cancer, AIDS, heart disease, chronic obstructive pulmonary disease and renal disease. *J Pain Symptom Manage* 2006; 31: 58–69.
40. Fortner BV, Neimeyer RA. Death anxiety in older adults: a quantitative review. *Death Stud* 1999; 23: 387–411.
41. Candy B, Jackson KC, Jones L, *et al.* Drug therapy for symptoms associated with anxiety in adult palliative care patients. *Cochrane Database Syst Rev* 2012; 10: CD004596.
42. Henderson M, MacGregor E, Sykes N, *et al.* The use of benzodiazepines in palliative care. *Palliat Med* 2006; 20: 407–412.
43. Poole P, Chong J, Cates CJ. Mucolytic agents versus placebo for chronic bronchitis or chronic obstructive pulmonary disease. *Cochrane Database Syst Rev* 2015; 7: CD001287.
44. Bolser DC. Cough suppressant and pharmacologic protussive therapy: ACCP evidence-based clinical practice guidelines. *Chest* 2006; 129: Suppl., 238S–249S.
45. Wee B, Browning J, Adams A, *et al.* Management of chronic cough in patients receiving palliative care: review of evidence and recommendations by a task group of the Association for Palliative Medicine of Great Britain and Ireland. *Palliat Med* 2012; 26: 780–787.
46. Cherny NI, Radbruch L. European Association for Palliative Care (EAPC) recommended framework for the use of sedation in palliative care. *Palliat Med* 2009; 23: 581–593.
47. Kehl KA. Moving toward peace: an analysis of the concept of a good death. *Am J Hosp Palliat Med* 2006; 23: 277–286.
48. Steinhauser KE, Christakis NA, Clipp EC, *et al.* Preparing for the end of life: preferences of patients, families, physicians, and other care providers. *J Pain Symp Manage* 2001; 22: 727–737.
49. Steinhauser K, Christakis N, Clipp E, *et al.* Factors considered important at the end of life by patients, family, physicians, and other care providers. *JAMA* 2000; 284: 2476–2482.
50. Virdun C, Luckett T, Davidson PM, *et al.* Dying in the hospital setting: a systematic review of quantitative studies identifying the elements of end-of-life care that patients and their families rank as being most important. *Palliat Med* 2015; 29: 774–796.

Disclosures: None declared.

Chapter 15

End-stage respiratory diseases and respiratory support

Paola Pierucci[1] and Annalisa Carlucci[2]

This chapter will focus on reviewing the current literature on care of dying patients with end-stage respiratory disorders in the last days of their life. First, the focus will be on recognising, assessing and relieving the most typical late-stage symptom: breathlessness (dyspnoea). Secondly, specific challenges to face when looking after these patients will be discussed: assisted breathing, oxygen use, mechanical ventilation withdrawal, medications and the role of palliative care. Lastly, ancillary topics will be covered, such as ethics, spiritual needs, and patients' and their families' perspectives.

The care of imminently dying patients unavoidably creates emotional and clinical challenges to the supporting team surrounding the patients and their families [1–3]. Training and experience in EOL care have now received appropriate recognition with the institution of palliative care as a specialty [4, 5]. However, much more remains to be done in order to improve the care of non-cancer patients who are dying, and to reach the goal of a higher standard of care that is already part of the routine care of people with advanced cancer. In fact, education in the assessment and management of the symptoms of end-stage respiratory diseases is needed as each of us as specialists face the potential death of our patients [6]. We therefore aim to review the current literature about the care of patients with end-stage respiratory disorders.

Dying from end-stage respiratory diseases

In 2012, the World Health Organization stated that COPD was the third leading cause of death globally, killing 3.1 million people [7]. A comparison of data over the past decade has shown no change in the number of people dying from COPD between 2000 and 2012, while a significant improvement was noted for the first two leading causes of death: ischaemic heart disease and stroke [7]. In addition, more than 50% of people affected by CRD live in low- and middle-income countries or deprived populations where whole populations are exposed to risk factors over their entire life span [7]. This poses questions on the real magnitude of the problem, as these numbers may be underestimated. The conclusion is that COPD-related deaths are expected to increase in the years ahead [7]. Interestingly, to date, only a few studies have focused their research on the care of people

[1]Dept of Respiratory Medicine, Concord Hospital, University of Sydney, NSW, Australia. [2]Pulmonary Rehabilitation Unit, IRCCS Fondazione S. Maugeri, Pavia, Italy.

Correspondence: Annalisa Carlucci, IRCCS Fondazione S. Maugeri, Via S. Maugeri 10, Pavia 27100, Italy. E-mail: annalisa.carlucci@fsm.it

 Print ISBN: 978-1-84984-071-2. Online ISBN: 978-1-84984-072-9. Print ISSN: 2312-508X. Online ISSN: 2312-5098.

dying from respiratory diseases [8–12]. To date, the majority of research has explored populations with cancer, including lung cancer. As expected, the last hours or days of patients' lives affected by respiratory diseases are usually characterised by several symptoms common to other pathologies: breathlessness (dyspnoea), fatigue, respiratory secretions (death rattle) and anxiety. However, delirium, confusion, loss of consciousness and severe pain are also experienced. Furthermore, depression and fear of imminent death appear to have a significant role in the complex picture of this group of dying people [8–11, 13–16].

Among patients with end-stage respiratory disorders, and in COPD patients in particular, breathlessness is the most prevalent symptom, affecting between 90% and 95% of people [13].

Over the last few years, many studies have tried to define breathlessness in patients with CRD. Thus, breathlessness can be further characterised as chronic, episodic or a 'breathlessness crisis' [6, 17, 18]. Chronic breathlessness persists despite treatments directed to address the underlying pathology, and is frequently encountered in patients affected by chronic cardiopulmonary diseases and lung cancer [17, 19]. A recent systematic review of the use of systematic opioids in COPD concluded that there was moderate benefit that was delivered safely in this population. The role of nebulised opioids required further research before it could be considered standard therapy [20]. Episodic breathlessness is defined as intermittent, short-term worsening of breathlessness beyond the usual chronic breathlessness that this patient type reports [18]. When episodic breathlessness episodes were observed in different patient populations, they were found to have a variable duration, being on average longer in people with COPD compared with people with lung cancer, with the majority of episodes lasting less than 20 min. These findings have opened a new line of enquiry as to how best to palliate this pattern of breathlessness, where current therapies may be inadequate, given the time until their onset of action [21]. A breathlessness crisis is, by definition of the American Thoracic Society (ATS) *ad hoc* committee, breathlessness near to death [6]. This separate entity is defined as "sustained and severe resting breathing discomfort that occurs in patients with advanced, often life-limiting illness and overwhelms the patient and caregivers' ability to achieve symptom relief". Using this definition, a breathlessness crisis embraces three main issues: acute worsening of the experience of breathlessness, a psychosocial/spiritual patient response, and a chaotic setting when sometimes caregivers are too overwhelmed to respond optimally. Not unexpectedly, patients will experience this as a distressing event, which in itself may worsen breathlessness, anxiety and fear, and may potentially worsen a range of other nonrespiratory symptoms. Hence, the challenge is to try to objectively measure a patient's discomfort, believe their assessments and respond to them appropriately [6, 10, 22–24].

The use of respiratory devices (*e.g.* oxygen mask, endotracheal tube, NIV mask, humidifier) can complicate things further in these patients. It also needs to be remembered that, when caring for people who are dying, the clinical scenario can change very quickly [6, 10].

Clearly, in the last days of life, it is highly relevant for the purpose of accurately assessing patients' breathlessness to distinguish between cognitively intact patients and those who are not, as different measurement tools will be necessary.

There are several tools to assess breathlessness in cognitively intact patients with chronic advanced disease. Usually, the VAS, NRS and modified Borg scale (mBORG) offer good available outcome measures, and they are the most commonly used in clinical practice [25,

26]. The VAS and NRS are used to evaluate a characteristic or attitude that is believed to range across a continuum of values, and both have been used to assess breathlessness. The NRS has been shown to be a more repeatable measure than the VAS, which is usually used for within-subject repeated measurements rather than for comparison between different patients, or between groups of patients. The mBORG scale, instead, was initially conceived to assess the intensity of exertion during exercise in healthy subjects, and was then modified and utilised to identify the intensity of breathlessness in patients with chronic lung disease; notably, it has the advantage that it can be used over the phone [19, 25, 26].

In theory, identical physiological changes that trigger distress in the patient with intact cognition will then produce similar distress when the patient experiences declining cognition. It should be noted that an inability to report symptom distress does not mean that the person is not experiencing suffering. This is of particular concern for symptoms such as breathlessness that are subjective. Some researchers have explored the topic and have proposed valid alternative measurement scales to quantify end-stage breathlessness in the context of impaired consciousness [27, 28]. These studies have clearly stated that, during these settings, a "yes" or "no" answer to the question "Are you short of breath?" may be the best guide to palliation, as trying to grade intensity may cause more distress. Observation and close monitoring of worsening signs of respiratory distress may be useful in this setting. A patient's family may also be of benefit at these stressful times [28].

Campbell *et al.* [29] have provided a Respiratory Distress Observation Scale. This scale is a behavioural assessment tool that focuses on eight parameters: heart rate, respiratory rate, accessory muscle use, paradoxical breathing pattern, restlessness, grunting at end-expiration, nasal flaring and a fearful facial display. Each parameter is scored from 0 to 2 points and the points are summed. Scale scores range from 0, signifying no distress, to 16, signifying the most severe distress. The purpose of this tool was to cover the gap in the knowledge of how to assess patients near to death with impaired consciousness who were vulnerable and unable to self-report breathlessness. Patients with neuromuscular damage and people experiencing locked-in syndrome or severe neuromuscular chest disorders are not suitable to be evaluated with this scale [29].

As mentioned previously, the ATS introduced in 2013 the concept of a breathlessness crisis, which highlights that respiratory symptoms play a key role in the last of days of life. In more detail, the consensus states that an important part of the problem is to address efficient communication, and care coordination. The COMFORT approach is an effective mnemonic tool offered, where C=call for help and calming voice and approach to patients and care givers; O=observe closely and assess breathlessness for ways to respond; M=medications to be tried; F=fan to face, which may decrease shortness of breath; O=oxygen therapy as previously found useful; R=reassure and use relaxation techniques; and T=timing and intervention to reduce breathlessness; work together, reassess and repeat.

An important part of the approach is not to underestimate the profound psychosocial downstream impact that breathlessness has on the quality of life of patients and their families. The ATS consensus stresses the point of maintaining a holistic approach in support of both patients and their families [6].

In this context, the *One Chance to Get it Right* document from the Leadership Alliance for the Care of Dying People [30] defined five priorities of care: 1) the possibility that a person may die within the coming days and hours is recognised and communicated clearly, decisions about care are made in accordance with the person's needs and wishes, and these are reviewed and revised regularly; 2) sensitive communication takes place between staff and the person who is dying and those important to them; 3) the dying person, and those identified as important to them, are involved in decisions about treatment and care; 4) the people important to the dying person are listened to and their needs are respected; and 5) care is tailored to the individual and delivered with compassion, with an individual care plan in place.

Davis and Tomas [31] reflected that: "No tool, irrespective of how well created or intended, could or should replace a values-based practice attending to a person, and the needs of his or her personhood." This article identified 10 facets of personhood to be considered at the EOL: spirituality, symptoms, expectation, emotions, legacy, sustenance, individuality, interaction, family, and dignity of self and others. Once again, this puts the accent on the global meaning of the word "care", which should never be discontinued, although other treatments may be. Moreover, the authors invoked the sunrise of the "professionalism" era and the sunset of the "paternalism" era. They suggested that, the sooner more literature on these topics appears, the sooner the paternalism attitude should be abandoned, so that enough space can be offered to education and professional standardised practice [31].

A recent Cochrane review also explored the effect of EOL care practice [32]. In this review, the use of an EOL pathway was compared with no pathway, as well as the use of one EOL pathway compared with another EOL pathway. Only one RCT was found, as none of the other studies met the inclusion criteria. The selected study by Costantini *et al.* [33] studied the Liverpool Care Pathway in eight Italian palliative care units, studying a population of people with cancer only [33]. This pathway, currently used in medical studies, showed no difference in key parameters between services that did and did not use the pathway. New RCTs, as suggested by the review's authors, will need to stratify participants in order to embrace the different care settings where these patients are cared for: emergency medicine, palliative care, intensive care, and general and specialist medicine.

Ongoing challenges

Supported breathing

The use of supported breathing aids in care of the dying with otherwise untreatable respiratory discomfort remains controversial. NIV has been suggested to be potentially useful during palliation as a measure to maximise comfort and minimise distress [34]. To date, only a small number of studies have addressed this topic. Although focused mainly on people with end-stage cancer, the use of NIV has shown some benefits. In fact, in a pilot study, it was demonstrated that its use in patients affected by end-stage solid cancer complicated by acute respiratory failure is feasible and, in a proportion of patients, is effective in providing a rapid improvement in breathlessness [35].

In a more structured, multicentre RCT by Nava *et al.* [36], which compared oxygen therapy with NIV in people with end-stage solid cancers, NIV reduced breathlessness and respiratory rate more quickly, with reduced morphine doses administered. In particular, when looking closely at the subpopulation of people with hypercapnia before applying NIV, these results reached statistical significance [36].

However, the use of NIV for pure palliation in people with non-cancer respiratory diseases is less certain. Before any decision making, as physicians, we should always refresh ourselves about the goal of care: *primum non nocere* ("first, do no harm"). Indeed, an inappropriate use of NIV in certain contexts could potentially mean an increased use of medical resources, prolongation of the dying process and intensification of suffering. In a recent document, the contribution that NIV could offer as a useful palliative tool to alleviate the burden of end-stage respiratory distress was outlined [34]. This requires active involvement of the patient and their family in decision making, often in more than one meeting with clinical staff [6]. Sometimes, NIV should be considered to relieve respiratory distress. This tool, by applying an inspiratory support, might temporarily assist fatigued respiratory muscles and reduce CO_2, thus allowing patients to breathe unsupported for the remaining time of their life [34–37].

Oxygen therapy

The use of oxygen in care of the dying has been explored in a few studies, with controversial results, in a small number of patients who were diagnosed with cancer or other life-limiting illness [38–44]. Two of these studies established that both oxygen and air administered intranasally improved the mean sensation of breathlessness for patients with advanced cancer. Notably, oxygen saturation measures did not correlate with ratings of breathlessness, which is in keeping with the knowledge that breathlessness in advanced cancer is the expression of multiple sensations and experiences, and is not simply related to oxygen tension [42, 44]. Moreover, LISS and GRANT [45] made an interesting point in a study in COPD patients. They showed that, in a population of COPD patients with mild hypoxia at rest, there was no breathlessness improvement with the use of supplemental oxygen when compared with the use of simple air [45]. Only one study, by CAMPBELL *et al.* [43], has specifically addressed the topic of using oxygen support in patients near to death. Their study sought to investigate whether, during their last days of life, patients with a wide range of life-limiting illnesses would benefit from oxygen flow compared with simple air flow or no air flow. 78% of patients involved in the study were affected by respiratory diseases (COPD, lung cancer or pneumonia) and 46% of all patients were already unconscious. Their respiratory status was assessed *via* the Respiratory Distress Observation Scale [29]. The authors concluded that, when the patient is comfortable and near to death, no further support is required: neither initiation nor continuation of oxygen therapy. Moreover, no significant changes in respiratory comfort were noticed over time when changing gas and/or flow conditions were applied. Three patients required oxygen after its withdrawal because of respiratory distress. Thus, most patients do not benefit from oxygen when imminently dying [43].

Another study showed a potential benefit from air flowing on to the face in the late stage of disease, and this could possibly be related to trigeminal nerve stimulation, thereby relieving breathlessness [46]. Following this idea, two different studies have explored the use of a hand-held fan directed towards the face as an aid to reduce breathlessness in people at the EOL [47, 48]. With no measurable harm, the use of a small battery-operated hand-held fan may offer good palliation to many people with breathlessness.

Recently, another relatively new system has found an application in people who are imminently dying. Humidified high-flow nasal oxygen (HFNO) is already known to reduce respiratory rate and the work of breathing. HFNO was shown to perform better than oxygen alone in do-not-intubate patients [49, 50]. Despite these promising results, the possible role of HFNO in people who are actively dying remains to be explored fully.

Withdrawal of mechanical ventilation

Ever since mechanical ventilation (MV) was first used, the question of when to stop it, if not successful, has been important [51]. Despite many research groups around the world trying to generate guidelines on this delicate topic, there is still a great variety of clinical approaches and uncertainty on how to proceed [6, 23, 52–54]. Many studies have pointed out the disparities of practice within different countries and within the same country between different ICUs. As such, there is no consensus, with factors such as economic, cultural, religious and legal differences, as well as personal attitudes, having to be taken into consideration when approaching this topic [53–62].

When patients are assessed for potential withdraw of MV, the first and most important issue is whether the patient is competent or not. This term refers to the patient's ability to fully understand, decide and communicate his or her decision regarding his or her own health after being provided with comprehensive information and prognosis. If the patient is competent and decides to forgo MV, then a psychiatry consult may be requested in some clinical settings, given that patients in this stage and location may experience depression, sleep deprivation and psychosis due to the surrounding environment or their medications. To respect the patient's autonomy is a fundamental ethical principle supported by ethical codes of national organisations, as well as from consensus statement of healthcare professionals [63–66]. However, despite the importance of the patient's decision, the family's support should be always sought for the patient's decision [67, 68]. In the case of a patient who is not competent, local laws and regulations will need to be followed. A frank but sensitive discussion is always required in this setting. For example, it is extremely relevant that, over the time spent with the patient and family, a clear assessment on whether or not to provide cardiopulmonary resuscitation should be gained. Also, different end-stage respiratory patterns after extubation should be described. Furthermore, the presence of airway secretions (death rattle), a protruding tongue and collapsing airways should be carefully considered as possible scenarios by the physician and the nurses caring for the patient. Families must be reassured that every possible measure will be put in place by the team to avoid the patient suffering [51–53, 63, 69].

Ideally, after a family meeting, a relatively short time frame should allow full assimilation of the information before starting any withdrawal procedure. Withdrawal from MV consists of discontinuing the breathing support to allow a so-called "natural death". MV may be withdrawn gradually (terminal weaning) or immediately. Currently, there is no right or wrong approach, and physicians are usually guided by personal experience, often favouring one over the other, based on the patient's status [52, 63]. Terminal weaning is usually achieved over a variable period, varying from hours to days. Usually, once there is an adequate environment and sufficient sedation to maintain the patient's comfort during the entire procedure, there are a few steps to follow. Initially, there is usually a gradual reduction in the positive end-expiratory pressure, as well as pressure support. Meanwhile, the inspiratory oxygen fraction (F_{IO_2}) should be reduced to room air. Close monitoring is essential to avoid a patient's distress at any time. Adjustment of sedation might be required during the process. Most patients will have died when they are no longer receiving any positive-pressure ventilatory support (which means when ventilator rate and pressure support rate is zero). If not, the mechanical ventilator is disconnected and the patient may be extubated. If the plan is not to extubate the patient, then further options include the connection to a T-tube or monitoring for signs of respiratory distress or discomfort, and addressing accordingly [53, 70]. After the patient's death, acute grief support should be a priority. Debriefing of the caring team should always be performed afterwards [53, 65].

On the same topic, Campbell *et al.* [71] recently published a pilot study for the feasibility of a nurse-led algorithm for terminally ill patients undergoing MV withdrawal. The study was designed as observational and prospective, with two groups of patients: "intervention (algorithmic process) compared with unstandardised usual care with at least 3 time periods of measuring patient respiratory distress". There is no mention of the patients' underlying diseases, and the number of patients involved was relatively small (14 patients in total: six intervention and eight usual care); however, the baseline characteristics were similar for age, gender, arterial oxygen saturation measured by pulse oximetry (S_{pO_2})/F_{IO_2} and Simplified Acute Physiology Score. This study demonstrated the feasibility of a nurse-led, multistep assessment that involved patient distress, medication use (in the intervention group, morphine was preferred to benzodiazepines), withdrawal method and extubation decision (with a cuff leak test done in all intervention patients) compared with a single-step approach conducted in the standard group. Significant differences were found between the groups for medications use, with benzodiazepines used more in the control group, and the onset of stridor in some of the control group's patients. Despite the fact that the numbers were small, this study is the first to have explored a potential nurse-led, multistep assessment plan. Further multicentre studies will be required to assess the matter in more detail.

Medications

There is still much controversy in the literature related to: 1) the timing of medications administration (anticipatory dosing or sedation in the terminal stages); 2) the types of medication that should address all the respiratory (excess secretion, death rattle, breathlessness, increased respiratory rate and stridor) and nonrespiratory (pain, vomiting, delirium, anxiety and fear) symptoms; and 3) dosing: large variations in doses have been published from various clinical settings (ICU, paediatric ICU, medical ICU, general ward and palliative care ward) [6, 16, 52, 53, 62, 69, 70, 72–79].

As mentioned previously, there is still a wide variation in practice in the medications used prior to and during withdrawal of MV. This reflects the lack of consensus on the topic and the urgent need to investigate further the pathophysiology of the mechanisms of symptomatic distress related to withdrawal.

Palliative care consultation

The palliative care specialty is now a well-recognised entity inside most hospitals around the world (*e.g.* www.capc.org/) [80–83]. In fact, palliative care has been proven to be effective in meeting the needs of bereaved family members whose relatives have died in the acute care hospital [84].

However, the recent literature indicates that there is still reticence in consulting a palliative care team, and within a suitable timeframe [74, 85, 86]. This is particularly true in nononcology specialties, such as respiratory medicine [85]. To counter this practice, there is a growing body of evidence that clearly shows how important palliative care referral is and how to choose the right time for such a referral. This is because palliative care aids communication and appropriate support to the families and improves the care of dying patients. This includes helping to determine when to cease futile treatments and implement appropriate EOL medication orders. In a recent study focused on patients in medical ICUs, it was shown that palliative care consults were associated with a reduced hospital length of stay and, as a consequence, reduced costs of care as well [80]. However, this result was obtained through better allocation of resources including fewer invasive procedures, not through hastened death. This demonstrated better patient care and better support for families [74, 80]. Moreover, as a collateral benefit, involvement of palliative care allows for modelling of good EOL care for nurses and doctors from other clinical teams, thereby providing ongoing education and support [83, 87, 88].

Additional considerations

Ethics in care of the dying

> "No right is held more sacred, or is more carefully guarded, by the common law, than the right of every individual to the possession and control of his own person, free from all restraint or interference of others, unless by clear and unquestionable authority of law." [65, 89]
>
> "The task of medicine is to cure sometimes, to relieve often, and to comfort always."
>
> Ambroise Paré (16th-century French surgeon).
>
> *Primum non nocere* ("First, do no harm").

These three sentences sum up the three most important medical ethics patient principles: autonomy, beneficence and nonmaleficence. Autonomy is the right of an individual to make decisions regarding his or her own body. Beneficence refers to achieving the best outcomes by acting in the patient's best interests. Nonmaleficence can best be explained by the Latin quote *primum non nocere*, which translates as "first, do no harm". However, in medical care, autonomy is often balanced against paternalism. The latter defines a situation in which healthcare professionals exercise unilateral authority over patients, acting with a patient as a father would with a child. This is based on a sense of superiority of understanding, knowledge, experience or training [65].

But is it true that we physicians are really more knowledgeable about the topic? What do we know about breathlessness in a person who is in the terminal phases of life?

Maybe the first step should be to try to clarify the pathophysiology of breathlessness. Hallenbeck [76] and Rady and Verheijde [90] tried to address this question, but they ended their articles with the awareness of a lack of knowledge and advised "the practicing clinician to consider what physiologic mechanisms may be at work in tailoring patient-specific therapeutic plans" [90]. On the same matter, Rady and Verheijde [91] drew our attention to two related ethical questions. 1) Could the withdrawal of mechanical positive-pressure ventilation harm patients despite our best intentions? 2) Is there sufficient evidence that opioids and benzodiazepines effectively suppress the nociception of breathlessness following the withdrawal of mechanical positive-pressure ventilation? These are important questions, and the answers are that we still do not know.

In their letter to the editor, Rady and Verheijde [91] posed an urgent call for research on the topic. There is an urgent need to understand "the pathophysiology and biologic mechanisms of alleviating [breathlessness], as well as the cognitive-affective processing of [breathlessness], which will ultimately enable physicians to optimise EOL care and good ethical decision making".

Spiritual needs

Respect for patients' dignity and their spiritual needs in their last days of life offers the physician and team a unique demand for consideration, especially when someone is facing the EOL.

Sulmasy [92] described in depth the origin of the word dignity. He states that Kant, in *The Metaphysics of Morals* [93], writes: "The respect I bear others or which another can claim from me (*osservantia aliis praestanda*) is the acknowledgement of the dignity (*dignitas*) of another man, *i.e.* a worth which has no price, no equivalent for which the object of valuation (*aestimii*) could be exchanged." He also states: "Humanity itself is a dignity" [93]. This Kantian idea of dignity was eventually borrowed as a Catholic Christian thought [92, 94]. This explains how the word "dignity" transcends a pure religious content to embrace a more universal value that should always remain the physician's first priority.

Facing death offers the opportunity for all human beings to raise questions about one's worth. Human dignity is an intrinsic concept, not bound by physical or cognitive dimensions. Sulmasy [92] also stated that respect for the person's intrinsic dignity also requires exploration of his or her spiritual needs, potentially allowing people the ability to grow further spiritually: "Death, indeed, has a powerful way of making clear what is really important, what really matters." Despite the value that patients put on faith or beliefs in their life, it is undoubtedly challenging to assess spiritual needs when they are dying. There are poor tools to evaluate unmet spiritual needs [95]. One tool to assess such needs has been validated only in cancer patients [96]. A proper spiritual screening, spiritual history, in-depth spiritual assessment and actively listening to patients' story have been suggested as part of the normal routine for dying patients. However, no consensus has yet been achieved in the palliative care community, reflecting the multifaceted aspects of this problem [95]. Other key factors to take into account are the clinical and cultural features of the population in which the outcome measures have been validated [97].

Spiritual needs, however, ought to be valued not just in the one-way direction of patient to physician. There are, in fact, many studies that have clearly underlined the strong relationships that tie physicians and nurses involved in care of the dying to their spirituality through their patients' care. Inevitably, caring for people who are dying may allow healthcare professionals, at any level, to ask themselves about the meaning and purpose of life at the same time that their patients are pondering these questions. This offers a unique opportunity to cultivate a deep sense of spirituality [1, 95, 98, 99].

Patients' and families' perspectives

Interestingly, patients affected by end-stage CRD often have a limited understanding of their stage of disease and the fact that death may be near. This occurs for many concomitant reasons: little or no EOL communication between respiratory care providers and patients about death and dying, poor advanced care planning and, at times, physicians' paternalistic behaviours [9, 12, 36, 100].

Something to consider carefully is the attitude of the relatives towards care of the dying. In fact, discrepancies have been highlighted between how people wish to be treated and how they believe others should be treated. We now know that patients with end-stage respiratory

Table 1. Key points in the care of patients dying from respiratory diseases

Breathlessness is experienced in up to 90–95% patients with end-stage respiratory disorders
NIV may be offered as a useful palliative tool, to alleviate the burden of end-stage respiratory distress
No unanimous consensus exists to date on when and how to withdraw patients from mechanical ventilation when this is deemed to be clinically futile treatment
Palliative care involvement is encouraged at an early stage in patients with end-stage respiratory diseases
Spiritual needs ought to be evaluated in people at the EOL
Clear and exhaustive communication on aspects of EOL care needs to be provided to patients and their families in order to provide optimal support

diseases may face a sudden fatal exacerbation. If this leads to intubation, patients may be unable to express their wishes, leaving the decision to family members (who should be asked what the patient would want in these circumstances) or physicians [101]. In these scenarios, relatives have shown the tendency to request more active treatment for their loved ones than the patient themselves would want [102]. Furthermore, surrogates are more likely to request life-prolonging interventions than patients [103]. They may also take decisions based on their own values, beliefs and, most importantly, insecurities [104, 105]. Specific training of caregivers in the field of care of the dying, by providing adequate family information and support, will play a key role. Advance directives, although limited in their influence on EOL decisions, may help bridge the gap between the wishes of patients with end-stage respiratory diseases and their relatives [36, 106–108]. Future studies to improve decision making should focus on enhancing communication and promoting more comprehensive advance care planning [82, 109].

Conclusion

In summary, despite all the recent attention and the studies that have sprung up on the topic of the last stages of life, there is much ahead that needs to be explored. EOL care is not synonymous with end of care. Patients with end-stage respiratory diseases deserve proper assessment and support akin to the care given more widely to people with advanced cancer (table 1). It is the commitment of every clinician to provide the best care for those who suffer, especially at such a vulnerable stage of their life. There is a need to promote further research to optimise patient's comfort and to reduce their fear of dying.

References

1. Sinclair S. Impact of death and dying on the personal lives and practices of palliative and hospice care professionals. *CMAJ* 2011; 183: 180–187.
2. Perez GK, Haime V, Jackson V, *et al.* Promoting resiliency among palliative care clinicians: stressors, coping strategies, and training needs. *J Palliat Med* 2015; 18: 332–337.
3. Kamal AH, Bull JH, Wolf SP, *et al.* Prevalence and predictors of burnout among hospice and palliative care clinicians in the U.S. *J Pain Symptom Manage* 2015; 51: 690–696.
4. Centeno C, Noguera A, Lynch T, *et al.* Official certification of doctors working in palliative medicine in Europe: data from an EAPC study in 52 European countries. *Palliat Med* 2007; 21: 683–687.
5. Blinderman CD, Billings JA. Comfort care for patients dying in the hospital. *N Engl J Med* 2015; 373: 2549–2561.
6. Mularski RA, Reinke LF, Carrieri-Kohlman V, *et al.* An official American Thoracic Society workshop report: assessment and palliative management of dyspnea crisis. *Ann Am Thorac Soc* 2013; 10: S98–S106.

7. World Health Organization. The Top 10 Causes of Death. www.who.int/mediacentre/factsheets/fs310/en/ Date last updated: May 2014. Date last accessed: June 11, 2016.
8. Morris D, Galicia-Castillo M. Dying with dyspnea in the hospital. *Am J Hosp Palliat Care* 2015; in press [DOI: 10.1177/1049909115604140].
9. Carlucci A, Vitacca M, Malovini A, *et al.* End-of-life discussion, patient understanding and determinants of the preferences in very severe COPD patients: a multicentric study. *COPD* 2016; 30: 1–7.
10. Campbell ML. Terminal dyspnea and respiratory distress. *Crit Care Clin* 2004; 20: 403–417.
11. Ekstrom M, Allingham SF, Eagar K, *et al.* Breathlessness during the last week of life in palliative care: an Australian prospective, longitudinal study. *J Pain Symptom Manag* 2016; 51: 816–823.
12. Carlucci A, Guerrieri A, Nava S. Palliative care in COPD patients: is it only an end-of-life issue? *Eur Respir Rev* 2012; 21: 347–354.
13. Solano JP, Gomes B, Higginson IJ. A comparison of symptom prevalence in far advanced cancer, AIDS, heart disease, chronic obstructive pulmonary disease and renal disease. *J Pain Symptom Manag* 2006; 31: 58–69.
14. Hall P, Schroder C, Weaver L. The last 48 hours of life in long-term care: a focused chart audit. *J Am Geriatr Soc* 2002; 50: 501–506.
15. Kehl KA, Kowalkowski JA. A systematic review of the prevalence of signs of impending death and symptoms in the last 2 weeks of life. *Am J Hosp Palliat Care* 2013; 30: 601–616.
16. Lokker ME, van Zuylen L, van der Rijt CC, *et al.* Prevalence, impact, and treatment of death rattle: a systematic review. *J Pain Symptom Manag* 2014; 47: 105–122.
17. Currow D, Johnson M, White P, *et al.* Evidence-based intervention for chronic refractory breathlessness: practical therapies that make a difference. *Br J Gen Pract* 2013; 63: 609–610.
18. Simon ST, Weingartner V, Higginson IJ, *et al.* Definition, categorization, and terminology of episodic breathlessness: consensus by an international Delphi survey. *J Pain Symptom Manag* 2014; 47: 828–838.
19. Dorman S, Jolley C, Abernethy A, *et al.* Researching breathlessness in palliative care: consensus statement of the National Cancer Research Institute Palliative Care Breathlessness Subgroup. *Palliat Med* 2009; 23: 213–227.
20. Ekstrom M, Nilsson F, Abernathy AP, *et al.* Effects of opioids on breathlessness and exercise capacity in chronic obstructive pulmonary disease. A systematic review. *Ann Am Thoracic Soc* 2015; 3: 12: 1079–1092.
21. Weingärtner V, Scheve C, Gerdes V, *et al.* Characteristics of episodic breathlessness as reported by patients with advanced chronic obstructive pulmonary disease and lung cancer: results of a descriptive cohort study. *Palliat Med* 2015; 29: 420–428.
22. American Thoracic Society. Dyspnea. Mechanisms, assessment, and management: a consensus statement. *Am J Respir Crit Care Med* 1999; 159: 321–340.
23. Parshall MB, Schwartzstein RM, Adams L, *et al.* An official American Thoracic Society statement: update on the mechanisms, assessment, and management of dyspnea. *Am J Respir Crit Care Med* 2012; 185: 435–452.
24. Campbell ML. Caring for dying patients in the intensive care unit: managing pain, dyspnea, anxiety, delirium, and death rattle. *AACN Adv Crit Care* 2015; 26: 110–120.
25. Gift AG, Narsavage G. Validity of the numeric rating scale as a measure of dyspnea. *Am J Crit Care* 1998; 7: 200–204.
26. Bausewein C, Farquhar M, Booth S, *et al.* Measurement of breathlessness in advanced disease: a systematic review. *Respir Med* 2007; 101: 399–410.
27. Campbell ML. Psychometric testing of a respiratory distress observation scale. *J Palliat Med* 2008; 11: 44–50.
28. Campbell ML, Templin T, Walch J. Patients who are near death are frequently unable to self-report dyspnea. *J Palliat Med* 2009; 12: 881–884.
29. Campbell ML, Templin T, Walch J. A Respiratory Distress Observation Scale for patients unable to self-report dyspnea. *J Palliat Med* 2010; 13: 285–290.
30. Leadership Alliance for the Care of Dying People. One chance to get it right Improving people's experience of care in the last few days and hours of life. www.gov.uk/government/uploads/system/uploads/attachment_data/file/323188/One_chance_to_get_it_right.pdf Date last updated: June 2014. Date last accessed: July 13, 2016.
31. Davis C, Tomas J. Care of the dying: how do we replace the Liverpool Care Pathway? *Br Med Bull* 2014; 112: 5–15.
32. Chan RJ, Webster J, Bowers A. End-of-life care pathways for improving outcomes in caring for the dying. *Cochrane Database Syst Rev* 2016; 2: CD008006.
33. Costantini M, Romoli V, Leo SD, *et al.* Liverpool Care Pathway for patients with cancer in hospital: a cluster randomised trial. *Lancet* 2014; 383: 226–237.
34. Curtis JR, Cook DJ, Sinuff T, *et al.* Noninvasive positive pressure ventilation in critical and palliative care settings: understanding the goals of therapy. *Crit Care Med* 2007; 35: 932–939.
35. Nava S, Cuomo AM. Acute respiratory failure in the cancer patient: the role of non-invasive mechanical ventilation. *Crit Rev Oncol Hematol* 2004; 51: 91–103.
36. Nava S, Ferrer M, Esquinas A, *et al.* Palliative use of non-invasive ventilation in end-of-life patients with solid tumours: a randomised feasibility trial. *Lancet Oncol* 2013; 14: 219–227.

37. Appendini L, Patessio A, Zanaboni S, *et al.* Physiologic effects of positive end-expiratory pressure and mask pressure support during exacerbations of chronic obstructive pulmonary disease. *Am J Respir Crit Care Med* 1994; 149: 1069–1076.
38. Uronis HE, Abernethy AP. Oxygen for relief of dyspnea: what is the evidence? *Curr Opin Support Palliat Care* 2008; 2: 89–94.
39. Abernethy AP, McDonald CF, Frith PA, *et al.* Effect of palliative oxygen *versus* room air in relief of breathlessness in patients with refractory dyspnoea: a double-blind, randomised controlled trial. *Lancet* 2010; 376: 784–793.
40. Bruera E, de Stoutz N, Velasco-Leiva A, *et al.* Effects of oxygen on dyspnoea in hypoxaemic terminal-cancer patients. *Lancet* 1993; 342: 13–14.
41. Bruera E, Schoeller T, MacEachern T. Symptomatic benefit of supplemental oxygen in hypoxemic patients with terminal cancer: the use of the N of 1 randomized controlled trial. *J Pain Symptom Manag* 1992; 7: 365–368.
42. Philip J, Gold M, Milner A, *et al.* A randomized, double-blind, crossover trial of the effect of oxygen on dyspnea in patients with advanced cancer. *J Pain Symptom Manag* 2006; 32: 541–550.
43. Campbell ML, Yarandi H, Dove-Medows E. Oxygen is nonbeneficial for most patients who are near death. *J Pain Symptom Manag* 2013; 45: 517–523.
44. Booth S, Kelly MJ, Cox NP, *et al.* Does oxygen help dyspnea in patients with cancer? *Am J Respir Crit Care Med* 1996; 153: 1515–1518.
45. Liss HP, Grant BJ. The effect of nasal flow on breathlessness in patients with chronic obstructive pulmonary disease. *Am Rev Respir Dis* 1988; 137: 1285–1288.
46. Schwartzstein RM, Lahive K, Pope A, *et al.* Cold facial stimulation reduces breathlessness induced in normal subjects. *Am Rev Respir Dis* 1987; 136: 58–61.
47. Bausewein C, Booth S, Gysels M, *et al.* Effectiveness of a hand-held fan for breathlessness: a randomised phase II trial. *BMC Palliat Care* 2010; 9: 22.
48. Galbraith S, Fagan P, Perkins P, *et al.* Does the use of a handheld fan improve chronic dyspnea? A randomized, controlled, crossover trial. *J Pain Symptom Manag* 2010; 39: 831–838.
49. Peters SG, Holets SR, Gay PC. High-flow nasal cannula therapy in do-not-intubate patients with hypoxemic respiratory distress. *Respir Care* 2013; 58: 597–600.
50. Epstein AS, Hartridge-Lambert SK, Ramaker JS, *et al.* Humidified high-flow nasal oxygen utilization in patients with cancer at Memorial Sloan-Kettering Cancer Center. *J Palliat Med* 2011; 14: 835–839.
51. Campbell ML. How to withdraw mechanical ventilation: a systematic review of the literature. *AACN Adv Crit Care* 2007; 18: 397–403.
52. Truog RD, Campbell ML, Curtis JR, *et al.* Recommendations for end-of-life care in the intensive care unit: a consensus statement by the American College [corrected] of Critical Care Medicine. *Crit Care Med* 2008; 36: 953–963.
53. Paruk F, Kissoon N, Hartog CS, *et al.* The Durban World Congress Ethics Round Table Conference Report: III. Withdrawing mechanical ventilation – the approach should be individualized. *J Crit Care* 2014; 29: 902–907.
54. Sprung CL, Woodcock T, Sjokvist P, *et al.* Reasons, considerations, difficulties and documentation of end-of-life decisions in European intensive care units: the ETHICUS Study. *Intensive Care Med* 2008; 34: 271–277.
55. van Beinum A, Hornby L, Ramsay T, *et al.* Exploration of withdrawal of life-sustaining therapy in Canadian intensive care units. *J Intensive Care Med* 2015; 31: 243–251.
56. Phua J, Joynt GM, Nishimura M, *et al.* Withholding and withdrawal of life-sustaining treatments in intensive care units in Asia. *JAMA Intern Med* 2015; 175: 363–371.
57. Toffart AC, Timsit JF. Is prolonged mechanical ventilation of cancer patients futile? *Crit Care* 2013; 17: 189.
58. Mark NM, Rayner SG, Lee NJ, *et al.* Global variability in withholding and withdrawal of life-sustaining treatment in the intensive care unit: a systematic review. *Intensive Care Med* 2015; 41: 1572–1585.
59. Collins N, Phelan D, Marsh B, *et al.* End-of-life care in the intensive care unit: the Irish Ethicus data. *Crit Care Resusc* 2006; 8: 315–320.
60. Ganz FD, Benbenishty J, Hersch M, *et al.* The impact of regional culture on intensive care end of life decision making: an Israeli perspective from the ETHICUS study. *J Med Ethics* 2006; 32: 196–199.
61. Sprung CL, Maia P, Bulow HH, *et al.* The importance of religious affiliation and culture on end-of-life decisions in European intensive care units. *Intensive Care Med* 2007; 33: 1732–1739.
62. Sprung CL, Cohen SL, Sjokvist P, *et al.* End-of-life practices in European intensive care units: the Ethicus Study. *JAMA* 2003; 290: 790–797.
63. Tasota FJ, Hoffman LA. Terminal weaning from mechanical ventilation: planning and process. *Crit Care Nurs Q* 1996; 19: 36–51.
64. American Thoracic Society. Withholding and withdrawing life-sustaining therapy. *Am Rev Respir Dis* 1991; 144: 726–731.
65. Szalados JE. Discontinuation of mechanical ventilation at end-of-life: the ethical and legal boundaries of physician conduct in termination of life support. *Crit Care Clin* 2007; 23: 317–337.
66. McGee A. Does withdrawing life-sustaining treatment cause death or allow the patient to die? *Med Law Rev* 2014; 22: 26–47.

67. Campbell ML. Case studies in terminal weaning from mechanical ventilation. *Am J Crit Care* 1993; 2: 354–358.
68. Campbell ML. Terminal weaning: it's not simply "pulling the plug". *Nursing* 1994; 24: 34–39.
69. Long AC, Muni S, Treece PD, *et al.* Time to death after terminal withdrawal of mechanical ventilation: specific respiratory and physiologic parameters may inform physician predictions. *J Palliat Med* 2015; 18: 1040–1047.
70. Truog RD, Brock DW, White DB. Should patients receive general anesthesia prior to extubation at the end of life? *Crit Care Med* 2012; 40: 631–633.
71. Campbell ML, Yarandi HN, Mendez M. A two-group trial of a terminal ventilator withdrawal algorithm: pilot testing. *J Palliat Med* 2015; 18: 781–785.
72. Pereira S, Kozikowski A, Pekmezaris R, *et al.* The relationship between the timing of a palliative care consult and utilization outcomes for ventilator-assisted intensive care unit patients. *Palliat Support Care* 2015; 13: 217–221.
73. O'Mahony S, McHugh M, Zallman L, *et al.* Ventilator withdrawal: procedures and outcomes. Report of a collaboration between a critical care division and a palliative care service. *J Pain Symptom Manag* 2003; 26: 954–961.
74. Lustbader D, Pekmezaris R, Frankenthaler M, *et al.* Palliative medicine consultation impacts DNR designation and length of stay for terminal medical MICU patients. *Palliat Support Care* 2011; 9: 401–406.
75. Kompanje EJ, van der Hoven B, Bakker J. Anticipation of distress after discontinuation of mechanical ventilation in the ICU at the end of life. *Intensive Care Med* 2008; 34: 1593–1599.
76. Hallenbeck J. Pathophysiologies of dyspnea explained: why might opioids relieve dyspnea and not hasten death? *J Palliat Med* 2012; 15: 848–853.
77. Edwards MJ. Opioids and benzodiazepines appear paradoxically to delay inevitable death after ventilator withdrawal. *J Palliat Care* 2005; 21: 299–302.
78. Deschepper R, Laureys S, Hachimi-Idrissi S, *et al.* Palliative sedation: why we should be more concerned about the risks that patients experience an uncomfortable death. *Pain* 2013; 154: 1505–1508.
79. Ellershaw J, Ward C. Care of the dying patient: the last hours or days of life. *BMJ* 2003; 326: 30–34.
80. McCarthy IM, Robinson C, Huq S, *et al.* Cost savings from palliative care teams and guidance for a financially viable palliative care program. *Health Serv Res* 2015; 50: 217–236.
81. Casarett D, Pickard A, Bailey FA, *et al.* Do palliative consultations improve patient outcomes? *J Am Geriatr Soc* 2008; 56: 593–599.
82. Lorenz KA, Lynn J, Dy SM, *et al.* Evidence for improving palliative care at the end of life: a systematic review. *Ann Intern Med* 2008; 148: 147–159.
83. Gade G, Venohr I, Conner D, *et al.* Impact of an inpatient palliative care team: a randomized control trial. *J Palliat Med* 2008; 11: 180–190.
84. Gelfman LP, Meier DE, Morrison RS. Does palliative care improve quality? A survey of bereaved family members. *J Pain Symptom Manag* 2008; 36: 22–28.
85. Le BH, Watt JN. Care of the dying in Australia's busiest hospital: benefits of palliative care consultation and methods to enhance access. *J Palliat Med* 2010; 13: 855–860.
86. Humphreys J, Harman S. Late referral to palliative care consultation service: length of stay and in-hospital mortality outcomes. *J Community Support Oncol* 2014; 12: 129–136.
87. Penrod JD, Deb P, Dellenbaugh C, *et al.* Hospital-based palliative care consultation: effects on hospital cost. *J Palliat Med* 2010; 13: 973–979.
88. Morrison RS, Penrod JD, Cassel JB, *et al.* Cost savings associated with US hospital palliative care consultation programs. *Arch Intern Med* 2008; 168: 1783–1790.
89. US Supreme Court. Union Pacific Railway Co. v. Botsford, 141 U.S. 250,251 (1891). No. 1375. Submitted January 6, 1891. Decided May 25, 1891.
90. Rady MY, Verheijde JL. Alleviating dyspnea and possible biologic mechanisms. *J Palliat Med* 2012; 15: 1056–1057.
91. Rady MY, Verheijde JL. The science and ethics of withdrawing mechanical positive pressure ventilatory support in the terminally ill. *J Palliat Med* 2013; 16: 828–830.
92. Sulmasy DP. Death and dignity in Catholic Christian thought. *Med Health Care Philos* 2016; in press [DOI: 10.1007/s11019-016-9690-9].
93. Kant I. The Metaphysics of Morals. Cambridge/New York, Cambridge University Press, 1996.
94. Catholic Church. Rerum novarum. Encyclical Letter of Pope Leo XIII on the Condition of Labor (with discussion club outline). New York, The Paulist Press, 1940.
95. Lunder U, Furlan M, Simonic A. Spiritual needs assessments and measurements. *Curr Opin Support Palliat Care* 2011; 5: 273–278.
96. Borneman T, Ferrell B, Puchalski CM. Evaluation of the FICA tool for spiritual assessment. *J Pain Symptom Manag* 2010; 40: 163–173.
97. Selman L, Harding R, Gysels M, *et al.* The measurement of spirituality in palliative care and the content of tools validated cross-culturally: a systematic review. *J Pain Symptom Manag* 2011; 41: 728–753.
98. Tornøe KA, Danbolt LJ, Kvigne K, *et al.* The challenge of consolation: nurses' experiences with spiritual and existential care for the dying – a phenomenological hermeneutical study. *BMC Nurs* 2015; 14: 62.
99. Boston PH, Mount BM. The caregiver's perspective on existential and spiritual distress in palliative care. *J Pain Symptom Manag* 2006; 32: 13–26.

100. Vitacca M, Comini L. How do patients die in a rehabilitative unit dedicated to advanced respiratory diseases? *Multidiscip Respir Med* 2012; 7: 18.
101. Berger JT, DeRenzo EG, Schwartz J. Surrogate decision making: reconciling ethical theory and clinical practice. *Ann Intern Med* 2008; 149: 48–53.
102. Sviri S, Garb Y, Stav I, *et al.* Contradictions in end-of-life decisions for self and other, expressed by relatives of chronically ventilated patients. *J Crit Care* 2009; 24: 293–301.
103. Libbus MK, Russell C. Congruence of decisions between patients and their potential surrogates about life-sustaining therapies. *Image J Nurs Sch* 1995; 27: 135–140.
104. Fagerlin A, Ditto PH, Danks JH, *et al.* Projection in surrogate decisions about life-sustaining medical treatments. *Health Psychol* 2001; 20: 166–175.
105. Vig EK, Taylor JS, Starks H, *et al.* Beyond substituted judgment: how surrogates navigate end-of-life decision-making. *J Am Geriatr Soc* 2006; 54: 1688–1693.
106. Feeg VD, Elebiary H. Exploratory study on end-of-life issues: barriers to palliative care and advance directives. *Am J Hosp Palliat Care* 2005; 22: 119–124.
107. Pautex S, Gamondi C, Philippin Y, *et al.* Advance directives and end-of-life decisions in Switzerland: role of patients, relatives and health professionals. *BMJ Support Palliat Care* 2015; in press [DOI: 10.1136/bmjspcare-2014-000730].
108. Pautex S, Herrmann FR, Zulian GB. Role of advance directives in palliative care units: a prospective study. *Palliat Med* 2008; 22: 835–841.
109. Teno J, Lynn J, Wenger N, *et al.* Advance directives for seriously ill hospitalized patients: effectiveness with the patient self-determination act and the SUPPORT intervention. SUPPORT Investigators. Study to Understand Prognoses and Preferences for Outcomes and Risks of Treatment. *J Am Geriatr Soc* 1997; 45: 500–507.

Disclosures: None declared.

Other titles in the series

ERS Monograph 72 – SARS, MERS and other Viral Lung Infections
David S. Hui, Giovanni A. Rossi and Sebastian L. Johnston

ERS Monograph 71 – Idiopathic Pulmonary Fibrosis
Ulrich Costabel, Bruno Crestani and Athol U. Wells

ERS Monograph 70 – Imaging
R. Graham Barr, David G. Parr and Jens Vogel-Claussen

ERS Monograph 69 – Controversies in COPD
Antonio Anzueto, Yvonne Heijdra and John R. Hurst

ERS Monograph 68 – Lung Cancer
Anne-Marie C. Dingemans, Martin Reck and Virginie Westeel

ERS Monograph 67 – Obstructive Sleep Apnoea
Ferran Barbé and Jean-Louis Pépin

ERS Monograph 66 – Pulmonary Complications of HIV
Charles Feldman, Eva Polverino and Julio A. Ramirez

ERS Monograph 65 – Respiratory Epidemiology
Isabella Annesi-Maesano, Bo Lundbäck and Giovanni Viegi

ERS Monograph 64 – Cystic Fibrosis
Marcus A. Mall and J. Stuart Elborn

ERS Monograph 63 – Community-Acquired Pneumonia
James D. Chalmers, Mathias W. Pletz and Stefano Aliberti

ERS Monograph 62 – Outcomes in Clinical Trials
Martin Kolb and Claus F. Vogelmeier